Advances in Surgery

Editor

LENA M. NAPOLITANO

CRITICAL CARE CLINICS

www.criticalcare.theclinics.com

Consulting Editor
JOHN A. KELLUM

April 2017 • Volume 33 • Number 2

ELSEVIER

1600 John F. Kennedy Boulevard • Suite 1800 • Philadelphia, Pennsylvania, 19103-2899

http://www.theclinics.com

CRITICAL CARE CLINICS Volume 33, Number 2
April 2017 ISSN 0749-0704, ISBN-13: 978-0-323-52400-1

Editor: Katie Pfaff
Developmental Editor: Casey Potter

Critical Care Clinics (ISSN: 0749-0704) is published quarterly by Elsevier Inc., 360 Park Avenue South, New York, NY 10010-1710. Months of issue are January, April, July, and October. Business and Editorial Offices: 1600 John F. Kennedy Blvd., Suite 1800, Philadelphia, PA 19103-2899. Customer Service Office: 6277 Sea Harbor Drive, Orlando, FL 32887-4800. Periodicals postage paid at New York, NY and additional mailing offices. Subscription prices are $221.00 per year for US individuals, $584.00 per year for US institution, $100.00 per year for US students and residents, $263.00 per year for Canadian individuals, $732.00 per year for Canadian institutions, $309.00 per year for international individuals, $732.00 per year for international institutions and $150.00 per year for Canadian and foreign students/residents. To receive student/resident rate, orders must be accompanied by name of affiliated institution, date of term, and the signature of program/residency coordinator on institution letterhead. Orders will be billed at individual rate until proof of status is received. Foreign air speed delivery is included in all *Clinics* subscription prices. All prices are subject to change without notice. POSTMASTER: Send address changes to *Critical Care Clinics*, Elsevier Periodicals Customer Service, 11830 Westline Industrial Drive, St. Louis, MO 63146. **Customer Service: 1-800-654-2452 (US). From outside of the US, call 1-314-447-8871. Fax: 1-314-447-8029. E-mail:** journalscustomerservice-usa@elsevier.com **(for print support) or** journalsonlinesupport-usa@elsevier.com **(for online support).**

Reprints. For copies of 100 or more of articles in this publication, please contact the Commercial Reprints Department, Elsevier Inc., 360 Park Avenue South, New York, NY 10010-1710. Tel.: 212-633-3874; Fax: 212-633-3820; E-mail: reprints@elsevier.com.

Critical Care Clinics is also published in Spanish by Editorial Inter-Medica, Junin 917, 1er A, 1113, Buenos Aires, Argentina.

Critical Care Clinics is covered in *MEDLINE/PubMed (Index Medicus), EMBASE/Excerpta Medica, Current Concepts/Clinical Medicine, ISI/BIOMED,* and *Chemical Abstracts.*

Contributors

CONSULTING EDITOR

JOHN A. KELLUM, MD, MCCM
Professor of Critical Care Medicine, Medicine, Bioengineering and Clinical & Translational Science, Director, Center for Critical Care Nephrology; Vice Chair for Research, Department of Critical Care Medicine, University of Pittsburgh School of Medicine, Pittsburgh, Pennsylvania

EDITOR

LENA M. NAPOLITANO, MD, FACS, FCCP, MCCM
Professor of Surgery, Division Chief, Acute Care Surgery [Trauma, Burn, Critical Care, Emergency Surgery], Associate Chair, Department of Surgery, Director, Trauma and Surgical Critical Care, University of Michigan Health System, Ann Arbor, Michigan

AUTHORS

AZRA BIHORAC, MD, MS
Associate Professor of Medicine, Department of Medicine, University of Florida, Gainesville, Florida

SCOTT C. BRAKENRIDGE, MD, MS, FACS
Assistant Professor, Department of Surgery, Sepsis and Critical Illness Research Center, University of Florida College of Medicine, Gainesville, Florida

DANIEL BRODIE, MD
Associate Professor of Medicine, Division of Pulmonary, Allergy & Critical Care Medicine, Columbia University Medical Center, New York, New York

JEREMY W. CANNON, MD, SM
Associate Professor of Surgery, Division of Trauma, Surgical Critical Care & Emergency Surgery, Perelman School of Medicine at the University of Pennsylvania, Philadelphia, Pennsylvania

MICHAEL W. CRIPPS, MD
Associate Professor, Department of Surgery, UT Southwestern, Dallas, Texas

E. WESLEY ELY, MD, MPH
Professor of Medicine and Critical Care, Associate Director of Aging Research, VA GRECC, Center for Health Services Research, Division of Allergy, Pulmonary and Critical Care Medicine, Vanderbilt University Medical Center, Nashville, Tennessee

BRADLEY D. FREEMAN, MD, FACS
Professor, Department of Surgery, Washington University School of Medicine, St Louis, Missouri

JACOB T. GUTSCHE, MD
Assistant Professor of Anesthesiology and Critical Care, Department of Anesthesiology and Critical Care, Perelman School of Medicine, University of Pennsylvania, Philadelphia, Pennsylvania

MICHAEL HEUNG, MD, MS
Clinical Associate Professor, Division of Nephrology, Department of Medicine, University of Michigan, Ann Arbor, Michigan

CHARLES HOBSON, MD, MHA
Department of Health Services Research, Management and Policy, University of Florida, Gainesville, Florida

RYAN T. HURT, MD, PhD
Associate Professor, Department of Medicine, Mayo Clinic, Rochester, Minnesota

LEWIS J. KAPLAN, MD, FACS, FCCM, FCCP
Section Chief, Surgical Critical Care, Corporal Michael J Crescenz VA Medical Center; Associate Professor of Surgery, Division of Trauma, Surgical Critical Care and Emergency Surgery, Perelman School of Medicine, University of Pennsylvania, Philadelphia, Pennsylvania

ANNACHIARA MARRA, MD, PhD(c)
Visiting Research Fellow, Center for Health Services Research, Division of Allergy, Pulmonary and Critical Care Medicine, Vanderbilt University Medical Center, University of Naples Federico II, Nashville, Tennessee

ROBERT G. MARTINDALE, MD, PhD
Professor of Surgery, Division of General Surgery, Department of Surgery, Oregon Health Sciences University, Portland, Oregon

STEPHEN A. McCLAVE, MD
Professor of Medicine, Division of Gastroenterology, University of Louisville, Louisville, Kentucky

CHRISTIAN T. MINSHALL, MD, PhD
Assistant Professor, Department of Surgery, UT Southwestern, Dallas, Texas

JUAN C. MIRA, MD
Post-Graduate Research Fellow, Department of Surgery, Sepsis and Critical Illness Research Center, University of Florida College of Medicine, Gainesville, Florida

LYLE L. MOLDAWER, PhD
Professor, Department of Surgery, Sepsis and Critical Illness Research Center, University of Florida College of Medicine, Gainesville, Florida

FREDERICK A. MOORE, MD, FACS, MCCM
Professor and Chief of Acute Care Surgery, Department of Surgery, Sepsis and Critical Illness Research Center, University of Florida College of Medicine, Gainesville, Florida

LENA M. NAPOLITANO, MD, FACS, FCCP, MCCM
Professor of Surgery, Division Chief, Acute Care Surgery [Trauma, Burn, Critical Care, Emergency Surgery], Associate Chair, Department of Surgery, Director, Trauma and Surgical Critical Care, University of Michigan Health System, Ann Arbor, Michigan

TIFFANY M. OSBORN, MD, MPH, FACEP
Professor of Surgery and Emergency Medicine, Section of Acute and Critical Care Surgery, Washington University School of Medicine, St Louis, Missouri

PRATIK P. PANDHARIPANDE, MD, MSCI, FCCM
Professor of Anesthesiology and Surgery, Chief, Division of Anesthesiology Critical Care Medicine, Department of Anesthesiology, Center for Health Services Research, Vanderbilt University Medical Center, Nashville, Tennessee

JAYSHIL J. PATEL, MD
Associate Professor of Medicine, Division of Pulmonary & Critical Care Medicine, Medical College of Wisconsin, Milwaukee, Wisconsin

MAYUR B. PATEL, MD, MPH, FACS
Assistant Professor of Surgery, Neurosurgery, Hearing and Speech Sciences, Division of Trauma, Surgical Critical Care and Emergency General Surgery, Section of Surgical Sciences, Department of Surgery, Center for Health Services Research, Vanderbilt University Medical Center, Nashville, Tennessee

RUPAM RUCHI, MD
Clinical Assistant Professor of Medicine, Department of Medicine, University of Florida, Gainesville, Florida

M. CHANCE SPALDING, DO, PhD
Trauma and Critical Care Surgeon, Department of Surgery, Grant Medical Center, Columbus, Ohio; Assistant Professor, Department of Surgery, Ohio University College of Osteopathic Medicine, Athens, Ohio

BRIAN WEISS, MD
Perelman School of Medicine, University of Pennsylvania, Philadelphia, Pennsylvania

LENAR YESSAYAN, MD, MS
Clinical Associate Professor, Division of Nephrology, Department of Medicine, University of Michigan, Ann Arbor, Michigan

Contents

The ABCDEF bundle represents an evidence-based guide for clinicians to approach the organizational changes needed for optimizing intensive care unit patient recovery and outcomes. This article reviews the core evidence and features behind the ABCDEF bundle. The bundle has individual components that are clearly defined, flexible to implement, and help empower multidisciplinary clinicians and families in the shared care of the critically ill. The ABCDEF bundle helps guide well-rounded patient care and optimal resource utilization resulting in more interactive intensive care unit patients with better controlled pain, who can safely participate in higher-order physical and cognitive activities at the earliest point in their critical illness.

Following advances in critical care, in-hospital multiple organ failure–related mortality is declining. Consequently, incidence of chronic critical illness is increasing. These patients linger in the intensive care unit, have high resource utilization, and poor long-term outcomes. Within this population, the authors propose that a substantial subset of patients have a new phenotype: persistent inflammation, immunosuppression, and catabolism syndrome. There is evidence that myelodysplasia with expansion of myeloid-derived suppressor cells, innate and adaptive immune suppression, and protein catabolism with malnutrition are major contributors. Optimal care of these patients will require novel multimodality interventions.

Acute respiratory distress syndrome (ARDS) occurs in more than 10% of intensive care unit admissions and in nearly 25% of ventilated patients. Mortality remains high at 40%, and, for patients who survive, recovery continues for months or even years. Early recognition and minimizing further lung injury remain essential to successful management of severe ARDS. Advanced treatment strategies, which complement lung protective ventilation, include short-term neuromuscular blockade, prone positioning, and extracorporeal membrane oxygenation. Alternative ventilator strategies include high-frequency ventilation and airway pressure release ventilation. This article reviews these options in patients with severe ARDS.

care for sepsis given these study findings? Furthermore, the definition of sepsis has now been updated. This article reviews key findings of these 3 trials and discusses these important issues in sepsis management.

Anemia is common in the intensive care unit (ICU), resulting in frequent administration of red blood cell (RBC) transfusions. Significant advances have been made in understanding the pathophysiology of anemia in the ICU, which is anemia of inflammation. This anemia is related to high hepcidin concentrations resulting in iron-restricted erythropoiesis, and decreased erythropoietin concentrations. A new hormone (erythroferrone) has been identified, which mediates hepcidin suppression to allow increased iron absorption and mobilization from iron stores. RBC transfusions are most commonly administered to ICU patients for treatment of anemia. All strategies to reduce anemia in the ICU should be implemented.

Acute kidney injury (AKI) is a common complication among critically ill patents, and 5% of intensive care unit (ICU) patients require initiation of renal replacement therapy (RRT). In recent years, clinical trials have provided evidence-based guidance for some important aspects of RRT management in patients with AKI, such as dialysis dosing and approaches to anticoagulation in patients undergoing continuous RRT. However, there remain many areas of uncertainty, and delivery of RRT in the ICU requires clinical judgment, flexibility, and an understanding of dialysis principles. This article reviews the components of RRT prescription and provides an update on best practices.

Acute kidney injury (AKI) is a common complication in surgical patients and is associated with increases in mortality, an increased risk for chronic kidney disease and hemodialysis after discharge, and increased cost. Better understanding of the risk factors that contribute to perioperative AKI has led to improved AKI prediction and will eventually lead to improved prevention of AKI, mitigation of injury when AKI occurs, and enhanced recovery in patients who sustain AKI. The development of advanced clinical prediction scores for AKI, new imaging techniques, and novel biomarkers for early detection of AKI provides new tools toward these ends.

The surgical critically ill patient is subject to a variable and complex metabolic response, which has detrimental effects on immunity, wound healing, and preservation of lean body muscle. The concept of nutrition support has evolved into nutrition therapy, whereby the primary objectives are to prevent oxidative cell injury, modulate the immune response, and attenuate the metabolic response. This review outlines the metabolic response to critical illness, describes nutritional risk; reviews the evidence for the role, dose, and timing of enteral and parenteral nutrition, and reviews the evidence for immunonutrition in the surgical intensive care unit.

CRITICAL CARE CLINICS

THE CLINICS ARE AVAILABLE ONLINE!
Access your subscription at:
www.theclinics.com

Preface

Advances in Surgical Critical Care 2017: Growing Population and Personalized Protocols

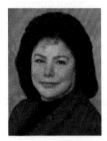

Lena M. Napolitano, MD, FACS, FCCP, MCCM
Editor

Critical care is a young specialty, initiated in 1953 when poliomyelitis patients required invasive mechanical ventilation, and even earlier for surgical patients recovering from anesthesia or traumatic injuries.[1,2] The burden of critical illness globally is high and has been increasing as our population ages.[3]

Paradoxically, critical care continues to grow in a shrinking hospital system. Although hospital beds decreased by 2.2% from 2000 to 2010 in the United States, critical care beds increased by 17.8%, with a 20.4% increase in the critical care medicine-to-hospital bed ratio (13.5%–16.2%). During this same time period, critical care costs nearly doubled (92.2%; $56–$108 billion) and the proportion of critical care cost to the gross domestic product increased by 32.1%.[4]

The provision of critical care globally is more variable, with a documented remarkable degree of variation in both the number of adult intensive care unit (ICU) beds (7-fold difference from least to greatest) and the volume of ICU admissions (10-fold difference) between seven different countries, but with a high inverse correlation between the number of ICU beds and hospital mortality for ICU patients.[5]

Use of critical care services for surgical patients is also widely variable, and significant variations in mortality in surgical critically ill patients have been reported.[6–8] Management of critically ill patients is challenging, and the field of critical care is undergoing rapid change. The population of critically ill patients is highly heterogeneous, with different comorbidities and varying types and degrees of organ dysfunction.

So how best can we improve the survival of critically ill patients in the context of these significant challenges? Intensivists must be knowledgeable about recent advances and randomized trials in the critically ill,[9] but must also be capable of providing personalized medicine to identify which patients can potentially benefit from new interventions that have been rigorously tested.[10]

Crit Care Clin 33 (2017) xiii–xv
http://dx.doi.org/10.1016/j.ccc.2017.01.001
0749-0704/17/© 2017 Published by Elsevier Inc.

This issue of *Critical Care Clinics* documents important progress made in the field of critical care and provides an update of the significant evidence-based advances in critical care that result in improved patient outcomes. In this issue, leading experts provide succinct reviews of important critical care advances in the broad areas of multidisciplinary patient care bundles, delirium, early mobility, airway, respiratory, renal, sepsis, transfusion, and nutrition support. They review cutting-edge advances and provide evidence-based recommendations for best practices in critical care.

I extend my deepest gratitude to our authors for their excellent contributions to this important issue on Advances in Critical Care, and to Richard W. Carlson, Patrick J. Manley, and Casey Potter and the entire editorial team.

We hope that this issue of *Critical Care Clinics* will assist in timely dissemination of critical care knowledge by providing the updated evidence base to ensure optimal care to all of our critically ill patients.

Lena M. Napolitano, MD, FACS, FCCP, MCCM
Division of Acute Care Surgery
[Trauma, Burns, Surgical Critical Care, Emergency Surgery]
Department of Surgery
University of Michigan Health System
Room 1C340A University Hospital
1500 East Medical Center Drive
Ann Arbor, MI 48109-5033, USA

E-mail address:
lenan@umich.edu

REFERENCES

1. Ibsen B. The anaesthetist's viewpoint on the treatment of respiratory complications in poliomyelitis during the epidemic in Copenhagen, 1952. Proc R Soc Med 1954;47:72–4.

2. Grenvik A, Pinsky MR. Evolution of the intensive care unit as a clinical center and critical care medicine as a discipline. Crit Care Clin 2009;25:239–50.

3. Adhikari NK, Fowler RA, Bhagwanjee S, et al. Critical care and the global burden of critical illness in adults. Lancet 2010;376(9749):1339–46.

4. Halpern NA, Goldman DA, Tan KS, et al. Trends in critical care beds and use among population groups and Medicare and Medicaid beneficiaries in the United States: 2000-2010. Crit Care Med 2016;44(8):1490–9.

5. Wunsch H, Angus DC, Harrison DA, et al. Variation in critical care services across North America and Western Europe. Crit Care Med 2008;36:2787–93.

6. Pearse RM, Moreno RP, Bauer P, et al, European Surgical Outcomes Study (EuSOS) group for the trials groups of the European Society of Intensive Care Medicine and the European Society of Anaesthesiology. Mortality after surgery in Europe: a 7 day cohort study. Lancet 2012;380(9847):1059–65.

7. International Surgical Outcomes Study Group. Global patient outcomes after elective surgery: prospective cohort study in 27 low-, middle- and high-income countries. Br J Anaesth 2016;117(5):601–9.

8. Gillies MA, Harrison EM, Pearse RM, et al. Intensive care utilization and outcomes after high-risk surgery in Scotland: a population-based cohort study. Br J Anaesth 2017;118(1):123–31.

9. Bellomo R, Landoni G, Young P. Improved survival in critically ill patients: are large RCTs more useful than personalized medicine? Yes. Intensive Care Med 2016;42(11):1775–7.

10. Vincent JL. Improved survival in critically ill patients: are large RCTs more useful than personalized medicine? No. Intensive Care Med 2016;42(11):1778–80.

The ABCDEF Bundle in Critical Care

Annachiara Marra, MD, PhD(c)[a], E. Wesley Ely, MD, MPH[b],
Pratik P. Pandharipande, MD, MSCI, FCCM[c], Mayur B. Patel, MD, MPH[d],*

KEYWORDS

- Pain • Spontaneous awakening trials • Spontaneous breathing trials • Sedation
- Analgesia • Delirium • Early mobility • Intensive care unit

KEY POINTS

- The ABCDEF bundle is an evidence-based guide for clinicians to coordinate multidisciplinary patient care in the intensive care unit (ICU).
- Assessment of pain is the first step before administering pain relief. The Behavioral Pain Scale (BPS) and the Critical-Care Pain Observation Tool (CPOT) are the most valid and reliable behavioral pain scales for ICU patients unable to communicate.

Continued

Disclosures and Funding Sources: E.W. Ely, P.P. Pandharipande, and M.B. Patel are supported by National Institutes of Health HL111111 and GM120484 (Bethesda, MD). E.W. Ely is supported by the Veterans Affairs Tennessee Valley Geriatric Research, Education and Clinical Center (Nashville, TN). E.W. Ely and P.P. Pandharipande are supported by the VA Clinical Science Research and Development Service (Washington, DC) and the National Institutes of Health AG027472 and AG035117 (Bethesda, MD). M.B. Patel is supported by the Vanderbilt Faculty Research Scholars Program. This project was supported by REDCap, a secure online database, supported in part by the National Institutes of Health TR000445. E.W. Ely has received honoraria from Abbott Laboratories, Hospira, Inc, and Orion Corporation, and research grants from Abbott Laboratories. P.P. Pandharipande and E.W. Ely have received research grants from Hospira, Inc. A. NIHMS: 834685. The authors have no other disclosures relevant to this article.
[a] Center for Health Services Research, Division of Allergy, Pulmonary and Critical Care Medicine, Vanderbilt University Medical Center, University of Naples Federico II, 1215 21st Avenue South, Medical Center East, Suite 6100, Nashville, TN 37232-8300, USA; [b] VA GRECC, Center for Health Services Research, Division of Allergy, Pulmonary and Critical Care Medicine, Vanderbilt University Medical Center, 1215 21st Avenue South, Medical Center East, Suite 6109, Nashville, TN 37232-8300, USA; [c] Division of Anesthesiology Critical Care Medicine, Department of Anesthesiology, Center for Health Services Research, Vanderbilt University Medical Center, 1211 21st Avenue South, Medical Arts Building, Suite 526, Nashville, TN 37212, USA; [d] Division of Trauma, Surgical Critical Care, and Emergency General Surgery, Section of Surgical Sciences, Department of Surgery, Center for Health Services Research, Vanderbilt University Medical Center, 1211 21st Avenue South, Medical Arts Building, Suite 404, Nashville, TN 37212, USA
* Corresponding author.
E-mail address: mayur.b.patel@Vanderbilt.Edu

Crit Care Clin 33 (2017) 225–243
http://dx.doi.org/10.1016/j.ccc.2016.12.005
0749-0704/17/Published by Elsevier Inc.

criticalcare.theclinics.com

Continued

- Coordination of spontaneous awakening trials (SAT) with spontaneous breathing trials (SBT) is associated with decreases in sedative use, delirium, time on mechanical ventilation, and ICU and hospital lengths of stay.
- Delirium monitoring and management is critically important because it is a strong risk factor for increased time on mechanical ventilation, length of ICU and hospital stay, cost of hospitalization, long-term cognitive impairment, and mortality.
- Early mobility is the only currently known intervention associated with a decrease in delirium duration. Physical therapy is safe and feasible in the ICU, even while on mechanical ventilation, renal-replacement therapy, and/or circulatory support.

With more than 4 million intensive care unit (ICU) admissions per year in the United States, there is increasing recognition of the long-term consequences of ICU care on the physical and mental health function of patients. An acute care hospitalization and critical illness has tangible consequences of cognitive decline,[1] posttraumatic stress disorder,[2] and depression.[3] In a multicenter cohort of 821 critically ill patients with respiratory failure or shock, our group demonstrated that one of four ICU patients had cognitive impairment after 12 months after critical illness that was similar in severity to that of patients with mild Alzheimer disease and moderate traumatic brain injury.[4] The largest risk factor for this ICU-related cognitive impairment was delirium. Disability associated with ICU care and hospitalization is an unfortunately common occurrence in older adults with significant consequences for patients and caregivers (Box 1).[5]

Box 1
Factors related to hospitalization-associated disability

Preillness determinants of functional reserve (vulnerability and capacity to recover)
- Age
- Poor mobility
- Cognitive function
- Activities of daily living and IADLs
- Geriatric syndrome (falls, incontinence)
- Social functioning
- Depression

Severity of acute illness

Hospitalization factors
- Environment
- Restricted mobility
- Undernutrition
- Enforced dependence
- Polypharmacy
- Little encouragement of independence

Posthospitalization factors
- Environment
- Resources
- Community supports
- Quality of discharge planning

Abbreviation: IADL, instrumental activities of daily living.
Data from Covinsky KE, Pierluissi E, Johnston CB. Hospitalization-associated disability: she was probably able to ambulate, but I'm not sure. JAMA 2011;306(16):1782–93.

ICU survivorship has become a top concern and methods to optimize patient recovery and outcomes are important objectives for the health provider, families, and researchers. In 2013, the American College of Critical Care Medicine, in collaboration with the Society of Critical Care Medicine and American Society of Health-System Pharmacists, updated the Clinical Practice Guidelines for the Management of Pain, Agitation, and Delirium in Adult Patients in the Intensive Care Unit (ICU PAD Guidelines) to provide recommendations for clinicians to better manage critically ill patients.[6] Many elements of the symptom-based ICU PAD guideline are implemented using an interdependent, multicomponent, evidence-based guide for the coordination multidisciplinary ICU care, the ABCDEF bundle. The ABCDEF bundle includes: *Assess, prevent, and manage pain; *Both spontaneous awakening trials (SAT) and spontaneous breathing trials (SBT); *Choice of analgesia and sedation; *Delirium: assess, prevent, and manage; *Early mobility and exercise; and *Family engagement and empowerment.

ASSESS, PREVENT, AND MANAGE PAIN

ICU patients commonly experience pain, with an incidence of up to 50% in surgical and medical patients. It is a major clinical symptom that requires systematic diagnosis and treatment.[7,8]

In a prospective, cross-sectional, multicenter, multinational study of pain intensity associated with 12 procedures, the Europain study, Puntillo and colleagues[9] showed that common ICU procedures induced a significant increase in pain, although no procedure caused severe pain. For the three most painful procedures (ie, chest tube removal, wound drain removal, and arterial line insertion) pain intensity more than doubled during the procedure compared with the preprocedural levels.

Assessment of pain is the first step before administering pain relief. Pain assessments are often only performed 35% of the time before ICU procedures.[7] Patient's self-report of pain using a 1 to 10 numerical rating scale is considered the gold standard and is highly recommended by many critical care societies.[6,8] Because of the high interrelation between delirium and pain,[8] assessing and treating pain could be important in the prevention and/or management of delirium.

In the absence of a patient's self-report, observable behavioral and physiologic indicators become important indices for the assessment of pain.[10] The Behavioral Pain Scale (BPS) and the Critical Care Pain Observation Tool (CPOT) are the most valid and reliable behavioral pain scales for ICU patients unable to communicate (Table 1). The BPS is composed of three subscales: (1) facial expression, (2) movement of the upper limbs, and (3) compliance with mechanical ventilation. Each subscale is scored from one (no response) to four (full response). A BPS score of five or higher is considered to reflect unacceptable pain. The CPOT has components: (1) facial expression, (2) body movements, (3) muscle tension, and (4) compliance with the ventilator for intubated patients or vocalization for extubated patients. Each component is scored from zero to two with a possible total score ranging from zero to eight. A CPOT greater than or equal to three indicates significant pain. Both the BPS and the CPOT provide guidance for the selection of pharmacologic interventions for pain and in the evaluation of their effectiveness.[11,12]

According to ICU PAD Guidelines, pain medications should be routinely administered in the presence of significant pain (ie, numerical rating scale ≥4, BPS >5, or CPOT ≥3) and before performing painful invasive procedures. Parenteral opioids are first-line pharmacologic agents for treating nonneuropathic pain in critically ill patients. All opioids have the potential to induce tolerance over time, resulting in the need

Table 1
Clinical Pain Observational Tool and Behavioral Pain Scale

Critical Pain Observational Tool (CPOT)

	Score
Facial expressions	
Relaxed, neutral	0
Tense	1
Grimacing	2
Body movements	
Absence of movements or normal position	0
Protection	1
Restlessness/agitation	2
Compliance with the ventilator (intubated patients)	
Tolerating ventilator or movement	0
Coughing but tolerating	1
Fighting ventilator	2
Vocalization (nonintubuted patients)	
Talking in normal tone or no sound	0
Sighing, moaning	1
Crying out sobbing	2
Muscle tension	
Relaxed	0
Tense, rigid	1
Very tense or rigid	2

Behavioral Pain Scale (BPS)

	Score
Facial expressions	
Relaxed	1
Partially tightened	2
Fully tightened	3
Upper limbs	
No movement	1
Partially bent	2
Fully bent with finger flexion	3
Permanently retracted	4
Compliance with ventilation	
Tolerating movement	1
Coughing but tolerating ventilation for most of the time	2
Fighting ventilator	3
Unable to control ventilation	4

BPS greater than five or CPOT greater than three indicate significant pain.
Adapted from Payen JF, Bru O, Bosson JL, et al. Assessing pain in critically ill sedated patients by using a behavioral pain scale. Crit Care Med 2001;29(12):2259.

for escalating doses to achieve the same analgesic effect. For the treatment of neuropathic pain in ICU patients, gabapentin or carbamazepine should be administered enterally, in addition to opioids. Nonopioid analgesics, such as acetaminophen, nonsteroidal anti-inflammatory drugs, or ketamine, should be used as adjunctive pain medications to reduce opioid requirements and opioid-related side effects. Use of regional analgesia in ICU patients is limited to the use of epidural analgesia in specific subpopulations of surgical patients, and in patients with traumatic rib fractures.[6] In managing pain in the ICU, nonpharmacologic methods are often effective and safe (eg, injury stabilization, patient repositioning, use of heat/cold).[13]

BOTH SPONTANEOUS AWAKENING TRIALS AND SPONTANEOUS BREATHING TRIALS

Daily SATs are the stopping of narcotics (as long as pain is controlled) and sedatives every day and, if needed, restarting either narcotics or sedatives at half the previous dose and titrating as need. Daily interruption of sedation shortens the duration of mechanical ventilation and the ICU length of stay. The 2013 ICU PAD Guidelines emphasize the importance of minimizing sedative use and maintaining a light level of sedation in patients, using either a daily sedative interruption strategy (ie, SAT), or by continuously titrating sedatives to maintain a light level of sedation (ie, targeted sedation strategy). Kress and colleagues[14] conducted a randomized, controlled trial involving 128 adult patients who were receiving mechanical ventilation and continuous infusions of sedative drugs in a medical ICU. In the intervention group, the sedative infusions were interrupted daily until the patients were awake; in the control group, the infusions were interrupted only at the discretion of the clinicians. In this study, daily interruption of the infusion of sedative drugs shortened the duration of mechanical ventilation by more than 2 days and the length of stay in the ICU by 3.5 days.[14] These data suggest that daily SAT uses less analgosedation while improving ICU outcomes.[14]

There is a consistent relationship between deeper sedation and worse ICU outcomes. Deep sedation in the first 48 hours of an ICU stay has been associated with delayed time to extubation, higher need for tracheostomy, increased risk of hospital, and long-term death.[15-17] Shehabi and colleagues[15] examined the relationships between early sedation and time to extubation, delirium, hospital, and 180-day mortality among ventilated critically ill patients in the ICU. Every additional Richmond Agitation-Sedation Score (RASS) assessment in the deep sedation range in the first 48 hours was associated with delayed time to extubation of 12.3 hours, a 10% increased risk of hospital death, and an 8% increased risk of death at 6 months. Balzer and colleagues[17] examined short- and long-term survival after deep sedation during the first 48 hours after ICU admission. In this study, 1884 patients receiving mechanical ventilation were grouped as either lightly or deeply sedated (light sedation, RASS −2 to 0; deep sedation, RASS −3 or less). Deep sedation (27.2%; n = 513) was associated with an in-hospital mortality hazard ratio of 1.661 (95% confidence interval [CI], 1.074–2.567; $P = .022$) and a 2-year hazard ratio of 1.866 (95% CI, 1.351–2.576; $P<.001$). In summary, deeply sedated patients had longer ventilation times, increased length of stay, and higher rates of mortality.[17] These studies show that early deep sedation is a modifiable risk factor and that the implementation of sedation protocols to achieve light sedation is feasible and reproducible in the early phase of ICU treatment.

Daily SBT has been proven to be effective and superior to other techniques to ventilator weaning. Numerous randomized trials support the use of ventilator weaning protocols that include daily SBTs as their centerpiece.[18,19] About two-thirds of the time on mechanical ventilation is spent during weaning, so anything that reduced this period would have a high likelihood of improving outcomes. Girard and colleagues[20] undertook the Awakening and Breathing Controlled (ABC) trial, a multicenter, randomized controlled trial to assess the efficacy and safety of a protocol of daily SATs paired with SBTs (intervention group, n = 168) versus a standard SBT protocol in patients receiving patient-targeted sedation as part of usual care (control group, n = 168). Patients in the intervention group (both SAT and SBT) spent more days breathing without assistance during the 28-day study period (14.7 days vs 11.6 days; mean difference, 3.1 days; 95% CI, 0.7–5.6; P = .02) and were discharged earlier from the ICU (median time in ICU, 9.1 days vs 12.9 days; P = .01) and earlier from the hospital (median hospital time, 14.9 days vs 19.2 days; P = .04).[20] During the year after enrollment, patients receiving SATs with SBTs (intervention) were less likely to die than were patients receiving only SBTs (control) (hazard ratio, 0.68; 95% CI, 0.50–0.92; P = 0.01). For every seven patients treated with the intervention, one life was saved (number needed to treat, 7.4; 95% CI, 4.2–35.5).[20] Conversely, the SLEAP trial (protocolized light sedation in combination with daily SAT vs protocolized light sedation alone) found no difference between the groups with regard to time to extubation, duration of ICU, and hospital stays.[21] One reason the SLEAP study might not have showed an effect is because both the treatment and control groups received high sedative doses that would result in moderate to deep levels, rather than light levels of sedation.[22]

No sedation has also been applied as a strategy in ICU patients. Strøm and colleagues[23] enrolled 140 critically ill adult patients who were undergoing mechanical ventilation and were expected to need ventilation for more than 1 day. Patients were randomly assigned in a 1:1 ratio (unblinded) to receive no sedation (n = 70 patients) or sedation (n = 70, control group). Patients receiving no sedation had significantly more days without ventilation (mean, 13.8 days [standard deviation, 11.0] vs mean, 9.6 days [standard deviation, 10.0]; mean difference, 4.2 days; 95% CI, 0.3–8.1; P = .0191) in a 28-day period, and reduced stays in the ICU and hospital. This study did find increased hyperactive delirium in the group receiving no sedation.[23]

Ultimately, the core features of the ABCDEF bundle involve coordination of SATs and SBTs emphasizing narcotic and sedation titration resulting in earlier liberation from mechanical ventilation, ICU, and hospitalization (Fig. 1).

CHOICE OF ANALGESIA AND SEDATION

The 2013 PAD guidelines emphasize the need for goal-directed delivery of psychoactive medications to avoid oversedation, to promote earlier extubation, and to help the medical team agree on a target sedation level by using sedation scales. Of the available reliable and valid sedation scales, the PAD guidelines recommend the use of the RASS and the Riker Sedation-Agitation Scale (SAS). Table 2 shows the psychometric properties of the RASS and SAS. The SAS has seven individual tiers ranging from unarousable (one) to dangerous agitation (seven).[24] RASS is a 10-point scale, with four levels of escalating agitation (RASS +1 to +4), one level denoting a calm and alert state (RASS 0), three levels of sedation (RASS −1 to −3), and two levels of coma (RASS −4 to −5). A unique feature of RASS is that it relies on the duration of eye contact following verbal stimulation. The RASS takes less than 20 seconds to perform with minimal training, and has shown high reliability among multiple types of health care providers and an excellent interrater reliability in a broad range of adult medical and surgical ICU patients.[25]

To maximize patient outcomes, it is essential to carefully choose sedatives and analgesic medications, and consider medication doses, titration, and discontinuation.[25] For example, there is a clear association between decreased exposure to

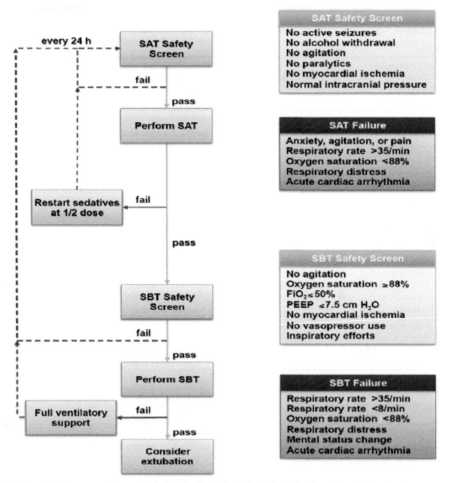

Fig. 1. "Wake up and breathe" protocol: SATs with SBTs. FiO₂, fraction of inspired oxygen; PEEP, positive end-expiratory pressure. (*From* ICU Delirium, Vanderbilt University. Available at: www.ICUdelerium.org.)

sedatives, particularly benzodiazepines, and improved patient outcomes.[15,17,26,27] Pandharipande and colleagues[28] evaluated 198 mechanically ventilated patients to determine the probability of daily transition to delirium, as a function of sedative and analgesic dose administration during the previous 24-hour period. They found that every unit dose of lorazepam was associated with a higher risk for daily transition to delirium (odds ratio, 1.2; 95% CI, 1.1–1.4; $P = .003$).[28] Similarly Seymour and colleagues[29] confirmed that benzodiazepines are an independent risk factor for development of delirium during critical illness even when given more than 8 hours before a delirium assessment. These results expand and support the recommendation made in the 2013 ICU PAD guidelines that nonbenzodiazepine sedative options may be preferred over benzodiazepine-based sedative regimens.[6]

Two major studies evaluated benzodiazepines against a novel α_2-agonist sedative, dexmedetomidine. The SEDCOM trial (Safety and Efficacy of Dexmedetomidine Compared with Midazolam) showed a reduction in the prevalence of delirium and in

Table 2
Richmond Agitation-Sedation Scale and Riker Sedation-Agitation Scale

RASS	SAS
+4 Combative Combative, violent immediate danger to staff	7 Dangerous agitation Pulling at ETT, trying to remove catheters, climbing over bedrail, striking at staff, trashing side-to-side
+3 Very agitated Pulls to remove tubes or catheters; aggressive	6 Very agitated Requiring restraint and frequent verbal reminding of limits, biting ETT
+2 Agitated Frequent nonpurposeful movement, fights ventilator	6 Very agitated Requiring restraint and frequent verbal reminding of limits, biting ETT
+1 Restless Anxious, apprehensive, movements not aggressive	5 Agitated Anxious or physically agitated, calms to verbal instructions
0 Alert and calm Spontaneously pays attention to caregiver	4 Calm and cooperative Calm, easily arousable, follows commands
−1 Drowsy Not fully alert, but has sustained awakening to voice: eye opening and contact >10 s	3 Sedated Difficult to arouse but awakens to verbal stimuli or gentle shaking, follows simple commands but drifts off again
−2 Light sedation Briefly awakens to voice: eyes open and contact <10 s	3 Sedated Difficult to arouse but awakens to verbal stimuli or gentle shaking, follows simple commands but drifts off again
−3 Moderate sedation Movement or eye opening to voice: no eye contact	3 Sedated Difficult to arouse but awakens to verbal stimuli or gentle shaking, follows simple commands but drifts off again
−4 Deep sedation No response to voice, but movement or eye opening to physical stimulation	3 Sedated Difficult to arouse but awakens to verbal stimuli or gentle shaking, follows simple commands but drifts off again 2 Very sedated Arouses to physical stimuli but does not communicate or follow commands, may move spontaneously
−5 Unarousable No response to voice or physical stimulation	1 Unarousable Minimal or no response to noxious stimuli, does not communicate or follow commands

Abbreviation: ETT, endotracheal tube.

From ICU Delirium, Vanderbilt University. Available at: www.ICUdelerium.org. Accessed December 29, 2016; and *Adapted from* Riker RR, Picard JT, Fraser GL. Prospective evaluation of the sedation-agitation scale for adult critically ill patients. Crit Care Med 1999;27(7):1327; and Sessler CN, Gosnell MS, Grap MJ, et al. The Richmond Agitation–Sedation Scale: validity and reliability in adult intensive care unit patients. Am J Respir Crit Care Med 2002;166:1339.

the duration of mechanical ventilation in patients sedated with dexmedetomidine compared with midazolam.[30] The MENDS study (Maximizing Efficacy of Targeted Sedation and Reducing Neurologic Dysfunction) evaluated the role of changing sedation paradigms on acute brain dysfunction, comparing dexmedetomidine with lorazepam.[31] The dexmedetomidine sedative strategy resulted in more days alive without delirium or coma, but without differences in mortality or ventilator-free days. Notably, the subgroup of patients with sepsis sedated with dexmedetomidine in the MENDS study had shorter durations of delirium and coma, lower daily probability of delirium, shorter time on the ventilator, and improved 28-day survival.[32] There is an ongoing trial (MENDS II study) to determine the best sedative medication to reduce delirium and improve survival and long-term brain function in the ventilated patient with sepsis (ClinicalTrials.gov Identifier: NCT01739933).

DELIRIUM—ASSESS, PREVENT, AND MANAGE

An important third element in the PAD guidelines is monitoring and management of delirium. Delirium is a disturbance in attention and awareness that develops over a short period of time, hours to days, and fluctuates over time.[33] More than 80% of patients developed delirium during their hospital stay, with most cases occurring in the ICU with an average time of onset between the second and the third day.

Several methods have been developed and validated to diagnose delirium in ICU patients but the Confusion Assessment Method for the Intensive Care Unit (CAM-ICU; Fig. 2A) and the Intensive Care Delirium Screening Checklist (ICDSC; Fig. 2B) are the most frequently used tools for this purpose.[34] The ICDSC checklist is an eight-item screening tool (one point for each item) that is based on Diagnostic and Statistical Manual criteria and applied to data that are collected through medical records or to information obtained from the multidisciplinary team.[34] The pooled values for the sensitivity and specificity of the ICDSC are 74% and 81.9%, respectively.[34] The CAM-ICU is composed by four features: (1) acute onset of mental status changes or fluctuating course, (2) inattention, (3) disorganized thinking, and (4) altered level of consciousness. The patient is considered CAM positive and thus delirious if he/she manifests both features one and two, plus either feature three or four.[35] Overall accuracy of the CAM-ICU is excellent, with pooled values for sensitivity and specificity of 80% and 95.9%, respectively.[34] The CAM-ICU has been modified and validated in pediatric, emergency department, and neurocritical care populations, and translated in more than 25 languages.[36–40]

Delirium can be categorized into subtypes according to psychomotor behavior. Hyperactive delirium (CAM positive, RASS positive range) is associated with a better overall prognosis and it is characterized by agitation, restlessness, and emotional lability.[41] Hypoactive delirium (CAM positive, RASS negative range), which is common and often more deleterious in the long term, is characterized by decreased responsiveness, withdrawal, and apathy and remains unrecognized in 66% to 84% of hospitalized patients.[42] Another categorization based on the ICDSC score assigns patients with a score of zero to have no delirium, those with a score greater than or equal to four to have clinical delirium, and those with a score of one to three to have subsyndromal delirium.[43] Whichever delirium metric is used, the best picture of the patient's mental status comes from assessing delirium serially throughout the day.

Evidence shows that delirium is a strong predictor of increased length of mechanical ventilation, longer ICU stays, increased cost, long-term cognitive impairment, and mortality (Fig. 3).[19,44–47] The cumulative effect of multiple days of delirium on mortality may be multiplicative, rather than additive.[48]

Numerous risk factors for delirium have been identified, including preexisting cognitive impairment; advanced age; use of psychoactive drugs; mechanical ventilation; untreated pain; and a variety of medical conditions, such as heart failure, prolonged immobilization, abnormal blood pressure, anemia, sleep deprivation, and sepsis.[42,49] The most frequent risk factor was the use of benzodiazepines or

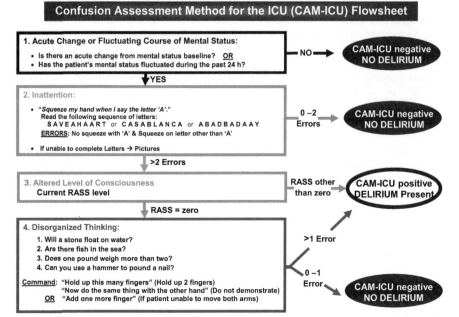

Fig. 2. (A) Confusion assessment method for the ICU (CAM-ICU). (B) Intensive Care Delirium Screening checklist. Normal, 0; delirium, 4–8; subsyndromal delirium, 1–3. Score your patient over the entire shift. Components do not all need to be present at the same time. Components 1 through 4 cannot be completed when the patient is deeply sedated or comatose (ie, SAS = 1 or 2; RASS = −4 or −5); Components 5 through 8 are based on observations throughout the entire shift. Information from the prior 24 hours should be obtained for components 7 and 8. ([A] *Courtesy of* E. Wesley, MD, MPH and Vanderbilt University, Nashville, TN; and [B] *Adapted from* Bergeron N, Dubois MJ, Dumont M, et al. Intensive care delirium screening checklist: evaluation of a new screening tool. Intensive Care Med 2001;27(5):859–64; and Ouimet S, Riker R, Bergeron N, et al. Sub-syndromal delirium in the ICU: evidence for a disease spectrum. Intensive Care Med 2007;33:1007–13.)

narcotics (98%).[44] The mean number of identified risk factors for delirium in these patients was 11 ± 4 with a range of 3 to 17 risk factors present. Patients with three or more risk factors were considered at high risk for delirium.[42,49,50] In delirious patients, a systematic protocolized search for all reversible precipitants is the first line of action and symptomatic treatment should be considered when available and not contraindicated (**Fig. 4**).[51]

Antipsychotics, especially haloperidol, are commonly administered for the treatment of delirium in critically ill patients. However, evidence for the safety and efficacy of antipsychotics in this patient population is lacking. Moreover, the 2013 PAD Guidelines include no specific recommendations for using any particular medication.[6] Ely and colleagues are conducting the MIND-USA (Modifying the Impact of ICU-Induced Neurologic Dysfunction-USA) Study (ClinicalTrials.gov Identifier NCT01211522) to define the role of antipsychotics in the management of delirium in vulnerable critically ill patients.

Delirium prophylaxis with medications is discouraged in the PAD guidelines. Recently, a prospective, randomized, multicenter trial compared a low-dose

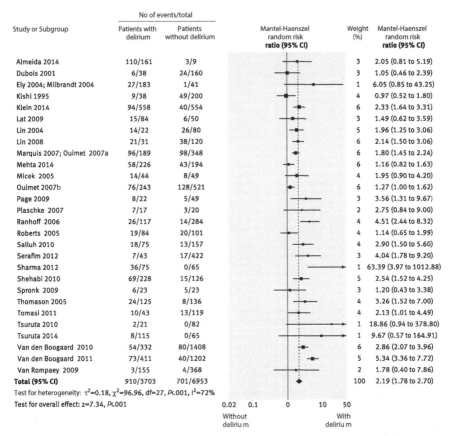

Study or Subgroup	No of events/total		Mantel-Haenszel random risk ratio (95% CI)	Weight (%)	Mantel-Haenszel random risk ratio (95% CI)
	Patients with delirium	Patients without delirium			
Almeida 2014	110/161	3/9		3	2.05 (0.81 to 5.19)
Dubois 2001	6/38	24/160		3	1.05 (0.46 to 2.39)
Ely 2004; Milbrandt 2004	27/183	1/41		1	6.05 (0.85 to 43.25)
Kishi 1995	9/38	49/200		4	0.97 (0.52 to 1.80)
Klein 2014	94/558	40/554		6	2.33 (1.64 to 3.31)
Lat 2009	15/84	6/50		3	1.49 (0.62 to 3.59)
Lin 2004	14/22	26/80		5	1.96 (1.25 to 3.06)
Lin 2008	21/31	38/120		6	2.14 (1.50 to 3.06)
Marquis 2007; Ouimet 2007a	96/189	98/348		6	1.80 (1.45 to 2.24)
Mehta 2014	58/226	43/194		6	1.16 (0.82 to 1.63)
Micek 2005	14/44	8/49		4	1.95 (0.90 to 4.20)
Ouimet 2007b	76/243	128/521		6	1.27 (1.00 to 1.62)
Page 2009	8/22	5/49		3	3.56 (1.31 to 9.67)
Plaschke 2007	7/17	3/20		2	2.75 (0.84 to 9.00)
Ranhoff 2006	26/117	14/284		4	4.51 (2.44 to 8.32)
Roberts 2005	19/84	20/101		4	1.14 (0.65 to 1.99)
Salluh 2010	18/75	13/157		4	2.90 (1.50 to 5.60)
Serafim 2012	7/43	17/422		3	4.04 (1.78 to 9.20)
Sharma 2012	36/75	0/65		1	63.39 (3.97 to 1012.88)
Shehabi 2010	69/228	15/126		5	2.54 (1.52 to 4.25)
Spronk 2009	6/23	5/23		3	1.20 (0.43 to 3.38)
Thomason 2005	24/125	8/136		4	3.26 (1.52 to 7.00)
Tomasi 2011	10/43	13/119		4	2.13 (1.01 to 4.49)
Tsuruta 2010	2/21	0/82		1	18.86 (0.94 to 378.80)
Tsuruta 2014	8/115	0/65		1	9.67 (0.57 to 164.91)
Van den Boogaard 2010	54/332	80/1408		6	2.86 (2.07 to 3.96)
Van den Boogaard 2011	73/411	40/1202		5	5.34 (3.36 to 7.72)
Van Rompaey 2009	3/155	4/368		2	1.78 (0.40 to 7.86)
Total (95% CI)	910/3703	701/6953		100	2.19 (1.78 to 2.70)

Test for heterogeneity: $\tau^2 = 0.18$, $\chi^2 = 96.96$, df=27, $P < .001$, $I^2 = 72\%$
Test for overall effect: z=7.34, $P < .001$

0.02   0.1   0   10   50
Without delirium   With delirium

Fig. 3. Impact of delirium on hospital mortality in critically ill patients. CI, confidence interval. (*From* Salluh JI, Wang H, Schneider EB, et al. Outcome of delirium in critically ill patients: systematic review and meta-analysis. BMJ 2015;350:h2538.)

haloperidol infusion administered for 12 hours (0.5-mg intravenous bolus injection followed by continuous infusion at a rate of 0.1 mg/h; n = 229 patients) with placebo (n = 228 patients) in the immediate postoperative period. This study provided evidence that haloperidol could reduce the incidence of delirium within the first 7 days postoperatively in patients undergoing noncardiac surgery (15.3% in the haloperidol group vs 23.2% in the control group; $P = .031$).[52] By contrast, another ICU study showed no benefit of early administration of intravenous haloperidol in a mixed population of medical and surgical adult ICU patients.[53] In this double-blinded, placebo-controlled randomized trial, 142 patients were randomized to receive haloperidol or placebo intravenously every 8 hours irrespective of coma or delirium status. Patients in the haloperidol group spent about the same number of days alive, without delirium or coma, as did patients in the placebo group (median, 5 days [interquartile range, 0–10] vs 6 days [0–11] days; $P = .53$).

The only strategy strongly recommended in the PAD Guidelines to reduce the incidence and duration of ICU delirium and to improve functional outcomes is promoting sleep hygiene to prevent sleep disruption and the use of early and progressive mobilization in these patients.

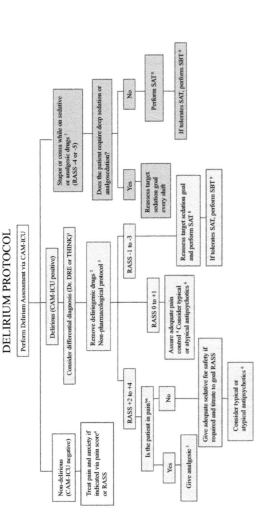

Fig. 4. Sample delirium protocol. CPAP, continuous positive airway pressure; EKG, electrocardiogram; PEEP, positive end-expiratory pressure; PS, Pressure Support. (*From* ICU Delirium, Vanderbilt University. Available at: www.ICUdelirium.org. Accessed December 29, 2016.)

EARLY MOBILITY

Early mobility is an integral part of the ABCDEF bundle and has been the only intervention resulting in a decrease in days of delirium.[54] During ICU stay critically ill patients can lose up to 25% peripheral muscle weakness within 4 days when mechanically ventilated and 18% in body weight by the time of discharge and this process is higher in the first 2 to 3 weeks of immobilization.[55] The consequence of physical dysfunction in critically ill patients is profound and long-term with significant reduction in functional status being observed even 1 year and 5 years after ICU discharge.[56–58]

ICU-acquired weakness is caused by many different pathophysiologic mechanisms that are not mutually exclusive given the diverse diseases that precipitate critical illness, the drugs used during its management, and the consequences of protracted immobility.[54] The reported incidence of ICU-acquired weakness ranges from 25% to 100%.[59,60] The diagnosis of ICU-acquired weakness is made by the Medical Research Council scale for grading the strength (ie, 0 [total palsy] to 5 [normal strength]) of various muscle groups in the upper and lower extremities. The scale ranges from 0 (complete tetraplegia) to 60 (normal muscle strength), with a score less than 48 diagnostic of ICU-acquired weakness.[61] Patients with ICU-acquired weakness should undergo serial evaluations, and if persistent deficits are noted, electrophysiologic studies, muscle biopsy, or both are warranted.[54]

Although clinical providers may have fears about early mobilization, there is good evidence regarding the strategy of minimizing sedation and increasing the physical activity of ICU patients to the point of getting up and out of bed.[54] Physical therapy has shown to be feasible and safe, even in the most complicated patients receiving the most advanced medical therapies (eg, continuous renal-replacement therapy, extracorporeal cardiopulmonary support).[62,63] Early activity can be done without increases in usual ICU staffing and with a low risk (<1%) of complications.[64] Studying patients early in the their course of mechanical ventilation (<3 days), Schweickert and colleagues[65] showed that a daily SAT combined with physical and occupational therapy, versus SAT alone, resulted in an improved return to independent functional status at hospital discharge, shorter duration of ICU-delirium, higher survival, and more days breathing without assistance. However, in a study where ICU patients were enrolled 4 days after the initiation of mechanical ventilation (average, 8 days), an intensive physical therapy program did not improve long-term physical functioning when compared with a standard of care program.[66] Although both these studies demonstrated feasibility of physical therapy, it may be more effective to embark on physical therapy early in the ICU course, rather than later when it is much more challenging to improve ICU-acquired weakness.[65,66]

The focus on rehabilitation of critically ill patients should begin in the ICU and continue all the way to recovery at home. The close collaboration and coordination with medicine, nursing, and physical therapists is fundamental for an efficacy and safe strategy.[62] This is particularly important because the burden of illness affects not only the patient but also his or her family or other caregivers.[54]

FAMILY ENGAGEMENT

The ABCDE bundle has evolved to include family engagement, because no ICU treatment plan is complete without incorporation of the family's wishes, concerns, questions, and participation. Family members and surrogate decision makers must become active partners in multiprofessional decision-making and treatment planning.

Through this partnership, patients' preferences are identified, the anxiety of families is lessened, and physicians can have appropriate input into decisions.[67]

Family presence on ICU rounds is beneficial, and it does not interfere with education and communication process.[68] Families have reported increased feelings of inclusion, respect, and having a better understanding of their loved one's care. Nurses have indicated satisfaction with team communication and facilitation of family relationships.[69] Several studies suggested that increased focus on communication with family members, through routine ICU family conferences, palliative care consultation, or ethics consultation, can reduce ICU length of stay for those patients whose trajectory is ultimately mortal.[70–73] One study of communication occurring during ICU family conferences sought to understand how ICU clinicians conduct communication concerning withdrawing life-sustaining treatments or the delivery of bad news, and how this communication might be improved.[74] Most clinicians failed to listen and respond appropriately, failed to acknowledge the expression of family members' emotions, and failed to explain key tenets of palliative care. An important missed opportunity when communicating with families is exploring patient treatment preferences that are key to clinical decision making in the ICU setting.[74]

Ethics and palliative care consultations have been introduced into the practice of medicine during the past several decades as a way to help health care professionals, patients, and surrogates come to a decision about medical treatment ensuring that the process of decision making is inclusive, educational, respectful of cultural values, and reflect appropriate resource utilization. When ethics consultation have been used, they have been associated with reductions in hospital and ICU lengths of stay, and more frequent decisions to forgo life-sustaining treatment.[72,75] When tackling treatment conflicts, most (87%) ICU physicians, nurses, and patients/surrogates agreed that ethics consultations are helpful. However, in a recent randomized study in four medical ICUs in those receiving mechanical ventilation for greater than 1 week, family discussions conducted by palliative care specialists (intervention) versus standard ICU-led family discussions (control) did not alter anxiety or depression symptoms in surrogate decision makers.[76]

Beyond sharing of communication, family presence has been encouraged in traumatizing medical events and procedures, such as cardiopulmonary resuscitation (CPR). In some studies, the family presence during CPR is associated with positive results on psychological variables, and did not interfere with medical efforts, increase stress in the health care team, or result in medicolegal conflicts. In fact, relatives who did not witness CPR had symptoms of anxiety and depression more frequently than those who did witness CPR.[77]

Critical illness usually impacts not only an individual, but their entire support system, which may or may not be their nuclear family, or some combination of family and friends or other caregivers who are actively engaged in supportive roles. In light of this, it is crucial not only to recognize the needs of the identified patient but also the needs of their family.

SUMMARY

The core evidence and features behind the ABCDEF bundle have been reviewed, which was created to combat the adverse effects of critical illness related to acute and chronic brain dysfunction. The ABCDEF bundle represents one method of approaching the organizational changes that create a culture shift in treatment of ICU patients. The multifold potential benefits of these recommended strategies outweigh minimal risks of costs and coordination. Ultimately, the ABCDEF bundle is one path to well-rounded patient care and optimal resource utilization resulting in more interactive ICU patients with better pain control, who can safely participate with their families and health care providers in higher-order physical and cognitive activities at the earliest point in their critical illness.

REFERENCES

1. Ehlenbach WJ, Hough CL, Crane PK, et al. Association between acute care and critical illness hospitalization and cognitive function in older adults. JAMA 2010; 303(8):763–70.
2. Patel MB, Jackson JC, Morandi A, et al. Incidence and risk factors for intensive care unit-related post-traumatic stress disorder in veterans and civilians. Am J Respir Crit Care Med 2016;193(12):1373–81.
3. Jackson JC, Pandharipande PP, Girard TD, et al. Depression, post-traumatic stress disorder, and functional disability in survivors of critical illness in the BRAIN-ICU study: a longitudinal cohort study. Lancet Respir Med 2014;2(5): 369–79.
4. Pandharipande PP, Girard TD, Jackson JC, et al. Long-term cognitive impairment after critical illness. N Engl J Med 2013;369(14):1306–16.
5. Covinsky KE, Pierluissi E, Johnston CB. Hospitalization-associated disability: "She was probably able to ambulate, but I'm not sure. JAMA 2011;306(16): 1782–93.
6. Barr J, Fraser GL, Puntillo K, et al. Clinical practice guidelines for the management of pain, agitation, and delirium in adult patients in the intensive care unit. Crit Care Med 2013;41(1):263–306.
7. Payen JF, Chanques G, Mantz J, et al. Current practices in sedation and analgesia for mechanically ventilated critically ill patients: a prospective multicenter patient-based study. Anesthesiology 2007;106(4):687–95.
8. Chanques G, Viel E, Constantin JM, et al. The measurement of pain in intensive care unit: comparison of 5 self-report intensity scales. Pain 2010;151(3):711–21.
9. Puntillo KA, Max A, Timsit JF, et al. Determinants of procedural pain intensity in the intensive care unit. The Europain(R) study. Am J Respir Crit Care Med 2014;189(1):39–47.
10. Gelinas C, Fillion L, Puntillo KA, et al. Validation of the critical-care pain observation tool in adult patients. Am J Crit Care 2006;15(4):420–7.
11. Chanques G, Jaber S, Barbotte E, et al. Impact of systematic evaluation of pain and agitation in an intensive care unit. Crit Care Med 2006;34(6):1691–9.
12. Payen JF, Bosson JL, Chanques G, et al. Pain assessment is associated with decreased duration of mechanical ventilation in the intensive care unit: a post hoc analysis of the DOLOREA study. Anesthesiology 2009;111(6):1308–16.
13. Erstad BL, Puntillo K, Gilbert HC, et al. Pain management principles in the critically ill. Chest 2009;135(4):1075–86.
14. Kress JP, Pohlman AS, O'Connor MF, et al. Daily interruption of sedative infusions in critically ill patients undergoing mechanical ventilation. N Engl J Med 2000; 342(20):1471–7.
15. Shehabi Y, Bellomo R, Reade MC, et al. Early intensive care sedation predicts long-term mortality in ventilated critically ill patients. Am J Respir Crit Care Med 2012;186(8):724–31.

16. Tanaka LM, Azevedo LC, Park M, et al. Early sedation and clinical outcomes of mechanically ventilated patients: a prospective multicenter cohort study. Crit Care 2014;18(4):R156.

17. Balzer F, Weiss B, Kumpf O, et al. Early deep sedation is associated with decreased in-hospital and two-year follow-up survival. Crit Care 2015;19:197.

18. Pandharipande P, Banerjee A, McGrane S, et al. Liberation and animation for ventilated ICU patients: the ABCDE bundle for the back-end of critical care. Crit Care 2010;14(3):157.

19. Ely EW, Baker AM, Dunagan DP, et al. Effect on the duration of mechanical ventilation of identifying patients capable of breathing spontaneously. N Engl J Med 1996;335(25):1864–9.

20. Girard TD, Kress JP, Fuchs BD, et al. Efficacy and safety of a paired sedation and ventilator weaning protocol for mechanically ventilated patients in intensive care (Awakening and Breathing Controlled trial): a randomised controlled trial. Lancet 2008;371(9607):126–34.

21. Mehta S, Burry L, Cook D, et al. Daily sedation interruption in mechanically ventilated critically ill patients cared for with a sedation protocol: a randomized controlled trial. JAMA 2012;308(19):1985–92.

22. Hughes CG, Girard TD, Pandharipande PP. Daily sedation interruption versus targeted light sedation strategies in ICU patients. Crit Care Med 2013;41(9 Suppl 1): S39–45.

23. Strøm T, Martinussen T, Toft P. A protocol of no sedation for critically ill patients receiving mechanical ventilation: a randomised trial. Lancet 2010;375(9713): 475–80.

24. Khan BA, Guzman O, Campbell NL, et al. Comparison and agreement between the Richmond agitation-sedation scale and the Riker Sedation-Agitation Scale in evaluating patients' eligibility for delirium assessment in the ICU. Chest 2012; 142(1):48–54.

25. Ely EW, Truman B, Shintani A, et al. Monitoring sedation status over time in ICU patients: reliability and validity of the Richmond Agitation-Sedation Scale (RASS). JAMA 2003;289(22):2983–91.

26. Kollef MH, Levy NT, Ahrens TS, et al. The use of continuous IV sedation is associated with prolongation of mechanical ventilation. Chest 1998;114(2):541–8.

27. Dale CR, Kannas DA, Fan VS, et al. Improved analgesia, sedation, and delirium protocol associated with decreased duration of delirium and mechanical ventilation. Ann Am Thorac Soc 2014;11(3):367–74.

28. Pandharipande P, Shintani A, Peterson J, et al. Lorazepam is an independent risk factor for transitioning to delirium in intensive care unit patients. Anesthesiology 2006;104(1):21–6.

29. Seymour CW, Pandharipande PP, Koestner T, et al. Diurnal sedative changes during intensive care: impact on liberation from mechanical ventilation and delirium. Crit Care Med 2012;40(10):2788–96.

30. Riker RR, Shehabi Y, Bokesch PM, et al. Dexmedetomidine vs midazolam for sedation of critically ill patients: a randomized trial. JAMA 2009;301(5):489–99.

31. Pandharipande PP, Pun BT, Herr DL, et al. Effect of sedation with dexmedetomidine vs lorazepam on acute brain dysfunction in mechanically ventilated patients: the MENDS randomized controlled trial. JAMA 2007;298(22):2644–53.

32. Pandharipande PP, Sanders RD, Girard TD, et al. Effect of dexmedetomidine versus lorazepam on outcome in patients with sepsis: an a priori-designed analysis of the MENDS randomized controlled trial. Crit Care 2010;14(2):R38.

33. American Psychiatric Association. Diagnostic and statistical manual of mental disorders: DSM-5. Washington, DC: American Psychiatric Association; 2013.

34. Gusmao-Flores D, Salluh JI, Chalhub RA, et al. The Confusion Assessment Method for the Intensive Care Unit (CAM-ICU) and Intensive Care Delirium Screening Checklist (ICDSC) for the diagnosis of delirium: a systematic review and meta-analysis of clinical studies. Crit Care 2012;16(4):R115.

35. Ely EW, Inouye SK, Bernard GR, et al. Delirium in mechanically ventilated patients: validity and reliability of the confusion assessment method for the intensive care unit (CAM-ICU). JAMA 2001;286(21):2703–10.

36. Mitasova A, Kostalova M, Bednarik J, et al. Poststroke delirium incidence and outcomes: validation of the Confusion Assessment Method for the Intensive Care Unit (CAM-ICU). Crit Care Med 2012;40(2):484–90.

37. Naidech AM, Beaumont JL, Rosenberg NF, et al. Intracerebral hemorrhage and delirium symptoms. Length of stay, function, and quality of life in a 114-patient cohort. Am J Respir Crit Care Med 2013;188(11):1331–7.

38. Han JH, Wilson A, Graves AJ, et al. Validation of the Confusion Assessment Method for the Intensive Care Unit in older emergency department patients. Acad Emerg Med 2014;21(2):180–7.

39. Smith HA, Boyd J, Fuchs DC, et al. Diagnosing delirium in critically ill children: validity and reliability of the pediatric confusion assessment method for the Intensive Care Unit. Crit Care Med 2011;39(1):150–7.

40. Smith HA, Gangopadhyay M, Goben CM, et al. The Preschool Confusion Assessment Method for the ICU: valid and reliable delirium monitoring for critically ill Infants and children. Crit Care Med 2016;44(3):592–600.

41. Pun BT, Ely EW. The importance of diagnosing and managing ICU delirium. Chest 2007;132(2):624–36.

42. Marcantonio ER, Goldman L, Mangione CM, et al. A clinical prediction rule for delirium after elective noncardiac surgery. JAMA 1994;271(2):134–9.

43. Ouimet S, Riker R, Bergeron N, et al. Subsyndromal delirium in the ICU: evidence for a disease spectrum. Intensive Care Med 2007;33(6):1007–13.

44. Ely EW, Shintani A, Truman B, et al. Delirium as a predictor of mortality in mechanically ventilated patients in the intensive care unit. JAMA 2004;291(14):1753–62.

45. Jackson JC, Hart RP, Gordon SM, et al. Six-month neuropsychological outcome of medical intensive care unit patients. Crit Care Med 2003;31(4):1226–34.

46. Lin SM, Liu CY, Wang CH, et al. The impact of delirium on the survival of mechanically ventilated patients. Crit Care Med 2004;32(11):2254–9.

47. Salluh JI, Wang H, Schneider EB, et al. Outcome of delirium in critically ill patients: systematic review and meta-analysis. BMJ 2015;350:h2538.

48. Pisani MA, Kong SY, Kasl SV, et al. Days of delirium are associated with 1-year mortality in an older intensive care unit population. Am J Respir Crit Care Med 2009;180(11):1092–7.

49. Inouye SK, Charpentier PA. Precipitating factors for delirium in hospitalized elderly persons. Predictive model and interrelationship with baseline vulnerability. JAMA 1996;275(11):852–7.

50. Inouye SK, Viscoli CM, Horwitz RI, et al. A predictive model for delirium in hospitalized elderly medical patients based on admission characteristics. Ann Intern Med 1993;119(6):474–81.

51. Ely EW, Gautam S, Margolin R, et al. The impact of delirium in the intensive care unit on hospital length of stay. Intensive Care Med 2001;27(12):1892–900.

52. Wang W, Li HL, Wang DX, et al. Haloperidol prophylaxis decreases delirium incidence in elderly patients after noncardiac surgery: a randomized controlled trial*. Crit Care Med 2012;40(3):731–9.

53. Page VJ, Ely EW, Gates S, et al. Effect of intravenous haloperidol on the duration of delirium and coma in critically ill patients (Hope-ICU): a randomised, double-blind, placebo-controlled trial. Lancet Respir Med 2013;1(7):515–23.

54. Kress JP, Hall JB. ICU-acquired weakness and recovery from critical illness. N Engl J Med 2014;371(3):287–8.

55. Morris PE. Moving our critically ill patients: mobility barriers and benefits. Crit Care Clin 2007;23(1):1–20.

56. Herridge MS, Cheung AM, Tansey CM, et al. One-year outcomes in survivors of the acute respiratory distress syndrome. N Engl J Med 2003;348(8):683–93.

57. Herridge MS, Tansey CM, Matte A, et al. Functional disability 5 years after acute respiratory distress syndrome. N Engl J Med 2011;364(14):1293–304.

58. Sacanella E, Perez-Castejon JM, Nicolas JM, et al. Functional status and quality of life 12 months after discharge from a medical ICU in healthy elderly patients: a prospective observational study. Crit Care 2011;15(2):R105.

59. De Jonghe B, Sharshar T, Lefaucheur JP, et al. Paresis acquired in the intensive care unit: a prospective multicenter study. JAMA 2002;288(22):2859–67.

60. Bednarik J, Vondracek P, Dusek L, et al. Risk factors for critical illness polyneuromyopathy. J Neurol 2005;252(3):343–51.

61. Kleyweg RP, van der Meche FG, Schmitz PI. Interobserver agreement in the assessment of muscle strength and functional abilities in Guillain-Barre syndrome. Muscle Nerve 1991;14(11):1103–9.

62. Dammeyer J, Dickinson S, Packard D, et al. Building a protocol to guide mobility in the ICU. Crit Care Nurs Q 2013;36(1):37–49.

63. Freeman R, Maley K. Mobilization of intensive care cardiac surgery patients on mechanical circulatory support. Crit Care Nurs Q 2013;36(1):73–88.

64. Bailey P, Thomsen GE, Spuhler VJ, et al. Early activity is feasible and safe in respiratory failure patients. Crit Care Med 2007;35(1):139–45.

65. Schweickert WD, Pohlman MC, Pohlman AS, et al. Early physical and occupational therapy in mechanically ventilated, critically ill patients: a randomised controlled trial. Lancet 2009;373(9678):1874–82.

66. Moss M, Nordon-Craft A, Malone D, et al. A randomized trial of an intensive physical therapy program for acute respiratory failure patients. Am J Respir Crit Care Med 2015;193(10):1101–10.

67. Davidson JE, Powers K, Hedayat KM, et al. Clinical practice guidelines for support of the family in the patient-centered intensive care unit: American College of Critical Care Medicine Task Force 2004-2005. Crit Care Med 2007;35(2):605–22.

68. Phipps LM, Bartke CN, Spear DA, et al. Assessment of parental presence during bedside pediatric intensive care unit rounds: effect on duration, teaching, and privacy. Pediatr Crit Care Med 2007;8(3):220–4.

69. Cameron MA, Schleien CL, Morris MC. Parental presence on pediatric intensive care unit rounds. J Pediatr 2009;155(4):522–8.

70. Lilly CM, De Meo DL, Sonna LA, et al. An intensive communication intervention for the critically ill. Am J Med 2000;109(6):469–75.

71. Campbell ML, Guzman JA. Impact of a proactive approach to improve end-of-life care in a medical ICU. Chest 2003;123(1):266–71.

72. Schneiderman LJ, Gilmer T, Teetzel HD, et al. Effect of ethics consultations on nonbeneficial life-sustaining treatments in the intensive care setting: a randomized controlled trial. JAMA 2003;290(9):1166–72.

73. Schneiderman LJ, Gilmer T, Teetzel HD. Impact of ethics consultations in the intensive care setting: a randomized, controlled trial. Crit Care Med 2000; 28(12):3920–4.

74. Curtis JR, Engelberg RA, Wenrich MD, et al. Missed opportunities during family conferences about end-of-life care in the intensive care unit. Am J Respir Crit Care Med 2005;171(8):844–9.

75. Dowdy MD, Robertson C, Bander JA. A study of proactive ethics consultation for critically and terminally ill patients with extended lengths of stay. Crit Care Med 1998;26(2):252–9.

76. Carson SS, Cox CE, Wallenstein S, et al. Effect of palliative care-led meetings for families of patients with chronic critical illness: a randomized clinical trial. JAMA 2016;316(1):51–62.

77. Jabre P, Belpomme V, Azoulay E, et al. Family presence during cardiopulmonary resuscitation. N Engl J Med 2013;368(11):1008–18.

Persistent Inflammation, Immunosuppression and Catabolism Syndrome

Juan C. Mira, MD[a], Scott C. Brakenridge, MD, MS[b],
Lyle L. Moldawer, PhD[b], Frederick A. Moore, MD, MCCM[b],*

KEYWORDS

- Shock • Multiple organ failure • Trauma • Sepsis • Chronic critical illness
- Cachexia • Myeloid-derived suppressor cells • PICS

KEY POINTS

- There has been a significant increase in patients with chronic critical illness (CCI): patients with prolonged hospitalizations, high resource utilization, and dismal long-term outcomes.
- Persistent inflammation, immunosuppression, and catabolism syndrome (PICS) describes a subgroup of patients with CCI who have experienced recurrent inflammatory insults.
- Prolonged expansion of myeloid-derived suppressor cells (MDSCs) provides a plausible mechanism for the pathobiology and poor outcomes observed in patients with PICS.
- MDSC expansion in emergency myelopoiesis can lead to chronic inflammation and suppression of adaptive immunity and predisposes patients to nosocomial infections.
- A combination of pharmacotherapy, physiotherapy, and nutritional support will be necessary to limit the progression of CCI into PICS.

Supported in part by grants P50 GM-111152-03, R01 GM-40586-24 and R01 GM-104481-04, awarded by the National Institute of General Medical Sciences (NIGMS), U.S.P.H.S. J.C. Mira was supported by a postgraduate training grant (T32 GM-08721) in burns, trauma, and perioperative injury by NIGMS.
Disclosure Statement: The authors have nothing to disclose.
^a Department of Surgery, Sepsis and Critical Illness Research Center, University of Florida College of Medicine, 1600 Southwest Archer Road, PO Box 100019, Gainesville, FL 32610-0019, USA; ^b Department of Surgery, Sepsis and Critical Illness Research Center, University of Florida College of Medicine, 1600 Southwest Archer Road, Room 6116, PO Box 100286, Gainesville, FL 32610-0286, USA
* Corresponding author.
E-mail address: Frederick.Moore@surgery.ufl.edu

Crit Care Clin 33 (2017) 245–258
http://dx.doi.org/10.1016/j.ccc.2016.12.001
0749-0704/17/© 2016 Elsevier Inc. All rights reserved.

INTRODUCTION

Multiple organ failure (MOF) has plagued surgical intensive care units (ICUs) for more than four decades, and its epidemiology has evolved because advances in care have allowed patients to survive previously lethal insults. Over the years, different predominant phenotypes of MOF have been described; all have consumed tremendous health care resources and have been associated with prolonged ICU stays and prohibitive mortality. The term *persistent inflammation, immunosuppression, and catabolism syndrome* (PICS) has been coined to describe the most recent observed phenotype of persistent inflammation, immune suppression, and protein catabolism, which the authors think represents the next challenge in surgical critical care. The purpose of this review is to describe the evolving epidemiology of MOF and the emergence of PICS, the PICS paradigm, the pathophysiology of PICS, and its clinical implications.

EVOLVING EPIDEMIOLOGY OF MULTIPLE ORGAN FAILURE AND EMERGENCE OF PERSISTENT INFLAMMATION, IMMUNOSUPPRESSION, AND CATABOLISM SYNDROME

MOF emerged in the early 1970s as a result of advances in ICU technology that allowed patients to survive single-organ failure (Fig. 1).[1] Early studies provided convincing evidence that MOF occurred as a result of uncontrolled sepsis leading to fulminant organ failure and early death, with the primary source being intra-abdominal infections (IAIs).[1] As a result, research efforts in the early 1980s were focused on the prevention/treatment of IAI and were effective in reducing this highly fatal phenotypic expression of MOF. However, in the mid-1980s, studies out of Europe reported that MOF frequently occurred after severe blunt trauma with no identifiable

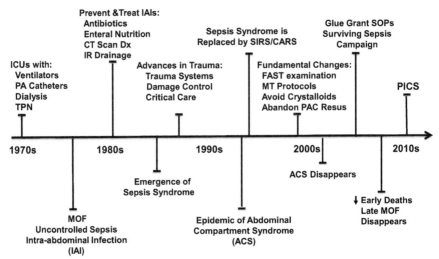

Fig. 1. Evolution of MOF. MOF evolves over 40 years, as does the clinical and surgical management of shock states. Paradigms to explain the developing phenotypes are adopted and discarded. The authors propose that PICS is the predominant phenotype resulting from CCI. CARS, compensatory antiinflammatory response syndrome; CT, computed tomography; Dx, diagnosis; FAST, focused assessment with sonography for trauma; IR, interventional radiology; MT, massive transfusion; PA, pulmonary artery; PAC, pulmonary artery catheter; SIRS, systemic inflammatory response syndrome; SOPs, standard operating procedures; TPN, total parenteral nutrition.

site of infection.[2,3] The term *sepsis syndrome* was popularized to describe this phenomenon. It became widely accepted that MOF could ensue after both infectious and noninfectious insults by a similar auto-destructive systemic inflammatory response syndrome (SIRS). Research focus in the late 1980s shifted to determining the underlying mechanisms of sepsis syndrome (eg, bacterial translocation, cytokine storm, ischemia reperfusion, and so forth). Simultaneously with these research efforts, tremendous independent advances in trauma care occurred that substantially reduced early deaths from bleeding but resulted in an epidemic of abdominal compartment syndrome (ACS) that emerged in the ICUs worldwide in the early 1990s.[4] Although clinical interest focused on understanding this as a new malignant MOF phenotype, epidemiology studies revealed that postinjury MOF was a bimodal phenomenon. Early MOF occurred after either an overwhelming insult (one-hit model) or sequential amplifying insults (2-hit model), whereas late MOF was precipitated by secondary nosocomial infections.[1]

The SIRS followed by a compensatory antiinflammatory response syndrome (CARS) was originally proposed to describe the pathophysiology and bimodal distribution of MOF. SIRS-induced early MOF was thought to occur as a result of exaggerated innate immunity (principally mediated by neutrophils), whereas CARS set the stage for immunosuppression-associated late infectious MOF.[5–8] The concept of CARS was initially based on trauma and sepsis studies that demonstrated that an early proinflammatory cytokine response was followed by an antiinflammatory cytokine response, the purpose of which was thought to restore immunologic homeostasis. However, basic immunologists focused their research efforts on characterizing CARS and expanded its definition to include multiple defects in the adaptive immunity (principally related to lymphocytes).[9–13] By the late 1990s, fundamental changes in the initial care of patients arriving with severe bleeding were widely implemented (that is, focused assessment with sonography for trauma, massive transfusion protocols, avoidance of excessive crystalloids and abandonment of pulmonary artery catheter directed resuscitation) and the epidemic of ACS virtually disappeared.[14–17] Concordantly, evidence-based medicine (EBM) became a health care mandate; through the 2000s it was a major driver for improved ICU care.

Two initiatives had notable impacts on the epidemiology of MOF. The first was the National Institutes of Health sponsored Glue Grant: Inflammation and the Host Response to Injury, which sought to characterize the genomic response to severe blunt trauma. To control the confounding effects of variable care, standard operating procedures (SOPs) for critical care were developed. Over the 6-year study period as a result of ongoing monitoring and improved SOP compliance, hospital mortality in the study cohort dropped from 22% to 11%.[16] The second major initiative was the *Surviving Sepsis Campaign*. Its rationale was based on the recognition that: the occurrence of sepsis in hospitalized patients was increasing, sepsis was and continues to be the most expensive condition treated in US hospitals, sepsis diagnosis was frequently delayed, and sepsis–directed SOPs were haphazardly delivered.[18–21] Implementation was an arduous process, but hospital mortality of severe sepsis has decreased from more than 35% to less than 15%.[22–24] As a result of these initiatives and others, there has been another striking change in the epidemiology of MOF. Early in-hospital mortality has decreased substantially, and the incidence of late-onset MOF deaths has largely disappeared. Unfortunately, a substantial portion of high-risk patients with MOF is surviving prolonged ICU stays; many are progressing into a new predominant MOF phenotype called PICS.

THE NEW PARADIGM OF PERSISTENT INFLAMMATION, IMMUNOSUPPRESSION, AND CATABOLISM SYNDROME

Based on recent laboratory and clinical research data, the following paradigm was proposed (Fig. 2).[5] Following an inflammatory insult (either trauma or sepsis), SIRS and CARS occur simultaneously. In some cases, SIRS can become overwhelming leading to an early MOF and fulminant death trajectory. Fortunately, modern ICU care is directed at early detection and prevention of this trajectory's fatal expression. If the severely insulted patients do not die of early MOF, there are two alternatives. Either their aberrant immunology rapidly recovers (ie, achieves homeostasis) or its dysfunction persists and they enter chronic critical illness (CCI, defined as >14 days in ICU with organ dysfunction). These patients with CCI experience ongoing immunosuppression (eg, lymphopenia) and inflammation (eg, neutrophilia) that is associated with a persistent acute phase response (eg, high C-reactive protein [CRP] levels) with ongoing somatic protein catabolism. Despite aggressive nutritional intervention, there is a tremendous loss of lean body mass and proportional decrease in functional status and poor wound healing. An estimated 30% to 50% of these patients with CCI progress into PICS. Readily available clinical biomarkers may be used to identify patients with PICS (Table 1). Clinically, patients with PICS have recurrent nosocomial infections and poor wound healing and are often discharged to long-term acute care facilities where they experience sepsis recidivism requiring rehospitalization, failure

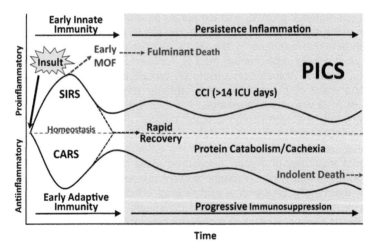

Time

Fig. 2. PICS paradigm. Following a major inflammatory insult (trauma, sepsis, burns, acute pancreatitis, and so forth), there is a simultaneous inflammatory and immunosuppressive response. Early deaths from acute MOF are now rare because of early recognition of shock and rapid implementation of supportive care thorough effective application of EBM and SOPs. Survivors may progress through two pathways: (a) patients readily return to immune homeostasis and achieve a rapid recovery or (b) patients smolder in the ICU with CCI and develop chronic inflammation, suppression of adaptive immunity, ongoing protein catabolism with cachectic wasting, and have recurrent nosocomial infections. These patients often have PICS, many of which fail to achieve functional independence, are discharged to long-term acute care facilities, have an extremely poor quality of life, and ultimately die an indolent death. (*Adapted from* Gentile LF, Cuenca AG, Efron PA, et al. Persistent inflammation and immunosuppression: a common syndrome and new horizon for surgical intensive care. J Trauma Acute Care Surg 2012;72(6):1491–501.)

Table 1
Persistent inflammation, immunosuppression, and catabolism syndrome biomarkers

PICS	Measurement
Critically ill patient	Admission to the ICU >14 d
Persistent inflammation	CRP >50 µg/dL
Persistent immunosuppression	Total lymphocyte count <0.80 × 10⁹/L
Catabolic state	Serum albumin <3.0 g/dL
	Prealbumin <10 mg/dL
	Creatinine height index <80%
	Weight loss >10% or BMI <18 during hospitalization

These markers are laboratory markers that are readily available in most clinical settings and can be used to identify patients with or at risk of PICS.
Abbreviation: BMI, body mass index.

to rehabilitate, and an indolent death.[5] As the population ages and perioperative care continues to improve, PICS will become the next challenging horizon in surgical critical care.

Dating back to the 1990s, there are reports describing CCI in ventilator-dependent patients. They primarily focused on describing the neuropathy and myopathy that caused significant long-term disability. More recently, the CCI literature has emphasized that ICU delirium contributes to long-term cognitive impairments.[25] These reports largely come from heterogeneous medical ICU patients and variably implicate different risk factors, including steroids, pharmacologic paralysis, immobilization, hyperglycemia, and benzodiazepines. Although these are likely operational in CCI related to PICS, the dominating risk factor for the PICS phenotype is recurrent inflammatory insults. This risk factor is not uncommon in surgical ICU patients who are exposed to an initial major insult (eg, surgery or trauma) and have recurrent inflammatory insults (operations, complications, and nosocomial infections) that set up a state of persistent low-grade inflammation, immunosuppression, and protein catabolism. Although not referred to as PICS, recent surgical literature documented improved early survival with poor long-term outcomes consistent with PICS after major burns (>30% of body surface area), major trauma (injury severity score >15), necrotizing pancreatitis, and surgical sepsis.[26-30]

As part of the authors' efforts to characterize PICS, they have prospectively studied 147 trauma and surgical ICU patients over the past two years who experienced severe sepsis and septic shock (Stortz J, unpublished data, 2017). A little more than half were male, with a mean age of 60 years. These patients were sick (mean Acute Physiology and Chronic Health Evaluation II = 23): 70% had major comorbidities, 80% required emergency surgery, and 55% presented in septic shock. Table 2 depicts biomarkers over 14 days consistent with PICS. Similarly, their clinical outcomes are consistent with PICS including low in-hospital mortality (13%), high rate of nosocomial infection (52%), few ventilator-free days (median 5, confidence interval [CI] 1–11), and few ICU-free days (median 5, CI 0–5). Eighty-four (58%) stayed in the ICU 14 or more days, and only 43 (29%) were discharged to home.

PATHOPHYSIOLOGY OF PERSISTENT INFLAMMATION, IMMUNOSUPPRESSION, AND CATABOLISM SYNDROME

Although other investigators have described the growing epidemic of CCI, glaringly absent is any unifying mechanistic explanation. The PICS paradigm was described

Table 2
Persistent inflammation, immunosuppression, and catabolism syndrome biomarkers over time

PICS	Marker	Sepsis Onset	Day 7	Day 14
Inflammation	CRP (mg/L)	206 ± 25	118 ± 58	86 ± 75
	Neutrophils (K/mm³)	15 ± 3	12 ± 6	10 ± 7
Immunosuppression	Lymphocytes (K/mm³)	0.6 ± 0.4	1.1 ± 1.3	1.0 ± 0.8
Catabolism	Albumin (g/dL)	2.3 ± 0	2.3 ± 0	2.5 ± 1.0
	Prealbumin (mg/L)	6 ± 2	7 ± 3	10 ± 5

Clinical biomarkers of PICS at 3 time points in chronically ill patients with severe sepsis/septic shock: sepsis onset, day 7, and day 14. These markers are consistent with the persistent inflammation, immune suppression, and catabolism seen in patients with PICS.

Abbreviations: CRP, C-reactive protein; g/dL, grams per deciliter; K/mm3, thousand per cubic millimeter; mg/L, milligrams per liter.

based on observed outcomes of surgical ICU patients who had a major inflammatory event (trauma/surgical sepsis) and who experienced recurrent insults (principally nosocomial infections). The authors propose a mechanism that can explain the persistent low-grade inflammation with the concurrent adaptive immune suppression and associated ongoing catabolism after a devastating injury or infection.

In response to sepsis or trauma, bone marrow granulocytes demarginate from the bone marrow to the site of injury/infection creating space for hematopoietic stem cell differentiation and repopulation of myeloid innate immune effector cells, a process termed emergency myelopoiesis.[31–34] Myeloid cell expansion predominates at the detriment of lymphopoiesis and erythropoiesis, promoting lymphopenia and anemia. Emergency myelopoiesis also results in the signal transducer and activator of transcription 3– and cyclooxygenase 2–mediated expansion of a heterogeneous population of inducible immature myeloid cells with immunosuppressive properties termed myeloid-derived suppressor cells (MDSCs).[35–38] The immunosuppressive activity to MDSCs has been attributed to several mechanisms and mediators described in both murine and human studies, including the upregulation of arginase 1 (ARG1) and nitric oxide synthase, increased interleukin (IL)-10 production and cell surface expression of programmed death-ligand 1 (PD-L1) and cytotoxic T-lymphocyte–associated antigen 4 (CTLA4), nitrosylation of major histocompatibility complex molecules preventing their appropriate interaction with the T-cell receptor (TCR) and coreceptors as well as promoting TCR dissociation, and promotion of regulatory T-cell expansion.[35,39–45] Although known for their adaptive immunosuppressive function, MDSCs also play an essential role in preserving innate immunity and producing inflammatory mediators, such as nitric oxide (NO), reactive oxygen species (ROS), tumor necrosis factor α (TNF α), regulated on activation normal T-cell expressed and secreted (RANTES), and macrophage inflammatory protein 1β.[46,47]

The emergency myelopoietic response and expansion of MDSCs in septic and trauma patients has been shown to be beneficial to the host by providing protection from early exuberant inflammation or from secondary infections.[33,39,48,49] Therefore, in addition to the contribution to systemic inflammation, emergency myelopoiesis is also important for early and late host protective immunity in the presence of suppressed adaptive immunity.

However, there is reason to think that emergency myelopoiesis is impaired in the elderly, the population recognized to be at higher risk for CCI and PICS. Recently, Efron and colleagues have shown that bone marrow progenitors in elderly mice fail to commence and conclude with an appropriate myelopoietic response, giving rise to myeloid cells with poor phagocytic and chemotactic function.[50] Additionally, in a subset of 72 patients with severe sepsis and septic shock described earlier, the authors observed that MDSC expansion persists in the first 28 days after sepsis onset (Fig. 3A).[51] Additionally, the normally high monocytic/granulocytic ratio of MDSCs is reversed after severe sepsis and septic shock (see Fig. 3B, C). The authors also showed that these MDCSs suppressed T lymphocyte proliferation in vitro and suppressed the release of T_{H1} and T_{H2} cytokines.[51] Finally, the authors showed that early

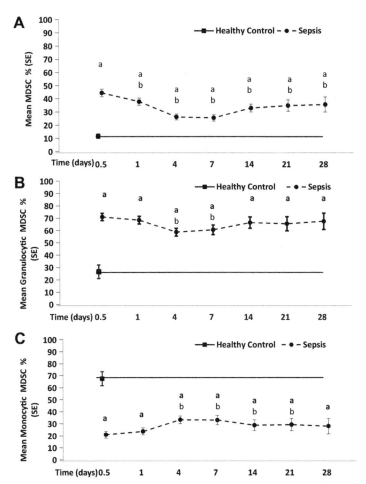

Fig. 3. MDSCs in PICS. Characterization of MDSCs (CD33+CD11b+HLA−DR−/low) in 72 trauma and surgical ICU patients with severe sepsis/septic shock (SS/SS).[51] (A) After sepsis onset, circulating MDSCs expand early and are persistently elevated by a significant margin over the first 28 days when compared with healthy controls (HC). (B, C) The commonly observed high ratio of monocytic/granulocytic MDSCs seen in healthy subjects is reversed in patients with SS/SS. [a] P<0.05 when compared with HC subjects. [b] P<0.05 when compared with patients with SS/SS at 12 hours. (From Mathias B, Delmas AL, Ozrazgat-Baslanti T, et al. Human myeloid-derived suppressor cells are associated with chronic immune suppression after severe sepsis/septic shock. Ann Surg 2016. [Epub ahead of print].)

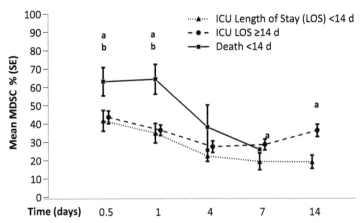

Fig. 4. MDSCs and ICU mortality/length of stay (LOS). Increase in circulating MDSCs correlates with early mortality and prolonged LOS. MDSC expansion was more significant in patients with early mortality (<14 days) than in patients who survived greater than 14 days at both 12 hours and 24 hours after sepsis onset. MDSC levels then decline until death. In patients with a prolonged ICU stay (>14 days), MDSCs are significantly elevated at 7 days and 14 days when compared with patients with and ICU LOS of less than 14 days. [a] P<0.05 when compared with patients with ICU LOS less than 14 days. [b] P<0.05 when compared with patients with ICU LOS 14 days or greater. (*From* Mathias B, Delmas AL, Ozrazgat-Baslanti T, et al. Human myeloid-derived suppressor cells are associated with chronic immune suppression after severe sepsis/septic shock. Ann Surg 2016. [Epub ahead of print].)

enhanced MDSC expansion was associated with early mortality (**Fig. 4**) and that persistent expansion was associated with prolonged ICU stays. Multivariate analysis demonstrated that MDSC expansion was a strong independent predictor of nosocomial infections and poor postdischarge disposition.[51] Thus, these data are supportive that prolonged expansion of MDSC after severe sepsis and septic shock contributes to outcomes consistent with the PICS phenotype.

In addition to MDSCs, patients with sepsis and trauma have significant tissue injury with release of damage-associated molecular patterns.[52,53] These endogenous alarmins may also contribute to the persistent inflammation in PICS[54,55]; their predominant sources are likely dysfunctional organs, such as the kidneys and lungs as well as the intestine.

CLINICAL IMPLICATIONS

Persistent inflammation, MDSC expansion, and suppression of protective immunity via anergy, lymphopenia, and dysfunctional innate effector cells predispose patients to reactivation of latent viral infections, nosocomial infections, continued protein catabolism, and malnutrition. This reactivation creates a propagating cycle whereby recurrent infections exacerbate inflammation driving aberrant myelopoiesis and continued expansion of MDSCs, which in turn induces suppression of adaptive immunity (**Fig. 5**).

Treatment must focus on interrupting this vicious cycle facing patients with CCI and PICS. Thus, treating PICS requires an understanding of the forces that drive the persistent inflammation, immunosuppression, and catabolism that manifests in these patients. Monotherapies will generally be ineffective unless they are pluripotent. Furthermore, most high-risk patients bring with them a significant number of comorbid diseases that all must be considered as part of the treatment plan.

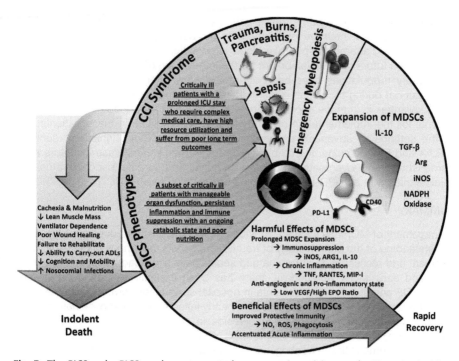

Fig. 5. The PICS cycle. PICS can be represented as a recurring, vicious cycle. First, the inciting inflammatory event stimulates an emergency myelopoietic response. Although the ensuing expansion of MDSC can be protective, prolonged expansion promotes suppression of adaptive immunity and chronic inflammation. Following this initial response, patients may convalesce or progress to CCI. In a subset of patients with CCI, PICS develops and is characterized by manageable organ dysfunction, ongoing inflammation and immune suppression, protein catabolism, muscle wasting, and unmet nutritional needs. This state predisposes patients for recurrent infections and recidivism of this cycle. ADLs, activities of daily living; Arg, arginase; EPO, erythropoietin; iNOS, inducible NO synthase; NADPH, nicotinamide adenine dinucleotide phosphate; TGF-β, transforming growth factor β; VEGF, vascular endothelial growth factor. (*Adapted from* Mira JC, Gentile LF, Mathias BJ, et al. Sepsis pathophysiology, chronic critical illness, and persistent inflammation-immunosuppression and catabolism syndrome. Crit Care Med 2017;45(2):253–62.)

Compliance with evidence-based management SOPs has significantly reduced in-hospital MOF deaths, and continued compliance in survivors is important to limit iatrogenic injury and reduce sepsis recidivism.[16,56] Early enteral nutrition has been shown to reduce nosocomial infections.[57] These diets should be supplemented with protein to insure 1.5 g/kg and even more for burn patients and those requiring dialysis. Although there is strong evidence supporting the use of immune-enhancing diets (IEDs) in trauma and perioperative patients, some have warned that the arginine in IEDs may cause harm in severe sepsis.[57] However, MDSC expansion in survivors of severe sepsis promotes immunosuppression via overexpression of *ARG1*, which depletes arginine and thereby impairs lymphocyte proliferation. Thus, arginine supplementation may be important in preventing the survivors from progressing into CCI and PICS. For patients who have failed to wean off the ventilator, inspiratory strength training exercises have been showed to improve outcomes.[58] Furthermore, other modes of physical therapy and mobilization, starting early in the ICU, have been shown to improve functional outcomes, decreased ICU and hospital stay, and improve quality of life.[59] Based on experience in severe burns, these patients will also likely benefit from receiving anabolic hormones, intensive insulin therapy, and beta-blockade.[60]

Despite failed attempts at pharmacologic intervention in trauma and sepsis, there is optimism on future drug development for the interruption of this cycle.[61] Most antiinflammatory modulations have been attempted early after the initial septic/trauma event but not during the continuing smoldering inflammation seen in PICS. Additionally, similarities in immune suppression seen in CCI and advanced cancer provide a rational for the implementation of immune system stimulants in these patients.[62,63] In the settings of advanced cancer, blockade of checkpoint inhibitors, such as CTLA4 and PD-L1, alone, in combination, or with methyltransferase inhibitors have demonstrated improvements in adaptive immunity and durable response rates.[64,65] Clinical trials with anti–PD-L1 in sepsis are currently underway (NCT02576457).

SUMMARY

Management of MOF has evolved significantly over the past four decades as has our understanding of the pathobiology of trauma and sepsis. Advances in the early management and resuscitation of trauma and sepsis have significant reduced early mortality and early MOF. Additionally, there has been a significant reduction in late-stage MOF and steady improvements in hospital survival for both entities. This successful recognition and management of the early inflammatory response has resulted in increased numbers of patients who reside in critical care units with persistent inflammation, adaptive immune suppression, defects in antigen presentation, protein catabolism, somatic tissue wasting, and dismal long-term outcomes. The authors provide a new terminology for this patient population, PICS, that recognizes the principal challenges to the successful management of these patients: management of their chronic inflammatory state, restoration of a more appropriate adaptive immune response, and protection against secondary nosocomial infections, as well as prevention or restoration of a cachectic, wasting syndrome. Furthermore, it recognizes that such patients have multiple, simultaneous immunologic and physiologic defects that require a multimodal therapeutic approach instead of single monotherapy treatment.

The authors think that MDSCs may play a significant role in the in the persistent inflammation, and immunosuppression, leading to detrimental long-term outcomes following severe trauma and sepsis. Furthermore, identifying MDSCs in humans as well as understanding their biological and immunologic contributions to the host during sepsis and trauma may not only offer a mechanism of this disease but also possible therapeutic targets to improve clinical outcomes. The PICS model argues that immunoadjuvants, such as anti–PD-L1 or IL-7, or drugs that can suppress the expansion of MDSCs, may benefit this population by reducing the likelihood of opportunistic infections or viral reactivation. In addition to supportive therapies aimed at reducing the likelihood of nosocomial infection, stimulation of anabolic signals with the implementation of early patient mobilization, resistance exercise, and optimization of nutritional support are suggested. Ultimately, it is a combination of pharmacotherapy, physiotherapy, and nutritional support that will most likely benefit these patients.

REFERENCES

1. Moore FA, Moore EE. Evolving concepts in the pathogenesis of postinjury multiple organ failure. Surg Clin North Am 1995;75(2):257–77.
2. Waydhas C, Nast-Kolb D, Jochum M, et al. Inflammatory mediators, infection, sepsis, and multiple organ failure after severe trauma. Arch Surg 1992;127(4): 460–7.

3. Faist E, Baue AE, Dittmer H, et al. Multiple organ failure in polytrauma patients. J Trauma 1983;23(9):775–87.
4. Balogh Z, McKinley BA, Cox CS Jr, et al. Abdominal compartment syndrome: the cause or effect of postinjury multiple organ failure. Shock 2003;20(6):483–92.
5. Gentile LF, Cuenca AG, Efron PA, et al. Persistent inflammation and immunosuppression: a common syndrome and new horizon for surgical intensive care. J Trauma Acute Care Surg 2012;72(6):1491–501.
6. Ward NS, Casserly B, Ayala A. The compensatory anti-inflammatory response syndrome (CARS) in critically ill patients. Clin Chest Med 2008;29(4):617–25, viii.
7. Rosenthal MD, Moore FA. Persistent inflammatory, immunosuppressed, catabolic syndrome (PICS): a new phenotype of multiple organ failure. J Adv Nutr Hum Metab 2015;1(1):e784.
8. Robertson CM, Coopersmith CM. The systemic inflammatory response syndrome. Microbes Infect 2006;8(5):1382–9.
9. Moldawer LL. Interleukin-1, TNF alpha and their naturally occurring antagonists in sepsis. Blood Purif 1993;11(2):128–33.
10. Rogy MA, Coyle SM, Oldenburg HS, et al. Persistently elevated soluble tumor necrosis factor receptor and interleukin-1 receptor antagonist levels in critically ill patients. J Am Coll Surg 1994;178(2):132–8.
11. Rogy MA, Oldenburg HS, Coyle S, et al. Correlation between Acute Physiology and Chronic Health Evaluation (APACHE) III score and immunological parameters in critically ill patients with sepsis. Br J Surg 1996;83(3):396–400.
12. MacLean LD, Meakins JL, Taguchi K, et al. Host resistance in sepsis and trauma. Ann Surg 1975;182(3):207–17.
13. Bone RC. Toward a theory regarding the pathogenesis of the systemic inflammatory response syndrome: what we do and do not know about cytokine regulation. Crit Care Med 1996;24(1):163–72.
14. Sauaia A, Moore EE, Johnson JL, et al. Temporal trends of postinjury multiple-organ failure: still resource intensive, morbid, and lethal. J Trauma acute Care Surg 2014;76(3):582–92 [discussion: 592–3].
15. Gonzalez EA, Moore FA. Resuscitation beyond the abdominal compartment syndrome. Curr Opin Crit Care 2010;16(6):570–4.
16. Cuschieri J, Johnson JL, Sperry J, et al. Benchmarking outcomes in the critically injured trauma patient and the effect of implementing standard operating procedures. Ann Surg 2012;255(5):993–9.
17. Sobrino J, Shafi S. Timing and causes of death after injuries. Proc (Bayl Univ Med Cent) 2013;26(2):120–3.
18. Torio CM, Andrews RM. National inpatient hospital costs: the most expensive conditions by payer, 2011: statistical brief #160. Rockville (MD): Healthcare Cost and Utilization Project (HCUP) Statistical Briefs; 2013.
19. Gaieski DF, Edwards JM, Kallan MJ, et al. Benchmarking the incidence and mortality of severe sepsis in the United States. Crit Care Med 2013;41(5):1167–74.
20. Dellinger RP, Carlet JM, Masur H, et al. Surviving Sepsis Campaign guidelines for management of severe sepsis and septic shock. Intensive Care Med 2004;30(4):536–55.
21. Dellinger RP, Levy MM, Rhodes A, et al. Surviving Sepsis Campaign: international guidelines for management of severe sepsis and septic shock: 2012. Crit Care Med 2013;41(2):580–637.
22. Rhodes A, Phillips G, Beale R, et al. The Surviving Sepsis Campaign bundles and outcome: results from the International Multicentre Prevalence study on Sepsis (the IMPreSS study). Intensive Care Med 2015;41(9):1620–8.

23. Gao F, Melody T, Daniels DF, et al. The impact of compliance with 6-hour and 24-hour sepsis bundles on hospital mortality in patients with severe sepsis: a prospective observational study. Crit Care 2005;9(6):R764–70.

24. Castellanos-Ortega A, Suberviola B, Garcia-Astudillo LA, et al. Impact of the Surviving Sepsis Campaign protocols on hospital length of stay and mortality in septic shock patients: results of a three-year follow-up quasi-experimental study. Crit Care Med 2010;38(4):1036–43.

25. Pandharipande PP, Girard TD, Jackson JC, et al. Long-term cognitive impairment after critical illness. N Engl J Med 2013;369(14):1306–16.

26. Davidson GH, Hamlat CA, Rivara FP, et al. Long-term survival of adult trauma patients. JAMA 2011;305(10):1001–7.

27. Callcut RA, Wakam G, Conroy AS, et al. Discovering the truth about life after discharge: long-term trauma-related mortality. J Trauma acute Care Surg 2016; 80(2):210–7.

28. Skouras C, Hayes AJ, Williams L, et al. Early organ dysfunction affects long-term survival in acute pancreatitis patients. HPB (Oxford) 2014;16(9):789–96.

29. Timmers TK, Verhofstad MH, Moons KG, et al. Long-term survival after surgical intensive care unit admission: fifty percent die within 10 years. Ann Surg 2011; 253(1):151–7.

30. Pavoni V, Gianesello L, Paparella L, et al. Outcome predictors and quality of life of severe burn patients admitted to intensive care unit. Scand J Trauma Resusc Emerg Med 2010;18:24.

31. Manz MG, Boettcher S. Emergency granulopoiesis. Nat Rev Immunol 2014;14(5): 302–14.

32. Furze RC, Rankin SM. Neutrophil mobilization and clearance in the bone marrow. Immunology 2008;125(3):281–8.

33. Scumpia PO, Kelly-Scumpia KM, Delano MJ, et al. Cutting edge: bacterial infection induces hematopoietic stem and progenitor cell expansion in the absence of TLR signaling. J Immunol 2010;184(5):2247–51.

34. Ueda Y, Kondo M, Kelsoe G. Inflammation and the reciprocal production of granulocytes and lymphocytes in bone marrow. J Exp Med 2005;201(11):1771–80.

35. Gabrilovich DI, Nagaraj S. Myeloid-derived suppressor cells as regulators of the immune system. Nat Rev Immunol 2009;9(3):162–74.

36. Dilek N, Vuillefroy de Silly R, Blancho G, et al. Myeloid-derived suppressor cells: mechanisms of action and recent advances in their role in transplant tolerance. Front Immunol 2012;3:208.

37. Bronte V. Myeloid-derived suppressor cells in inflammation: uncovering cell subsets with enhanced immunosuppressive functions. Eur J Immunol 2009;39(10): 2670–2.

38. Talmadge JE, Gabrilovich DI. History of myeloid-derived suppressor cells. Nat Rev Cancer 2013;13(10):739–52.

39. Cuenca AG, Delano MJ, Kelly-Scumpia KM, et al. A paradoxical role for myeloid-derived suppressor cells in sepsis and trauma. Mol Med 2011;17(3–4):281–92.

40. Popovic PJ, Zeh HJ 3rd, Ochoa JB. Arginine and immunity. J Nutr 2007;137(6 Suppl 2):1681S–6S.

41. Heim CE, Vidlak D, Kielian T. Interleukin-10 production by myeloid-derived suppressor cells contributes to bacterial persistence during Staphylococcus aureus orthopedic biofilm infection. J Leukoc Biol 2015;98(6):1003–13.

42. Lei GS, Zhang C, Lee CH. Myeloid-derived suppressor cells impair alveolar macrophages through PD-1 receptor ligation during Pneumocystis pneumonia. Infect Immun 2015;83(2):572–82.

43. Bunt SK, Sinha P, Clements VK, et al. Inflammation induces myeloid-derived suppressor cells that facilitate tumor progression. J Immunol 2006;176(1):284–90.
44. Nagaraj S, Gupta K, Pisarev V, et al. Altered recognition of antigen is a mechanism of CD8+ T cell tolerance in cancer. Nat Med 2007;13(7):828–35.
45. Youn JI, Nagaraj S, Collazo M, et al. Subsets of myeloid-derived suppressor cells in tumor-bearing mice. J Immunol 2008;181(8):5791–802.
46. Delano MJ, Scumpia PO, Weinstein JS, et al. MyD88-dependent expansion of an immature GR-1(+)CD11b(+) population induces T cell suppression and Th2 polarization in sepsis. J Exp Med 2007;204(6):1463–74.
47. Noel JG, Osterburg A, Wang Q, et al. Thermal injury elevates the inflammatory monocyte subpopulation in multiple compartments. Shock 2007;28(6):684–93.
48. Noel G, Wang Q, Osterburg A, et al. A ribonucleotide reductase inhibitor reverses burn-induced inflammatory defects. Shock 2010;34(5):535–44.
49. Sander LE, Sackett SD, Dierssen U, et al. Hepatic acute-phase proteins control innate immune responses during infection by promoting myeloid-derived suppressor cell function. J Exp Med 2010;207(7):1453–64.
50. Nacionales DC, Szpila B, Ungaro R, et al. A detailed characterization of the dysfunctional immunity and abnormal myelopoiesis induced by severe shock and trauma in the aged. J Immunol 2015;195(5):2396–407.
51. Mathias B, Delmas AL, Ozrazgat-Baslanti T, et al. Human myeloid-derived suppressor cells are associated with chronic immune suppression after severe sepsis/septic shock. Ann Surg 2016. [Epub ahead of print].
52. Yamanouchi S, Kudo D, Yamada M, et al. Plasma mitochondrial DNA levels in patients with trauma and severe sepsis: time course and the association with clinical status. J Crit Care 2013;28(6):1027–31.
53. Gao S, Yang Y, Fu Y, et al. Diagnostic and prognostic value of myeloid-related protein complex 8/14 for sepsis. Am J Emerg Med 2015;33(9):1278–82.
54. Kang JW, Kim SJ, Cho HI, et al. DAMPs activating innate immune responses in sepsis. Ageing Res Rev 2015;24(Pt A):54–65.
55. Timmermans K, Kox M, Scheffer GJ, et al. Danger in the intensive care unit: damps in critically ill patients. Shock 2016;45(2):108–16.
56. Levy MM, Rhodes A, Phillips GS, et al. Surviving Sepsis Campaign: association between performance metrics and outcomes in a 7.5-year study. Crit Care Med 2015;43(1):3–12.
57. McClave SA, Taylor BE, Martindale RG, et al. Guidelines for the provision and assessment of nutrition support therapy in the adult critically ill patient: Society of Critical Care Medicine (SCCM) and American Society for Parenteral and Enteral Nutrition (A.S.P.E.N.). JPEN J Parenter Enteral Nutr 2016;40(2):159–211.
58. Martin AD, Smith BK, Davenport PD, et al. Inspiratory muscle strength training improves weaning outcome in failure to wean patients: a randomized trial. Crit Care 2011;15(2):R84.
59. Kayambu G, Boots R, Paratz J. Physical therapy for the critically ill in the ICU: a systematic review and meta-analysis. Crit Care Med 2013;41(6):1543–54.
60. Jeschke MG, Chinkes DL, Finnerty CC, et al. Pathophysiologic response to severe burn injury. Ann Surg 2008;248(3):387–401.
61. Fink MP, Warren HS. Strategies to improve drug development for sepsis. Nat Rev Drug Discov 2014;13(10):741–58.
62. Hotchkiss RS, Opal S. Immunotherapy for sepsis–a new approach against an ancient foe. N Engl J Med 2010;363(1):87–9.
63. Hotchkiss RS, Moldawer LL. Parallels between cancer and infectious disease. N Engl J Med 2014;371(4):380–3.

64. Ott PA, Hodi FS, Robert C. CTLA-4 and PD-1/PD-L1 blockade: new immunotherapeutic modalities with durable clinical benefit in melanoma patients. Clin Cancer Res 2013;19(19):5300–9.
65. Redman JM, Gibney GT, Atkins MB. Advances in immunotherapy for melanoma. BMC Med 2016;14(1):20.

Optimal Strategies for Severe Acute Respiratory Distress Syndrome

Jeremy W. Cannon, MD, SM[a],*, Jacob T. Gutsche, MD[b],
Daniel Brodie, MD[c]

KEYWORDS

- Acute respiratory distress syndrome • Lung protective ventilation
- High-frequency oscillatory ventilation • Neuromuscular blockade • Prone positioning
- Pulmonary vasodilators • Extracorporeal membrane oxygenation
- Physical conditioning

KEY POINTS

- Acute respiratory distress syndrome (ARDS) occurs in more than 10% of intensive care unit admissions and nearly 25% of ventilated patients.
- Low-volume, low-pressure lung protective ventilation remains the mainstay of ARDS management.
- In severe ARDS, early use of neuromuscular blockade and prone positioning improve survival.
- High-frequency oscillatory ventilation has no clear mortality benefit and may harm some patients.
- Extracorporeal membrane oxygenation consultation should be obtained early to permit initiation in appropriate patients before multisystem organ failure and severe musculoskeletal deconditioning occur.

The opinions expressed in this document are solely those of the authors and do not represent an endorsement by or the views of the United States Air Force, the Department of Defense, or the United States government.

Disclosure: Dr D. Brodie is currently on the medical advisory boards of ALung Technologies and Kadence. All compensation for these activities is paid to Columbia University. Drs J.W. Cannon and J.T. Gutsche report nothing to disclose.

[a] Division of Trauma, Surgical Critical Care & Emergency Surgery, The Perelman School of Medicine at the University of Pennsylvania, 51 North 39th Street, MOB Suite 120, Philadelphia, PA 19104, USA; [b] Department of Anesthesiology and Critical Care, The Perelman School of Medicine at the University of Pennsylvania, 51 North 39th Street, Philadelphia, PA 19104, USA; [c] Division of Pulmonary, Allergy, & Critical Care Medicine, Columbia University Medical Center, 622 West 168 Street, PH 8 East, Room 101, New York, NY 10032, USA
* Corresponding author.
E-mail address: jeremy.cannon@uphs.upenn.edu

INTRODUCTION

Much has transpired in the 5 years since a volume of this publication was dedicated to acute respiratory failure.[1] The most significant developments include:

- A new definition of acute respiratory distress syndrome (ARDS), termed the Berlin definition
- Numerous landmark clinical trials in ventilator and nonventilator management strategies for ARDS
- The reincarnation of the ARDS Network (ARDSNet) research network as the PETAL (Prevention and Early Treatment of Acute Lung Injury) Network
- A commitment by the European Society of Intensive Care Medicine to study ARDS globally

The consensus-based Berlin definition of ARDS (Box 1) has allowed investigators and clinicians to more readily identify patients with ARDS in order to optimize management and design impactful clinical trials.[2] This definition has been quickly and comprehensively applied across numerous intensive care unit (ICU) populations to further the understanding of this challenging clinical syndrome. It also provides a framework for matching treatment strategies to severity of ARDS (Fig. 1).

Concurrent with the development and dissemination of this new definition, several important clinical trials (Table 1) and systematic reviews on various aspects of ARDS management have been or will soon be published. The results of these trials and their practical application are discussed at length in this article.

In addition, the future of ARDS research in both the United States and abroad has been well funded, in keeping with the burdens of both morbidity and mortality that result from ARDS. The ARDSNet research network has transformed to include many of the original centers along with several new centers, and these have established a reputation for providing new insights into the diagnosis and management of ARDS. Funded by the National Heart, Lung, and Blood Institute (NHLBI) of the National Institutes of Health (NIH), this new consortium has been termed the Prevention and Early Treatment of Acute Lung Injury (PETAL) Network.[3,4] Similarly, the European Society of Intensive Care Medicine (ESICM) has shown a commitment to supporting ARDS research, as manifested by the recently published LUNG SAFE (Large Observational Study to Understand the Global Impact of Severe Acute Respiratory Failure)

Box 1
Berlin definition of acute respiratory distress syndrome

Respiratory failure within 1 week of a known clinical insult or new/worsening respiratory symptoms

Bilateral opacities on CXR or chest CT not fully explained by effusions, lobar/lung collapse, or nodules

Respiratory failure not fully explained by cardiac failure or fluid overload (need objective assessment [eg, echocardiography] to exclude hydrostatic edema if no risk factor present)

Mild	PFR 201–300 mm Hg with PEEP or CPAP $\geq$5 cm H_2O
Moderate	PFR 101–200 mm Hg with PEEP $\geq$5 cm H_2O
Severe	PFR $\leq$100 mm Hg with PEEP $\geq$5 cm H_2O

Abbreviations: CPAP, continuous positive airway pressure; CT, computed tomography; CXR, chest radiograph; PEEP, positive end-expiratory pressure; PFR, Pao_2/fraction of inspired oxygen ratio.

From Ranieri VM, Rubenfeld GD, Thompson BT, et al. Acute respiratory distress syndrome: the Berlin definition. JAMA 2012;307(23):2526–33.

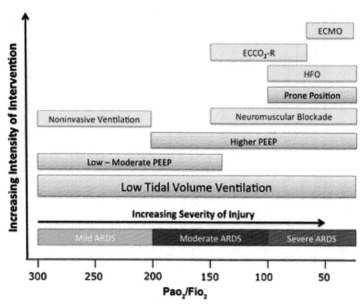

Fig. 1. Therapies for treatment of ARDS matched to severity of ARDS. ECCO2-R, extracorporeal CO2 removal; ECMO, extracorporeal membrane oxygenation; Fio2, fraction of inspired oxygen, HFO, high-frequency oscillation; PEEP, positive end-expiratory pressure. (*From* Ferguson ND, Fan E, Camporota L, et al. The Berlin definition of ARDS: an expanded rationale, justification, and supplementary material. Intensive Care Med 2012;38(10):1573–82; with permission of Springer.)

observational study results.[5] This and future planned studies by this group will doubtless shape the understanding and management of ARDS for years to come.

A useful framework for conceptualizing ARDS management aligns interventions with the severity of illness. Diaz and colleagues[6] provided practical guidance using such an approach in 2010. A similar framework has now been published by the creators of the Berlin definition.[7] Most patients with mild ARDS and many with moderate ARDS can be safely managed with well-established ventilator-based strategies. However, as the hypoxemia and resulting tissue hypoxia worsen, advanced maneuvers may be required.[8] This article focuses specifically on the safe application of these advanced ventilator and adjunctive management approaches typically reserved for patients with severe ARDS.

EPIDEMIOLOGY OF SEVERE ACUTE RESPIRATORY DISTRESS SYNDROME

The review of acute lung injury (ALI) and ARDS epidemiology by Blank and Napolitano[9] summarized the most current trends in respiratory survival development and outcomes in modern ICU care. These investigators made the following observations:

- This is a heterogeneous condition that occurs in heterogeneous ICU populations
- The incidence of ALI/ARDS is declining because of a decrease in hospital-acquired respiratory failure
- The mortality associated with ARDS remains high at 20% to 25% in randomized controlled trials and 40% outside of clinical trials

The newly established Berlin definition of ARDS (see Box 1) is now widely accepted for diagnosing ARDS and for prognostication.[2] Most significantly, this definition

Table 1
Landmark trials and publications in severe acute respiratory distress syndrome management 2012 to 2016

Authors	Study Name/Subject	Population (n)	Main Findings
Bellani et al,[5] 2016	LUNG SAFE/ARDS incidence and outcomes	All patients admitted to an ICU over a 4-wk period (29,144) including 3022 with ARDS	ARDS occurs in 10.4% of ICU admissions and in 23.4% of ventilated patients. ARDS is underdiagnosed and lung protective ventilator settings are underused. Hospital mortality is 40%
Young et al,[30] 2013	OSCAR/HFOV	Patients with a PFR ≤200 mm Hg: HFOV (398) vs usual ventilation support (397)	30-d mortality no different between the HFOV vs usual ventilation support groups (41.7% vs 41.1%)
Ferguson et al,[31] 2013	OSCILLATE/HFOV	Patients with a PFR ≤200 mm Hg and an Fio_2 ≥0.5: HFOV (275) vs pressure control ventilation (273)	Study stopped early because of worse in-hospital mortality in HFOV vs pressure control ventilation (47% vs 35%)
Papazian et al,[41] 2010	ACURASYS Study/NMB	Patients with a PFR <150 mm Hg, PEEP ≥5 cm H_2O and V_T 6–8 mL/kg PBW: NMB (178) vs placebo (162)	After a preplanned adjustment for baseline PFR, P_{PLAT}, and APACHE II to ensure matched patient groups, 90-d mortality was improved with NMB (OR, 0.68; 95% CI, 0.48–0.98). 28-d unadjusted mortality was 23.7% with NMB vs 33.3% with placebo ($P = .05$)
Guerin et al,[43] 2013	PROSEVA/proning	Patients with a PFR <150 mm Hg: prone (237) vs supine (229)	28-d and 90-d mortality were decreased in the prone vs supine groups (28-d 16.0% vs 32.8% and 90-d 23.6% vs 41.0%)
Schmidt et al,[58] 2014	RESP score/ECMO prognosis	Adult patients with severe ARDS on ECMO in the ELSO registry (2355) externally validated on 140 patients	The RESP score can accurately predict ECMO survival (c = 0.74), which was externally validated with excellent discrimination (c = 0.92)
Combes et al,[60] 2014	ECMO Net/consensus statement	Patients with severe ARDS on VV ECMO	ECMO should be conducted in high-volume regional centers that support the community with an ECMO transport program
International ECMO Network[71]	EOLIA/early VV ECMO	Patients with PFR <80 mm Hg	Trial ongoing

Abbreviations: CI, confidence interval; ECMO, extracorporeal membrane oxygenation; ELSO, extracorporeal life support organization; Fio_2, fraction of inspired oxygen; HFOV, high-frequency oscillatory ventilation; ICU, intensive care unit; LUNG SAFE, Large Observational Study to Understand the Global Impact of Severe Acute Respiratory Failure; NMB, neuromuscular blockade; OR, odds ratio; OSCAR, oscillation in ARDS; OSCILLATE, oscillation for acute respiratory distress syndrome treated early; PBW, predicted body weight; PFR, Pao_2/Fio_2 ratio; P_{PLAT}, plateau pressure; PROSEVA, proning severe ARDS patients; RESP, Respiratory Extracorporeal Membrane Oxygenation Survival Prediction; V_T, tidal volume; VV, venovenous.

incorporates ventilator settings as an important determinant of ARDS severity classification. Some clinicians argue that classification of ARDS should be made with the ventilator adjusted to a positive end-expiratory pressure (PEEP) of exactly 5 cm H_2O rather than at higher levels of PEEP to avoid underestimating the patient's severity of respiratory failure.[10] This approach is not always safe or practical, especially in patients with tenuous oxygenation on high levels of PEEP.

A recently completed international observational study (Large Observational Study to Understand the Global Impact of Severe Acute Respiratory Failure [LUNG SAFE]) of nearly 30,000 ICU admissions used automated metrics to identify patients who met ARDS criteria.[5] By the Berlin definition of ARDS, 10.4% of patients admitted to ICUs and 23.4% on mechanical ventilation develop ARDS at some point during their stay. Patients with ARDS required a median of 8 days of ventilator support and remained in the ICU for a median of 10 days. The incidence of ARDS varied by geographic region, with the highest rates in Oceana (0.57 cases per bed every 4 weeks), Europe (0.48 cases per bed every 4 weeks), and North America (0.46 cases per bed every 4 weeks). The distribution of ARDS severity included 30% mild, 46.6% moderate, and 23.4% severe. Of the patients with mild ARDS, 4.5% progressed to severe ARDS, whereas 12.7% of those with moderate ARDS progressed to severe ARDS. Hospital mortality increased significantly with ARDS severity: mild ARDS, 34.9% mortality; moderate ARDS, 40.3%; and severe ARDS, 46.1%.

In addition to these demographics, this study revealed that ARDS is frequently underdiagnosed and that potentially beneficial, well-established therapies are thus not applied even when indicated. At the time ARDS criteria were first met, only 34% of cases were clinician recognized, and only 60.2% were clinician recognized at some point during the patient's ICU course. The rate of recognition increased in mechanically ventilated patients and with increasing ARDS severity but still was only recognized 78.5% of the time in severe ARDS. Similarly, therapies with potential benefit, such as neuromuscular blockade, prone positioning, and extracorporeal membrane oxygenation (ECMO), were infrequently used (Table 2). Tidal volume did not change with clinical recognition of ARDS, whereas PEEP and the use of neuromuscular blockade and prone position all increased with ARDS recognition.

Table 2
Clinician recognition and application of adjunctive therapies in patients with acute respiratory distress syndrome

	Total MV + ARDS (n = 2377)	Severe ARDS (n = 729)
Clinician Recognition	1525 (64.2%)	437 (78.5%)
Recruitment Maneuver	496 (20.9%)	238 (32.7%)
HFOV	28 (1.2%)	11 (1.5%)
Neuromuscular Blockade	516 (21.7%)	274 (37.8%)
Prone Positioning	187 (7.9%)	119 (16.3%)
Inhaled Vasodilators	182 (7.7%)	95 (13.0%)
ECMO	76 (3.2%)	48 (6.6%)
Any of the Above	946 (39.8%)	445 (61.0%)

Abbreviation: MV, mechanical ventilation.

Adapted from Bellani G, Laffey JG, Pham T, et al. Epidemiology, Patterns of care, and mortality for patients with acute respiratory distress syndrome in intensive care units in 50 countries. JAMA 2016;315(8):788.

The mechanisms whereby ARDS causes death are myriad, but, in patients with severe ARDS, hypoxemia resulting in an accumulating oxygen debt[11,12] as well as cytokine release from lung injury (both iatrogenic and disease related) are all likely contributing factors.[13–15] Although conventional wisdom holds that most patients with ARDS die with ARDS rather than from ARDS, this likely does not hold true in those with severe ARDS. Thus, clinicians should identify patients with severe and rapidly progressive respiratory failure early and ensure that supportive measures and interventions with a demonstrated benefit are safely applied. A range of therapies that should be considered in patients with severe ARDS are reviewed later.

VENTILATOR MANAGEMENT
Standard Ventilator Management

The goal of the management of severe ARDS is to safely support gas exchange without further injuring the patient's lungs.[16] The optimal initial approach seems to be a low-volume, low-pressure ventilation strategy with volume control ventilation, which showed a survival benefit in the ARDSNet ARMA (Ventilation with Lower Tidal Volumes as Compared with Traditional Tidal Volumes for Acute Lung Injury and the Acute Respiratory Distress Syndrome) trial.[17] This lung protective strategy limits the patient's tidal volume (V_T) to 4 to 8 mL/kg predicted body weight (PBW) combined with some level of PEEP, which keeps the plateau pressure (P_{PLAT}) less than or equal to 30 cm H_2O.[17,18] During the initial management, a V_T of 8 mL/kg may be used, but this should be decreased to 6 mL/kg within 2 to 4 hours. If the P_{PLAT} remains greater than 30 cm H_2O, the tidal volume can be further reduced to 4 mL/kg while concomitantly increasing the respiratory rate to afford adequate ventilation.[6,17] Gas exchange goals should include oxygen saturation greater than or equal to 88% to 95% and pH greater than or equal to 7.3 with a normal lactate level and base excess showing adequate end-organ oxygen delivery.

PEEP can be adjusted by one of the ARDSNet PEEP/fraction of inspired oxygen (Fio_2) tables,[19] by titrating based on measured transpulmonary pressures,[20] or by using a pressure-volume curve.[21] The ARDSNet tables include one with lower PEEP/higher Fio_2 and another with higher PEEP/lower Fio_2.[19] The risks of using this protocolized approach to PEEP adjustment include excessive PEEP resulting in both inadequate venous return leading to hypoperfusion and barotrauma in those patients with poorly recruitable lungs.[22] Furthermore, there does not seem to be a clear benefit of one table rather than the other,[19] although there is a trend toward improved mortality using the high-PEEP table in patients with moderate to severe ARDS.[23] A clinical trial that examined a so-called open-lung approach by adding recruitment maneuvers and higher PEEP levels to a low-tidal-volume strategy did not show an improved all-cause mortality (36.4% open lung vs 40.4% control; $P = .19$).[24] However, there were lower incidences of refractory hypoxemia and death with refractory hypoxemia with the open-lung strategy. Another trial that adjusted PEEP to target a P_{PLAT} of 28 to 30 cm H_2O similarly showed no significant mortality benefit.[25] However, this approach did result in more ventilator-free days and less multiorgan failure. Looking at this another way, minimizing the driving pressure (P_{PLAT} – PEEP) may optimize the patient's chances of survival.[26]

Deviating from this approach risks further lung injury through what is likely the combined mechanisms of barotrauma (P_{PLAT} >30 cm H_2O or peak inspiratory pressure >35 cm H_2O), volutrauma (V_T >6–8 mL/kg PBW), atelectrauma (low or no PEEP resulting in repeated opening and closing of alveolar units in the setting of injured lungs), and inflammatory biotrauma from various injury mechanisms.[16] Notwithstanding, adherence to these ventilator parameters in modern ICUs by clinicians familiar with ARDS and its poor outcomes remains surprisingly low, as described earlier.[5] In particular, with regard to ventilator management, recognition of ARDS did not result in significant changes in ventilator management. In this study, 35% of patients with severe ARDS were managed with a V_T of greater than 8 mL/kg PBW, whereas the median PEEP in this group was 10 cm H_2O, and only 40% of patients with ARDS had a measured P_{PLAT} during the course of their ICU stay. The mainstay of hypoxemia management seemed to be increased Fio_2. More than a decade and a half following publication of the ARDSNet ARMA trial, there remains significant room for improvement in applying these fundamental ventilator management principles to patients with ARDS.

Alternative Ventilator Strategies

The standard approach to lung protective ventilation established by the ARDSNet ARMA trial is volume-controlled ventilation. Alternative ventilator strategies include pressure-controlled ventilation, pressure-regulated volume-cycled ventilation, inverse ratio ventilation, high-frequency ventilation, airway pressure release ventilation (APRV), and neurally adjusted ventilator assist. All of these modes can be adjusted to minimize iatrogenic ventilator-associated lung injury; however, most have not been thoroughly evaluated in patients with ARDS to fully elucidate their role in managing these patients. A detailed review of all of these modes of ventilation is beyond the scope of this article but significant developments in several of these modes are highlighted.

In patients with severe ARDS doing poorly on volume-controlled ventilation, lung protective ventilation can be achieved using other modes of ventilation.[27] Triggers that may lead clinicians to consider another ventilator approach include patient dyssynchrony refractory to deep sedation, air trapping and auto-PEEP from a high respiratory rate, or patient discomfort. In patients with refractory hypoxemia, before changing ventilator modes, the authors advocate for PEEP optimization as discussed earlier, consideration of neuromuscular blockade, and prone positioning (discussed later). A so-called low-level recruitment maneuver can also be considered. This maneuver is performed by holding a pressure of 40 cm H_2O for 40 seconds.[8] Before this maneuver, the physician must prepare to manage unstable hemodynamics from decreased venous return. After this maneuver, the patient's oxygenation status can be reevaluated. If the oxygenation improves, this suggests that the patient still has recruitable lung and may benefit from a higher PEEP level.[28] If none of these maneuvers improve the patient's oxygenation, alternative ventilator modes or ECMO should be pursued (Fig. 2).

High-frequency ventilation

High-frequency ventilation can be provided in several different forms. The most common types in an ICU setting are either high-frequency oscillatory ventilation (HFOV) or high-frequency percussive ventilation (HFPV). Some enthusiasm for HFOV in the adult critical care specialties began when Derdak and colleagues[29] published a multicenter randomized controlled trial in patients with moderate to severe ARDS comparing conventional ventilation (CV) (V_T 6–10 mL/kg) with HFOV. Oxygenation improved within 24 hours in the HFOV group, and there was a trend toward improved 30-day (63% HFOV vs 48% CV) and 90-day (53% vs 41%) survival, although neither reached statistical significance.

However, 2 recent clinical trials, Oscillation in ARDS (OSCAR)[30] and Oscillation for Acute Respiratory Distress Syndrome Treated Early (OSCILLATE),[31] failed to show any mortality benefit for HFOV compared with conventional ventilation with either usual ventilator management modeled after ARDSNet ARMA (OSCAR) or a pressure-controlled lung protective strategy (OSCILLATE) in moderate to severe

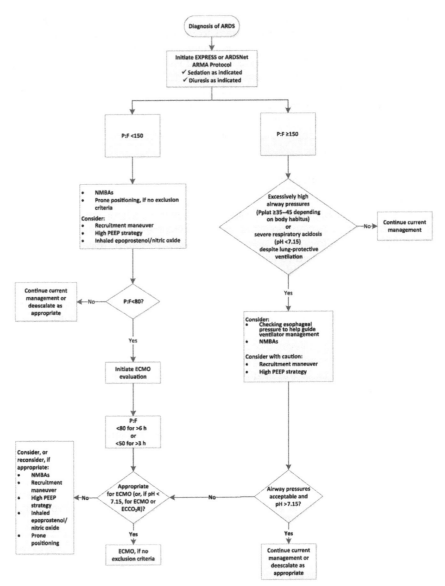

Fig. 2. Stepwise management of patients with moderate to severe ARDS, showing the sequential application of therapies up to and including venovenous ECMO. NMBA, neuromuscular blocking agents. EXPRESS, expiratory pressure study group; P:F, Pao2/fraction of inspired oxygen ratio. (*Adapted from* Brodie D, Guérin C. Rescue therapy for refractory ARDS should be offered early: no. Intensive Care Med 2015;41(5):926–9.)

ARDS. OSCILLATE was terminated early because of increased mortality in the HFOV arm. Thus, the role for HFOV in managing severe ARDS remains unclear. In our practice, the ready availability of ECMO in circumstances in which traditional management is failing largely removes the need for HFOV.

HFPV is a pressure-regulated ventilatory mode that provides oscillatory ventilation around 2 different set pressures. This mode of ventilation effectively mobilizes secretions, thus it is widely used in patients with inhalation injury and those with tenacious, purulent secretions.[32,33] Its role in patients with ARDS outside these specific populations remains ill defined,[34] although HFPV was shown to improve oxygenation at lower peak and mean airway pressures in 1 small study of patients with ARDS.[35]

Airway pressure release ventilation

APRV is a form of inverse ratio pressure-controlled ventilation applied with a special release valve that allows patients to exhale at any time during the respiratory cycle.[36] Thus, this mode of ventilation allows patients to autoregulate their degree of stretch, thereby theoretically limiting the possibility of overdistending normal portions of the diseased lung while optimally recruiting other areas. APRV has been advocated by clinicians who believe that low-volume volume-controlled ventilation underemphasizes lung recruitment and leads to continued ventilation-perfusion mismatching as a result, whereas APRV is thought to reduce so-called alveolar microstrain or dynamic alveolar heterogeneity.[37,38]

Clinical studies of APRV have yet to fully delineate its role in the management of ARDS. One small randomized controlled trial in patients with trauma in which a small minority had moderate to severe ARDS showed no significant differences in outcomes between APRV and low-tidal-volume ventilation.[39] A more recent retrospective study suggests that early application of APRV may reduce the progression to ARDS in high-risk patients with trauma compared with conventional ventilation.[40] In our practice, ideal patients for APRV include those who are stable enough to not require deep sedation and neuromuscular blockade but who have evidence of recruitable lung on chest radiograph in the setting of moderate to severe ARDS. Theoretically, on APRV, sedation can be lightened and the patient may be able to participate in physical therapy activities while still receiving the benefit of lung recruitment. Furthermore, ventilator support can easily be weaned on APRV by slowly decreasing the inspiratory pressure and lengthening the time at this pressure until the patient is on straight continuous positive airway pressure.

ADVANCES IN NONVENTILATOR MANAGEMENT

Nonventilatory adjunctive therapies also play an important role in the management of patients with moderate to severe ARDS. In recent years, important studies have shown a potential survival benefit with the use of these therapies, whereas others have not been proved beneficial or have even been found to be associated with harm. The roles of neuromuscular blockade, prone positioning, and inhaled pulmonary vasodilators in patients with severe ARDS are discussed later in this article.

Neuromuscular Blockade

Neuromuscular blockade has been associated with ICU-acquired weakness. However, in patients with severe forms of ARDS or rapidly worsening ARDS, a short course (48 hours) of neuromuscular blockade may facilitate the application of lung protective ventilator settings while eliminating such problems as ventilator dyssynchrony. One randomized controlled clinical trial of early neuromuscular blockade (within 48 hours of ARDS diagnosis) showed no crude mortality benefit in patients with moderate to severe ARDS (Pao_2/Fio_2 ratio [PFR] <150 mm Hg), but, after making prespecified adjustments for differences in severity of illness, plateau pressure, and PFR, a benefit was shown. A mortality benefit was also identified in a prespecified subgroup with worse hypoxemia (PFR <120 mm Hg).[41] Cisatracurium (Nimbex) was used in this study and does not require dose adjustment in renal or hepatic insufficiency[42]; thus we preferentially use this agent in patients with ARDS. The PETAL Network is currently conducting the Reevaluation of Systemic Early Neuromuscular Blockade (ROSE) trial (https://clinicaltrials.gov/ct2/show/NCT02509078) to reexamine the efficacy of this strategy.

Prone Positioning

If the patient's disease is primarily in the lower lobes (based on chest radiograph or computed tomography findings), a trial of prone positioning for 2 to 6 hours should be performed and the patient's clinical response assessed. This repositioning improves lower lobe aeration, thereby optimizing ventilation-perfusion matching, among other potential benefits (Fig. 3). The PROSEVA (Proning Severe ARDS Patients) trial enrolled patients with moderate to severe ARDS (PFR <150 mm Hg) and showed a mortality benefit to prone positioning protocolized to a minimum of 16 h/d.[43] Other investigators have shown that this technique can be performed in and may have benefits for a range of ICU patients, including patients with burns[44] and even patients receiving ECMO.[45]

This approach is best implemented in the setting of specific training for clinicians performing the prone positioning.[45] This should include education on the indications and contraindications, training on the proper technique for prone positioning (see online video Prone Positioning of Patients with the Acute Respiratory Distress Syndrome, available at http://www.nejm.org/doi/full/10.1056/NEJMoa1214103#t=article), an overview of routine nursing care of prone patients, and a review of emergency procedures (ie, response to patients who develop unstable cardiac rhythms).

Pulmonary Vasodilators

Inhaled pulmonary vasodilators, including inhaled nitric oxide (iNO) and inhaled prostacyclins, afford the theoretic benefit of optimizing ventilation-perfusion matching by specifically dilating pulmonary vascular beds within aerated lung regions.[46] These therapies typically improve oxygenation in patients with severe ARDS.[47,48] However, showing further outcomes benefits to these therapies has proved elusive. iNO has recently been associated with increased acute kidney injury presumably caused by systemic effects on renal perfusion.[47] Initiation of these agents can be used to trigger an evaluation for ECMO because they can potentially signify patients with refractory hypoxemia more reliably than ventilator settings and PFR. In our practice, these agents are used for short-term rescue in patients with rapidly progressive hypoxemic respiratory failure until more labor-intensive therapies, such as prone positioning or ECMO, can be instituted.

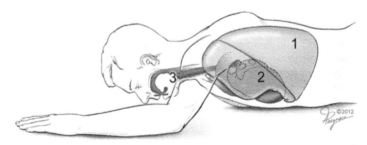

Fig. 3. The benefits of prone positioning for patients with severe ARDS. Benefits include (*1*) improved ventilation to the lower lobes, which reduces ventilation-perfusion mismatch; (*2*) reduced compression of the lower lungs by the heart; and (*3*) postural drainage of secretions. (*From* James MM, Beilman GJ. Mechanical ventilation. Surg Clin North Am 2012;92(6):1463–74. *Courtesy of* Joseph A. Pangrace, DO, MPH, Minneapolis, MN.)

EXTRACORPOREAL MEMBRANE OXYGENATION

Venovenous ECMO (VV ECMO) has assumed an important role in the management of patients with severe ARDS (Fig. 4). In the past decade, the number of adults with severe ARDS managed with ECMO and the number of self-identifying adult ECMO centers has increased greatly.[49,50] The landmark Conventional Ventilation or ECMO for Severe Adult Respiratory Failure (CESAR) trial and the influenza A (H1N1) pandemic served to raise awareness of the technologic advances in this field and of the excellent outcomes that could potentially be achieved with good patient selection and careful management.[51,52] Since that time, several small studies and 1 large clinical trial (ECMO to Rescue Lung Injury in Severe ARDS [EOLIA], ClinicalTrials.gov identifier NCT01470703) have been conducted to further elucidate the role of ECMO in managing patients with severe ARDS. The most significant insights gained in this field since 2009 are summarized later. For further detailed reading, several excellent reviews[53–55] and a monograph on ECMO[56] are available.

Patient Selection

Making the decision to proceed with ECMO requires a careful assessment of the risks and benefits associated with this support modality in each center or region. General guidance has been published[57] and remains useful for establishing local practices. However, these guidelines do not account for the heterogeneity of severe ARDS by cause and pattern of illness, the trajectory of individual patients, or the experience and qualifications of the ECMO team, and are not evidence based. In the landmark CESAR trial, which compared referral of patients with severe ARDS to a regional ECMO center in the UK versus usual care in conventional management centers, patients randomized to be considered for ECMO had a mean PFR of 76 mm Hg, PEEP of 14 cm H_2O, pH of 7.1, and an ALI score of 3.5 out of 4. Note that very few received a trial of high-frequency ventilation (7%), prone positioning (4%), or iNO (10%).[51] In our practice, we undertake a brief trial of the ventilator-based and non–ventilator-based therapies described earlier in patients with severe ARDS. If the patient's oxygenation status and hemodynamics stabilize with these maneuvers,

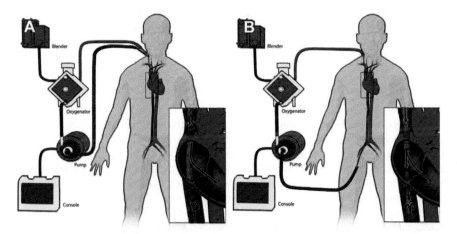

Fig. 4. VV ECMO cannulation options. (*A*) Double-lumen venous cannula (27–31 Fr) for single-site VV ECMO support. (*B*) Two single-lumen cannulas used for femoral venous drainage and internal jugular blood return. (*Reprinted from* https://collectedmed.com/.)

they are continued. However, if the patient remains unstable in any respect or shows progressive hypoxia despite optimal application of these measures, we initiate VV ECMO (see Fig. 2).

The only absolute contraindication to ECMO for severe ARDS is a preexisting condition incompatible with patient recovery. Relative contraindications that may warrant consideration include advanced physiologic age, poor preexisting functional status, and high mechanical ventilation settings for more than 7 days. The recently developed Respiratory Extracorporeal Membrane Oxygenation Survival Prediction (RESP) score can be used to determine a patient's projected survival on ECMO, although it does not provide a comparison with survival without ECMO.[58] This score ranges from −22 (poor prognosis) to +15 (good prognosis), with a score of 0 representing a predicted survival of approximately 50%. It accounts for patient features, the cause of respiratory failure, and the particulars of pre-ECMO care. An online calculator is available for quick reference (http://www.respscore.com/). Because this tool provides no estimate of the patient's outcome without ECMO,[59] careful judgment and a thoughtful discussion with the patient's family or representative are required any time ECMO is undertaken.

Regionalization and Transport

ECMO should be performed by physicians and teams experienced in the many nuances of long-term extracorporeal care. If ECMO is initiated urgently in a low-volume center, measures should be taken to transfer the patient to a high-volume regional center. These principles were affirmed in a recent consensus statement by global ECMO leaders.[60] In summary, ECMO for adult respiratory failure should be performed by centers that maintain a minimum case volume of 20 patients per year with at least 12 patients managed on ECMO for respiratory failure. In general, a population base of 2 million to 3 million patients is required for 1 ECMO center. Subsequent analysis of the Extracorporeal Life Support Organization (ELSO) registry showed improved outcomes in adult centers with more than 30 annual ECMO cases (of all types) compared with those with fewer than 6.[61]

Regional ECMO transport teams can help ensure that patients with severe ARDS do not become marooned in centers that are unable to provide ECMO support.[60,62,63] In addition, ECMO centers should register with ELSO and submit registry data to help optimize patient selection and outcomes. The authors also believe that regional centers should seek designation as ELSO centers of excellence, which requires a rigorous review of site-specific policies, practices, and outcomes, similar to trauma center verification by the American College of Surgeons.

Ventilator Management During Extracorporeal Membrane Oxygenation

ECMO does not intrinsically provide any therapy to patients with severe ARDS. Instead, it permits safe gas exchange while allowing the reduction of ventilator settings to less injurious levels and potentially permitting the elimination of rescue therapies, such as neuromuscular blockade and deep sedation, that may contribute to the poor long-term functional outcomes experienced by patients with severe ARDS.[64,65] However, to date, the optimal approach to ventilator management in patients with ARDS receiving ECMO has not been determined. A recent study has shown that survival is independently associated with higher levels of PEEP during the first 3 days of ECMO support.[66] This finding might be balanced by rapidly decreasing the driving pressure, thereby restoring a safe level of open-lung ventilator support, which does not rely on the lungs for gas exchange. Other unproven measures that may hasten lung recovery during ECMO include frequent bronchoscopy, early tracheotomy, and

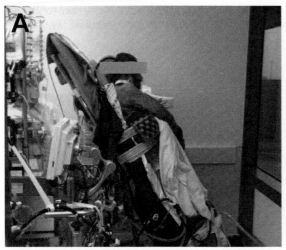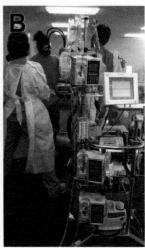

Fig. 5. Physical conditioning in patients on ECMO. This conditioning may include a tilt table in patients with continued lower extremity weakness (*A*) or even walking on a treadmill before lung transplant (*B*).

aggressive elimination of extravascular lung water with diuresis (combined with albumin if the patient is malnourished) or renal replacement therapy with hemofiltration.

Physical Conditioning

The major long-term morbidity of severe ARDS is neurologic and/or musculoskeletal disability related to prolonged inactivity.[64,65] Consequently, the authors advocate a daily awakening trial[67] once the patient has been stabilized on ECMO as well as an aggressive program of early mobilization (Fig. 5). These reconditioning programs involve multidisciplinary support and consist of a staged approach beginning with passive range of motion (performed multiple times daily by providers, nurses, therapists, coworkers, and family) and then progressing to sitting up at the side of the bed, moving from bed to chair, and ambulating with assistance.[68,69] Some limited data suggest that such aggressive physical therapy measures can safely be applied in ECMO patients.[70]

SUMMARY

Several insights into the clinical entity of ARDS have been gleaned over the past several years even as the care of these patients has continued to advance in many ways. Nonetheless, much work is still required to promote early diagnosis of ARDS and the application of evidence-based ventilator management principles in these patients. High-frequency ventilation has not shown a clear benefit in patients with severe ARDS, but other modes of ventilator support, such as APRV, may have a continued role in select patients. Nonventilator adjuncts, such as neuromuscular blockade and prone positioning, should be applied early in patients with severe forms of ARDS even as ECMO is being considered. ECMO should ideally be performed in high-volume centers, which should support the surrounding region with a transport program. During ECMO support, safer ventilator settings can be restored and physical reconditioning can be initiated to improve functional survival in these critically ill patients. Results of the EOLIA trial, which should be published soon, may further illuminate the role of ECMO in the management of patients with severe ARDS.

REFERENCES

1. Raghavendran K, Napolitano LM. ALI and ARDS: challenges and advances. Crit Care Clin 2011;27(3):xiii–xiv.
2. Ranieri VM, Rubenfeld GD, Thompson BT, et al. Acute respiratory distress syndrome: the Berlin definition. JAMA 2012;307(23):2526–33.
3. PETAL Network [Internet]. Available at: http://petalnet.org/. Accessed July 18, 2016.
4. Brown SM, Grissom CK, Moss M, et al. Non-linear imputation of PaO_2/FIO_2 from SpO_2/FIO_2 among patients with acute respiratory distress syndrome. Chest 2016; 150(2):307–13.
5. Bellani G, Laffey JG, Pham T, et al. Epidemiology, patterns of care, and mortality for patients with acute respiratory distress syndrome in intensive care units in 50 countries. JAMA 2016;315(8):788.
6. Diaz JV, Brower R, Calfee CS, et al. Therapeutic strategies for severe acute lung injury. Crit Care Med 2010;38(8):1644–50.
7. Ferguson ND, Fan E, Camporota L, et al. The Berlin definition of ARDS: an expanded rationale, justification, and supplementary material. Intensive Care Med 2012;38(10):1573–82.
8. Hemmila MR, Napolitano LM. Severe respiratory failure: advanced treatment options. Crit Care Med 2006;34(Suppl 9):S278–90.
9. Blank R, Napolitano LM. Epidemiology of ARDS and ALI. Crit Care Clin 2011; 27(3):439–58.
10. Caironi P, Carlesso E, Cressoni M, et al. Lung recruitability is better estimated according to the Berlin definition of acute respiratory distress syndrome at standard 5 cm H_2O rather than higher positive end-expiratory pressure: a retrospective cohort study. Crit Care Med 2015;43(4):781–90.
11. Rixen D, Raum M, Holzgraefe B, et al. A pig hemorrhagic shock model: oxygen debt and metabolic acidemia as indicators of severity. Shock 2001;16(3):239–44.
12. Shoemaker WC, Appel PL, Kram HB. Role of oxygen debt in the development of organ failure sepsis, and death in high-risk surgical patients. Chest 1992;102(1): 208–15.
13. Donnelly SC, Strieter RM, Reid PT, et al. The association between mortality rates and decreased concentrations of interleukin-10 and interleukin-1 receptor antagonist in the lung fluids of patients with the adult respiratory distress syndrome. Ann Intern Med 1996;125(3):191–6.
14. Zhang R, Pan Y, Fanelli V, et al. Mechanical stress and the induction of lung fibrosis via the midkine signaling pathway. Am J Respir Crit Care Med 2015; 192(3):315–23.
15. Butt Y, Kurdowska A, Allen TC. Acute lung injury: a clinical and molecular review. Arch Pathol Lab Med 2016;140(4):345–50.
16. Slutsky AS, Ranieri VM. Ventilator-induced lung injury. N Engl J Med 2013; 369(22):2126–36.
17. Brower RG, Matthay MA, Morris A, et al. Ventilation with lower tidal volumes as compared with traditional tidal volumes for acute lung injury and the acute respiratory distress syndrome. N Engl J Med 2000;342(18):1301–8.
18. Petrucci N, De Feo C. Lung protective ventilation strategy for the acute respiratory distress syndrome. Cochrane Database Syst Rev 2013;(2):CD003844.

19. Brower RG, Lanken PN, MacIntyre N, et al. Higher versus lower positive end-expiratory pressures in patients with the acute respiratory distress syndrome. N Engl J Med 2004;351(4):327–36.
20. Talmor D, Sarge T, Malhotra A, et al. Mechanical ventilation guided by esophageal pressure in acute lung injury. N Engl J Med 2008;359(20):2095–104.
21. Siegel MD, Hyzy RC. Mechanical ventilation of adults in acute respiratory distress syndrome. UpToDate 2016.
22. Kallet RH, Branson RD. Do the NIH ARDS clinical trials network PEEP/FIO$_2$ tables provide the best evidence-based guide to balancing PEEP and FIO$_2$ settings in adults? Respir Care 2007;52(4):461–77.
23. Briel M, Meade M, Mercat A, et al. Higher vs lower positive end-expiratory pressure in patients with acute lung injury and acute respiratory distress syndrome: systematic review and meta-analysis. JAMA 2010;303(9):865–73.
24. Meade MO, Cook DJ, Guyatt GH, et al. Ventilation strategy using low tidal volumes, recruitment maneuvers, and high positive end-expiratory pressure for acute lung injury and acute respiratory distress syndrome: a randomized controlled trial. JAMA 2008;299(6):637–45.
25. Mercat A, Richard J-CM, Vielle B, et al. Positive end-expiratory pressure setting in adults with acute lung injury and acute respiratory distress syndrome: a randomized controlled trial. JAMA 2008;299(6):646–55.
26. Amato MBP, Meade MO, Slutsky AS, et al. Driving pressure and survival in the acute respiratory distress syndrome. N Engl J Med 2015;372(8):747–55.
27. Chacko B, Peter JV, Tharyan P, et al. Pressure-controlled versus volume-controlled ventilation for acute respiratory failure due to acute lung injury (ALI) or acute respiratory distress syndrome (ARDS). Cochrane Database Syst Rev 2015;(1):CD008807.
28. Fan E, Wilcox ME, Brower RG, et al. Recruitment maneuvers for acute lung injury: a systematic review. Am J Respir Crit Care Med 2008;178(11):1156–63.
29. Derdak S, Mehta S, Stewart TE, et al. High-frequency oscillatory ventilation for acute respiratory distress syndrome in adults: a randomized, controlled trial. Am J Respir Crit Care Med 2002;166(6):801–8.
30. Young D, Lamb SE, Shah S, et al. High-frequency oscillation for acute respiratory distress syndrome. N Engl J Med 2013;368(9):806–13.
31. Ferguson ND, Cook DJ, Guyatt GH, et al. High-frequency oscillation in early acute respiratory distress syndrome. N Engl J Med 2013;368(9):795–805.
32. Chung KK, Wolf SE, Renz EM, et al. High-frequency percussive ventilation and low tidal volume ventilation in burns: a randomized controlled trial. Crit Care Med 2010;38(10):1970–7.
33. Hall JJ, Hunt JL, Arnoldo BD, et al. Use of high-frequency percussive ventilation in inhalation injuries. J Burn Care Res 2007;28(3):396–400.
34. Hurst JM, Branson RD, Davis K, et al. Comparison of conventional mechanical ventilation and high-frequency ventilation. A prospective, randomized trial in patients with respiratory failure. Ann Surg 1990;211(4):486–91.
35. Hurst JM, Branson RD, DeHaven CB. The role of high-frequency ventilation in post-traumatic respiratory insufficiency. J Trauma 1987;27(3):236–42.
36. Maung AA, Kaplan LJ. Airway pressure release ventilation in acute respiratory distress syndrome. Crit Care Clin 2011;27(3):501–9.
37. Kollisch-Singule M, Jain S, Andrews P, et al. Effect of airway pressure release ventilation on dynamic alveolar heterogeneity. JAMA Surg 2016;151(1):64.

38. Kollisch-Singule M, Emr B, Smith B, et al. Mechanical breath profile of airway pressure release ventilation: the effect on alveolar recruitment and microstrain in acute lung injury. JAMA Surg 2014;149(11):1138.

39. Maxwell RA, Green JM, Waldrop J, et al. A randomized prospective trial of airway pressure release ventilation and low tidal volume ventilation in adult trauma patients with acute respiratory failure. J Trauma 2010;69(3):501–10 [discussion: 511].

40. Andrews PL, Shiber JR, Jaruga-Killeen E, et al. Early application of airway pressure release ventilation may reduce mortality in high-risk trauma patients: a systematic review of observational trauma ARDS literature. J Trauma Acute Care Surg 2013;75(4):635–41.

41. Papazian L, Forel JM, Gacouin A, et al. Neuromuscular blockers in early acute respiratory distress syndrome. N Engl J Med 2010;363(12):1107–16.

42. Murray MJ, Cowen J, DeBlock H, et al. Clinical practice guidelines for sustained neuromuscular blockade in the adult critically ill patient. Crit Care Med 2002; 30(1):142–56.

43. Guérin C, Reignier J, Richard J-C, et al. Prone positioning in severe acute respiratory distress syndrome. N Engl J Med 2013;368(23):2159–68.

44. Hale DF, Cannon JW, Batchinsky AI, et al. Prone positioning improves oxygenation in adult burn patients with severe acute respiratory distress syndrome. J Trauma Acute Care Surg 2012;72(6):1634–9.

45. Dickinson S, Park PK, Napolitano LM. Prone-positioning therapy in ARDS. Crit Care Clin 2011;27(3):511–23.

46. Levy SD, Alladina JW, Hibbert KA, et al. High-flow oxygen therapy and other inhaled therapies in intensive care units. Lancet 2016;387(10030):1867–78.

47. Adhikari NKJ, Dellinger RP, Lundin S, et al. Inhaled nitric oxide does not reduce mortality in patients with acute respiratory distress syndrome regardless of severity: systematic review and meta-analysis. Crit Care Med 2014;42(2):404–12.

48. van Heerden PV, Barden A, Michalopoulos N, et al. Dose-response to inhaled aerosolized prostacyclin for hypoxemia due to ARDS. Chest 2000;117(3):819–27.

49. Extracorporeal Life Support Organization (ELSO) Registry International Summary [Internet]. Available at: https://www.elso.org/Registry/Statistics/International Summary.aspx. Accessed July 30, 2016.

50. Karagiannidis C, Brodie D, Strassmann S, et al. Extracorporeal membrane oxygenation: evolving epidemiology and mortality. Intensive Care Med 2016; 42(5):889–96.

51. Peek GJ, Mugford M, Tiruvoipati R, et al. Efficacy and economic assessment of conventional ventilatory support versus extracorporeal membrane oxygenation for severe adult respiratory failure (CESAR): a multicentre randomised controlled trial. Lancet 2009;374(9698):1351–63.

52. Davies A, Jones D, Bailey M, et al. Extracorporeal membrane oxygenation for 2009 influenza A(H1N1) acute respiratory distress syndrome. JAMA 2009; 302(17):1888–95.

53. Park PK, Napolitano LM, Bartlett RH. Extracorporeal membrane oxygenation in adult acute respiratory distress syndrome. Crit Care Clin 2011;27(3):627–46.

54. Brodie D, Bacchetta M. Extracorporeal membrane oxygenation for ARDS in adults. N Engl J Med 2011;365(20):1905–14.

55. Ventetuolo CE, Muratore CS. Extracorporeal life support in critically ill adults. Am J Respir Crit Care Med 2014;190(5):497–508.

56. Annich G, Lynch W, MacLaren G, et al. ECMO: extracorporeal cardiopulmonary support in critical care. 4th edition. Ann Arbor (MI): ELSO; 2012.

57. Extracorporeal Life Support Organization (ELSO) guidelines for adult respiratory failure, version 1.3 [Internet]. 2013. Available at: http://www.elso.org/Portals/0/IGD/Archive/FileManager/989d4d4d14cusersshyerdocumentselsoguidelinesfor adultrespiratoryfailure1.3.pdf. Accessed July 24, 2016.
58. Schmidt M, Bailey M, Sheldrake J, et al. Predicting survival after extracorporeal membrane oxygenation for severe acute respiratory failure. The Respiratory Extracorporeal Membrane Oxygenation Survival Prediction (RESP) score. Am J Respir Crit Care Med 2014;189(11):1374–82.
59. Goligher EC, Douflé G, Fan E. Update in mechanical ventilation, sedation, and outcomes 2014. Am J Respir Crit Care Med 2015;191(12):1367–73.
60. Combes A, Brodie D, Bartlett R, et al. Position paper for the organization of extracorporeal membrane oxygenation programs for acute respiratory failure in adult patients. Am J Respir Crit Care Med 2014;190(5):488–96.
61. Barbaro RP, Odetola FO, Kidwell KM, et al. Association of hospital-level volume of extracorporeal membrane oxygenation cases and mortality. Analysis of the extracorporeal life support organization registry. Am J Respir Crit Care Med 2015; 191(8):894–901.
62. Cannon JW, Allan PF, Osborn EC, et al. Transport of the ECMO patient from concept to implementation. In: Annich GM, Lynch WR, MacLaren G, et al, editors. ECMO Extracorporeal cardiopulmonary support in critical care, 4th edition. Ann Arbor (MI): ELSO; 2012. p. 451–78.
63. Javidfar J, Brodie D, Takayama H, et al. Safe transport of critically ill adult patients on extracorporeal membrane oxygenation support to a regional extracorporeal membrane oxygenation center. ASAIO J 2011;57(5):421–5.
64. Herridge MS, Cheung AM, Tansey CM, et al. One-year outcomes in survivors of the acute respiratory distress syndrome. N Engl J Med 2003;348(8):683–93.
65. Herridge MS, Tansey CM, Matte A, et al. Functional disability 5 years after acute respiratory distress syndrome. N Engl J Med 2011;364(14):1293–304.
66. Schmidt M, Stewart C, Bailey M, et al. Mechanical ventilation management during extracorporeal membrane oxygenation for acute respiratory distress syndrome: a retrospective international multicenter study. Crit Care Med 2015;43(3):654–64.
67. Kress JP, Pohlman AS, O'Connor MF, et al. Daily interruption of sedative infusions in critically ill patients undergoing mechanical ventilation. N Engl J Med 2000; 342(20):1471–7.
68. Pohlman MC, Schweickert WD, Pohlman AS, et al. Feasibility of physical and occupational therapy beginning from initiation of mechanical ventilation. Crit Care Med 2010;38(11):2089–94.
69. Schweickert WD, Pohlman MC, Pohlman AS, et al. Early physical and occupational therapy in mechanically ventilated, critically ill patients: a randomised controlled trial. Lancet 2009;373(9678):1874–82.
70. Abrams D, Javidfar J, Farrand E, et al. Early mobilization of patients receiving extracorporeal membrane oxygenation: a retrospective cohort study. Crit Care 2014;18(1):R38.
71. International ECMO Network: Current Projects [Internet]. Available at: http://www.internationalecmonetwork.org/current_projects/. Accessed July 24, 2016.

Ventilator-Associated Pneumonia: New Definitions

M. Chance Spalding, DO, PhD[a,b,*], Michael W. Cripps, MD[c],
Christian T. Minshall, MD, PhD[c]

KEYWORDS

- Ventilator-associated pneumonia • Sepsis • Nosocomial infection • Critical care

KEY POINTS

- New NHSN definition for ventilator-associated events (VAE) replaces previous definition of pneumonia.
- Clear, defined objective criteria for each category of VAE eliminates subjectivity of previous definition.
- Shifts focus of reportable events from pneumonia to broader classification of respiratory deterioration.
- May underestimate the rate of clinical pneumonia, but captures other noninfectious causes of respiratory compromise in ventilated patients.
- Definition may need to be modified to account for specific patient populations and alternative modes of ventilation.

INTRODUCTION

Ventilator-associated pneumonia (VAP) remains one of the most common nosocomial infections in the intensive care unit (ICU) affecting one-third of patients that require mechanical ventilation during a noninfectious admission.[1] Despite having a significant attributable mortality (4.6%), VAP remains a single a component of a larger constellation of adverse events, such as aspiration, atelectasis, pulmonary edema, venous thromboembolic event, delirium, and acute respiratory distress syndrome (ARDS), which potentially increase the morbidity, mortality, hospital length of stay (LOS), and cost of care in mechanically ventilated patients. This broader view of complications that arise in patients requiring ventilator support provides the framework for the new

Disclosure Statement: This paper comprises original work created by the authors and they have no commercial or financial conflicts of interest to disclose.

[a] Department of Surgery, Grant Medical Center, 111 South Grant Avenue, Columbus, OH 43215, USA; [b] Department of Surgery, Ohio University College of Osteopathic Medicine, 35 West Green Drive, Athens, OH 45701, USA; [c] Department of Surgery, UT Southwestern, 5323 Harry Hines Boulevard, Dallas, TX 75390, USA
* Corresponding author.
E-mail address: Chance.Spalding@ohiohealth.com

quality metrics put forth by the Centers for Disease Control and Prevention (CDC) for ventilated patients.

In 2011, CDC a workgroup encompassing physician leaders from multiple professional societies (eg, American College of Chest Physicians, American Thoracic Society, Society of Critical Care Medicine, Infectious Diseases Society of America) in conjunction with representatives of the US Department of Health and Human Services, Office of Disease Prevention and Heath Promotion, National Institutes of Health, and the CDC met to create a new definition of VAP that improves diagnosis, the reliability and validity of surveillance, and create a reporting algorithm for the National Healthcare Safety Network (NHSN).[2] The final product of this workgroup resulted in a tiered system that encompasses the broader classification of ventilator-associated events (VAE), subcategorized by objective criteria for infection-related ventilator-associated condition (IVAC) and then more specifically by possible- and probable-VAP (Fig. 1).

This article reviews the criteria for ventilator-associated condition (VAC) and IVAC, including the classifications of probable- or possible-VAP; compares how the tiered definition of pneumonia contrasts to the previous NHSN definition; summarizes the studies validating its application; and explores its utility in surgical patients.

NEW DEFINITION

In 2013, NHSN supplanted the previous definition of pneumonia with the working group's classification of VAE (Table 1). The intent is to cast a wider net using defined, objective criteria that captures all potentially preventable complications from data available in the electronic medical record (EMR) in most institutions. Automated surveillance directly from EMR is thought to decrease reporting bias by eliminating subjectivity from the analysis.

VAC is defined as a sustained increase in oxygen requirements in a ventilated patient over a period of 2 days. Sustained oxygen requirement is defined as an increase in the daily minimum positive end-expiratory pressure (PEEP) of greater than or equal to 3 cm H_2O or an increase in the daily minimum fraction of inspired oxygen (FIO_2) of greater than or equal to 20 points for 2 days. To qualify as a VAC, the patient must have had a minimum of 2 days of mechanical ventilation with stable or decreasing oxygen requirements before the days of increased oxygenation.

The progression from VAC to IVAC depends on timing in relation to the increased oxygenation requirements that define a VAC, clinical signs of infection, and treatment of the patient with antibiotics by the ICU team. Patients must be mechanically ventilated a minimum of 3 days and have signs of infection in the 2 days before or 2 days after the diagnosis of VAC. In addition, the patient must have a low-grade fever (>38°C) or hypothermia (<36°C) or leukocytosis ($\geq$12,000 cells/mm^3) or leukopenia ($\leq$4000 cells/mm^3) and be started on a new antimicrobial agent for greater than or equal to 4 days. IVAC suggests a causal relationship between infectious cause and VAC.

In the new classification of VAE, patients that meet the criteria for VAC and IVAC are further characterized with the diagnosis of VAP according to the type of evidence available from their sputum assessment. Possible-VAP requires either a qualitative sputum analysis demonstrating purulent respiratory secretions defined as greater than or equal to 25 neutrophils and less than or equal to 10 squamous cells per low-power field or a positive qualitative, semiquantitative, or quantitative culture obtained from the lungs, bronchi, or trachea. Probable-VAP requires the presence of purulent secretions and specific cutoffs for the number of colony-forming units identified

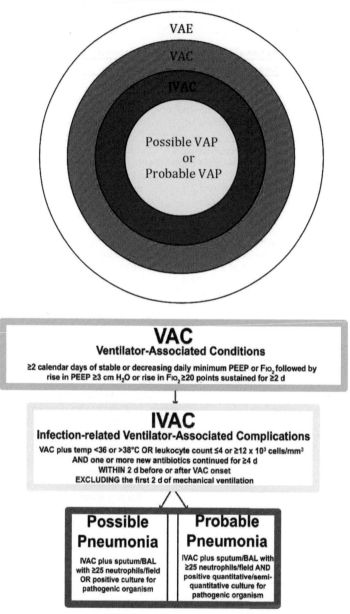

Fig. 1. Targeting VAE. Broad description of ventilator-related complications is more narrowly defined by each tier of the new CDC definition: VAC, IVAC, possible- or probable-VAP. F_{IO_2}, fraction of inspired oxygen; PEEP, positive end-expiratory pressure.

in culture that are determined by what level of the airway the sputum sample was obtained (see Table 1). Any of the following results may supplant the presence of purulent sputum in the diagnosis of probable-VAP: positive pleural fluid culture, positive lung histopathology, positive diagnostic test for legionella, or the presence of common respiratory viral pathogens in sputum.

Table 1
NHSN VAE criteria

NHSN Surveillance Guidelines for Diagnosis of VAE		
Name: Description	Dependent Qualification	Definition
VAC: new respiratory deterioration	≥2 calendar days of stable or decreasing daily minimum PEEP or daily minimum F$_{IO_2}$	Followed by a daily Minimum PEEP of ≥3 cm H$_2$O OR Minimum F$_{IO_2}$ by >20 points sustained for ≥2 calendar days
iVAC: VAC + clinical signs of infection	Within 2 calendar days before or after onset of a VAC Excludes the first 2 d of mechanical ventilation	Temperature: <36°C or >38°C OR Leukocyte count: ≤4000 or ≥12,000 cells/mm^3 AND One or more new antibiotics continued for ≥4 d
Possible VAP: IVAC + qualitative evidence of pulmonary infection	Within 2 calendar days before or after onset of a VAC Excludes the first 2 d of mechanical ventilation	Gram staining of endotracheal aspirate or BAL showing ≥25 neutrophils and ≤10 epithelial cells per low-power field OR Positive culture from sputum, endotracheal aspirate, BAL, lung tissue
Probable VAP: IVAC + quantitative evidence of pulmonary infection	Within 2 calendar days before or after onset of a VAC Excludes the first 2 d of mechanical ventilation	Positive culture of endotracheal aspirate ≥10^5 CFU/mL, or positive BAL culture with ≥10^4 CFU/mL, or positive culture of protected specimen brush ≥10^3 CFU/mL OR One of the following (without requirement for purulent secretions) Positive pleural fluid culture (where specimen was obtained during thoracentesis or initial placement of chest tube and NOT from indwelling chest tube) Positive lung histopathology Positive diagnostic test for legionella Positive diagnostic test on respiratory secretions for influenza virus, respiratory syncytial virus, adenovirus, parainfluenza virus, rhinovirus, human metapneumovirus, coronavirus

Highlights the stepwise respiratory deterioration associated with VAC, iVAC, possible pneumonia, and probable pneumonia with specific, objective criteria that define each category.

Sputum cultures excludes the following: normal respiratory/oral flora, mixed respiratory/oral flora or equivalent; *Candida* species or yeast not otherwise specified; coagulase-negative *Staphylococcus* species; *Enterococcus* species.

Abbreviations: BAL, bronchoalveolar lavage; CFU, colony-forming unit; F$_{IO_2}$, fraction of inspired oxygen; PEEP, positive end-expiratory pressure.

The diagnosis of VAP is not easily established but is clearly defined within the new surveillance criteria of VAE. The mechanically ventilated patient must have a period of stability followed by deterioration and increased support (VAC), a suspected infectious cause (IVAC), and finally meet the confirmatory criteria for either possible-VAP or probable-VAP. Each tier has specific and clearly defined, objective criteria that must be met to qualify for the next level. This system is substantially different from the previous NHSN definition of VAP (PNU1), which was more subjective with many of the parameters not clearly stipulated. The PNU1 diagnosis was made when a patient met radiographic, systemic, and pulmonary function criteria. The guidelines were less precise allowing significant leeway in the interpretation, which led to high degree of variability between providers in defining when a patient had pneumonia. One ramification of the interobserver variability was that it limited the ability to compare reporting within institutions and across hospital systems. To highlight how the new diagnosis of VAP differs, we next review the three categories comprising the diagnosis of PNU1 (Box 1).

OLD VERSUS NEW

PNU1 definition required radiologic evaluation with two or more serial studies that demonstrated a new, progressive, or persistent infiltrate, consolidation, or cavitation. The current VAE criteria do not have a radiographic component. Although radiographic evaluation may be helpful in identifying causes for worsening pulmonary function, a finding on plain chest radiograph may easily be interpreted as an infiltrate, atelectasis, effusion, or pneumonia between providers and frequently may not manifest until well after a patient with pulmonary dysfunction has clinically improved. Radiographic studies are an adjunct to the diagnosis of pneumonia but are not required and have been eliminated from VAE surveillance criteria.

The systemic component of the PNU1 definition required the patient to have at least one of the following criteria: fever with temperature greater than 38°C, leukopenia ($\leq$4000 cells/mm^3) or leukocytosis ($\geq$12,000 cells/mm^3), or altered mental status in patients who are greater than or equal to 70 years of age with no other identified cause. These criteria are similar to the standards that determine when a patient has an IVAC, except there is not a stipulation regarding hypothermia, temperature less than 36°C in

---

Box 1
NHSN PNU1 definition

Radiologic criteria ($\geq$2 serial radiographs with at least one of the following)

1. New or progressive infiltrate

2. Consolidation

3. Cavitation

Systemic criteria (at least one of the following)

1. Fever (>38°C or >100.4°F)

2. Leukopenia (<4000 white blood cell/mm^3) or leukocytosis ($\geq$12,000 white blood cell/mm^3)

3. For adults $\geq$70 years old, altered mental status with no other recognized cause

Pulmonary criteria (at least two of the following)

1. New onset of purulent sputum, or change in character of sputum, or increased respiratory secretions, or increased suctioning requirements

2. Worsening gas exchange (eg, desaturations, increased requirements, or increased ventilator demands)

3. New-onset or worsening cough, or dyspnea, or tachypnea

4. Rails or bronchial breath sounds

the PNU1 definition. Conversely, the IVAC definition does not have a component that accounts for altered mental status in elderly patients.

To fulfill the pulmonary component of PNU1, patients must meet at least two of four criteria. New onset of purulent sputum, change in the character of the sputum, or need for more frequent suctioning were considered one element but there were no specific cutoffs leaving the evaluation of purulent, character, or frequency purely subjective. The new VAP definition has defined qualitative and quantitative values of neutrophil count and colony-forming units that must be met to establish possible-VAP and probable-VAP. The second of the four pulmonary criteria vaguely defined worsening gas exchange. However, these criteria were described as desaturations, increased oxygen requirements, or increased ventilator demand but did not define the increment or duration of time. In comparison the diagnosis of VAP is contingent on the patient having met the criteria of a VAC. The VAC criteria clearly establish minimum increases in FiO_2 and/or PEEP and stipulate the duration of time relative to a previous period of stability and to the diagnosis of VAP. The two remaining pulmonary criteria for PNU1 were comprised of patient symptoms: worsening cough, dyspnea, or tachypnea; and patient examination findings, such as rales or bronchial breath sounds. In contrast, the VAE surveillance definition does not use any symptoms or examination findings as criteria for defining VAP.

WHAT'S THE POINT?

The new characterization of VAE allows for multiple novel opportunities that were not accounted for by solely focusing on VAP and the PNU1 definition. Most (75%) patients that meet criteria for VAE have a noninfectious cause responsible for their respiratory setback (Fig. 2). Clinical complications, such as venous thromboembolic event, pulmonary edema, aspiration, and ARDS, can adversely affect the duration of mechanical ventilation; ICU LOS; increase mortality; and further convolute other important aspects of care, such as sedation, prevention of ICU delirium, and early mobility. Objectively identifying VAEs provides a wider vantage point that can promulgate performance improvement for all patients that require support with mechanical ventilation.

The benefit of defining specific criteria that identify VAE and eliminates subjectivity is readily apparent. It allows for the creation of programs to identify these searchable elements from the EMR, which simplifies reporting and reduces variability. The data within institutions, between health care systems, and even across borders can now be collected and compared in an easy, efficient manner. This cross-comparison at multiple levels would allow for identification of effective patterns of care that could potentially be shared within and across health care systems.

SUMMARY OF STUDIES EVALUATING THE PRACTICALITY OF THE VENTILATOR-ASSOCIATED EVENTS CRITERIA

Since the introduction of the VAE surveillance criteria multiple studies have been performed to validate its clinical applicability (Table 2). One of the first studies to evaluate how the surveillance criteria for VAE could be used to identify patient complications used retrospective data collected from three academic medical centers in different regions of the United States. Each unit submitted 100 patients that were mechanically ventilated 2 to 7 days and 100 patients that ventilated for greater than 7 days. Each patient was independently assessed using the VAC criteria and according to the PNU1 definition. This study demonstrated that patients who met criteria for VAC and PNU1 had a longer duration of mechanical ventilation, ICU LOS, and hospital LOS. VAC diagnosis was associated with increased mortality, whereas PNU1

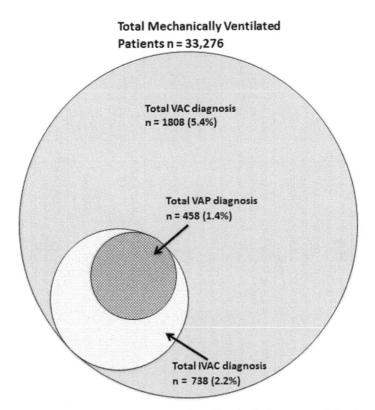

Total Mechanically Ventilated
Patients n = 33,276

Total VAC diagnosis
n = 1808 (5.4%)

Total VAP diagnosis
n = 458 (1.4%)

Total IVAC diagnosis
n = 738 (2.2%)

Fig. 2. Diagram summarizing cumulative number of patients that met VAC, iVAC, and both possible- and probable-VAP criteria from the published studies summarized in Table 2.

diagnosis was not, and VAC assessment was considerably less time consuming for the assessors to perform compared with evaluation with the PNU1 criteria.[3] Another early study performed in 11 ICUs in Canada and the United States prospectively evaluated 1320 patients using VAC, IVAC, and PNU1 criteria.[4] This study demonstrated that patients meeting criteria for VAC and IVAC had increased mortality compared with patients diagnosed with VAP using PNU1. The results also highlight the importance of the subjective surveillance definition, because there was a poor correlation agreement between patients that met the criteria for VAC or IVAC and patients diagnosed with VAP using the PNU1 definition. Similarly, another retrospective study from a tertiary, teaching hospital in Australia evaluated 543 patients intubated greater than or equal to 2 days, using the VAC surveillance criteria, and demonstrated patients with VAC had increased duration of mechanical ventilation, ICU LOS, and duration of antibiotic therapy.[5]

In 2014, a group from the Netherlands published results from a prospective evaluation of the EMR from patients in two tertiary care centers from 2011 to 2012. This study reviewed ventilator settings, microbiology, and clinical data from 2080 patients who were mechanically ventilated for greater than 2 consecutive days. In addition to screening the EMR with the VAE surveillance criteria, the authors also developed clinical definition of prospective VAP, which used the VAE criteria for possible-VAP and the radiographic evidence from PNU1. The results of this study demonstrated that patients with VAC diagnosis have an increased mortality compared with those without

Table 2
Summary of studies that evaluated patients using NHSN VAE criteria

	Emphasis	Design/Population	Summary	VAE Rates n (%)
Klompas et al,[7] 2014	Epidemiology and morbidity of VAE	Retrospective review at an academic medical center studying adult patients on MV over 5 y	20,356 patients studied over 5 y showing VAEs corresponded with three times longer to extubate patients, increased hospital LOS by 50%, and doubled the risk of death compared with those that did not meet the criteria for VAE. Most frequent organisms were *Staphylococcus aureus* (29%), *Pseudomonas aeruginosa* (14%), and *Enterobacter* species (7.9%).	VAC 1141 (5.61) IVAC 431 (2.12) pVAP 139 (0.68) prVAP 127 (0.62)
Klouwenberg et al,[6] 2014	Novel electronic surveillance mechanism to identify VAE	Multi-institutional prospective cohort study on mixed ICU patients	2080 patients ventilated for >2 d. The VAE algorithm detected 32% of clinical VAP patients. Most VAC patients had volume overload and infections, but not necessarily VAP. Concordance between VAE algorithm and clinical VAP was poor.	VAC 158 (7.60) IVAC 66 (3.17) p/prVAP 51 (2.45)
Boyer et al,[11] 2015	Prospectively evaluate VAE and VAC rates and preventability	Prospective cohort study at an academic medical center studying adult medical and surgical ICU patients	1209 patients studied. Most common cause of VAC were IVACs (50.7%), ARDS (16.4%), pulmonary edema (14.9%), and atelectasis (9%). 37.3% of VACs were determined to be potentially preventable. The sensitivity of NHSN criteria for detecting VAP determined to be 25.9%.	VAC 77 (6.37) iVAC 34 (2.81) pVAP 6 (0.49) prVAP 15 (1.24)
Stoeppel et al,[14] 2014	Applicability of NHSN VAE definitions in surgical ICU patients	Prospective cohort study at an academic medical center studying adult surgical and ICU patients	437 surgical ICU patients of which only 37 met VAE criteria. Of the 400 other patients who did not meet VAE criteria, 111 (28%) had respiratory deterioration, 99 patients had clinical pneumonia. Most of these patients (58%) had <2 d of respiratory deterioration. Agreement between prVAP and clinical VAP was 77.3%.	VAC 37 (8.47) IVAC 31 (7.09) p/prVAP 22 (5.03)
Lewis et al,[17] 2014	Evaluate risk factors for VAE	Retrospective case-controlled study at an academic medical center studying adult medical, surgical, cardiac, and neuroscience patients	2990 patients analyzed and 110 case matched to control subjects showing significant risk factors in developing a VAE were mandatory modes of ventilation, positive fluid balance, starting benzodiazepines before intubation, total opioid exposure, and use of paralytic medications.	VAC 172 (5.75) IVAC 70 (2.34)

Study	Purpose	Study design and population	Findings	Results
Lilly et al,[9] 2014	Prevalence and characteristics of VAE	Prospective cohort study at two academic medical centers studying adult medical, surgical, cardiovascular, and neurologic ICU patients	8408 MV patients discharged from ICU. NHSN VAE guidelines had a poor predictive value (0.07) of patients with clinically determined VAP. Most patients (71%) who met VAE/VAC criteria were diagnosed with ARDS.	VAC – 13.8/1000 MV days / IVAC – 8.8/1000 MV days / VAP – 2.96/1000 MV days
Resetar et al,[18] 2014	Use of automated electronic surveillance to detect VAE from EMR data	Retrospective review at an academic medical center studying adult medical, surgical, cardiac, cardiothoracic, and neurologic ICU patients	3691 patients with 19,105 MV days. Electronic VAE surveillance is a significant clinical and technical investment. The greatest cost was implementation and testing.	VAC 62 (1.67) / IVAC 35 (0.94) / pVAP 14 (0.38) / prVAP 10 (0.27)
Stevens et al,[8] 2014	Validation of automated algorithm to detect VAE	Retrospective cohort analysis at a tertiary care hospital studying adult medical and surgical ICU patients	426 patients validated by human abstractor. The electronic algorithm had a net sensitivity of 93.5% and specificity of 100% and accuracy of 99.5% compared with the human reviewer. Algorithm took 0.16 s per patient compared with 17–30 min per patient for the human reviewer.	VAC 19 (4.46) / IVAC 3 (0.70) / pVAC 6 (1.41) / prVAC 0 (0)
McMullen et al,[15] 2015	Retrospective evaluation with an automated algorithm compared with prospective clinical evaluation	Retrospective review and prospective cohort study at an academic medical center studying adult medical and surgical patients	1209 patients evaluated with both automated algorithms and prospective clinical evaluation showed good agreement between clinicians using NHSN definitions and automated algorithms to detect VAEs.	VAC 37 (3.06) / IVAC 19 (1.57) / pVAC 8 (0.66) / prVAC 5 (0.41)
Nuckchady et al,[19] 2015	Accuracy of automated surveillance techniques for VAE	Retrospective review at an academic medical center studying MV patients >48 h	192 patients identified by billing records who were analyzed with an automated algorithm to detect VAE per the NHSN definitions. Sensitivity, specificity, PPV, and NPV all >93% and reduced the time spent on detection of VAEs by >90%.	VAC 44 (22.92) / IVAC 22 (11.46) / pVAC 12 (6.25) / prVAC 1 (0.52)

(continued on next page)

Table 2
(continued)

	Emphasis	Design/Population	Summary	VAE Rates n (%)
Zhu et al,[20] 2015	Impact of VAE surveillance on clinical outcomes	Multi-institutional prospective cohort study on adult medical and surgical patients	2356 patients received MV for 8438 d. Compared with patients without VAEs those with VACs had longer ICU LOS (6.2 d), longer duration of MV (7.7 d), and higher hospital mortality rate (50% vs 27.3%). Patients with IVAC had longer duration of MV and increased LOS compared with those with VAC alone.	VAC 94 (3.99) IVAC 31 (1.32) pVAC 16 (0.68) prVAP 0 (0)
Klompas et al,[3] 2011	Validation of a novel surveillance paradigm to identify complications of MV	Retrospective review at an academic medical center studying adult medical and surgical patients	597 patients evaluated showing that VAP and VAC patients had prolonged intubation, ICU LOS, and hospital LOS. VAC was associated with increased mortality, but not VAP.	VAC 137 (23) VAP 56 (9.3)[a]
Prospero et al,[21] 2012	Characterizing VAE rates	Prospective cohort study at an academic medical center studying adult MV patients	127 patients analyzed with a significant increase in days of MV, ICU LOS, and mortality for those patients diagnosed with VAC compared VAC-negative patients. VAP patients showed increased mortality compared with non-VAP patients.	VAC 19 (15) VAP 2 (1.57)[a]
Muscedere et al,[4] 2013	Impact and preventability of VAC	Multi-institutional retrospective study on adult medical, surgical, and trauma ICU patients	1320 patients studied with an agreement between clinically diagnosed VAP and VAC of 0.18, VAP and IVAC and 0.19. Patients with VAC or IVAC had more ventilator days, hospital days, antibiotic days, and higher hospital mortality. Although the agreement between clinically diagnosed VAP and VAC/IVAC is poor these NHSN criteria define potential useful quality indicators.	VAC 139 (10.53) IVAC 65 (4.92) VAP 26 (1.97)[a]
Dessap et al,[22] 2014	Evaluation of depletive fluid management on rates of VAC	Multi-institutional randomized controlled trial of adult ICU patients	304 patients evaluated from the B-type Natriuretic Peptide for the Fluid Management of Weaning (BMC) trial showing that depletive fluid management was associated with significantly reduced rates of VAC and VAP.	VAC 40 (13.16) VAP 17 (5.60)[a]

Abbreviations: MV, mechanical ventilation; NPV, negative predictive value; PPV, positive predictive value; prVAP, probable VAP; pVAP, possible VAP.
[a] VAP diagnosis made using additional clinical findings not specified in the NHSN surveillance guidelines.

VAC. This was similar to the patients diagnosed with prospective VAP. VAE surveillance criteria only detected 32% of prospectively diagnosed VAP.[6]

The Dutch study was the first to demonstrate the complexity involved in applying the surveillance criteria to EMR data. The authors identified that using the minimum Fio_2 and PEEP settings recorded daily in the respiratory flow-rows frequently identified the values recorded during the spontaneous breathing trial (SBT) and were not the true baseline levels of oxygen support. Transitions from the Fio_2 and PEEP during SBT back to the baseline levels when patient completed their trial but were not extubated resulted in an erroneous identification of VAE. The authors realized that establishing a surveillance programs that does not accommodate for similar variations in support will likely result in overestimating patients with respiratory deterioration and can significantly effect VAE reporting.

Two large retrospective studies were published in 2014 that used automated data analysis to review the EMR of patients, based on VAE surveillance criteria, and provide descriptive epidemiology of VAE. The first study reviewed the charts of 20,356 mechanically ventilated patients and found a low overall rate of VAC (5.6%) with low rates of IVAC (2.1%) and even lower rates of possible- (0.7%) and probable-VAP (0.6%). The median day to the onset of VAC was 6, and was more common in medical, surgical, and thoracic units.[7] The other study reviewed the records from 10,998 patients and identified a lower overall rate of VAE (3%). This study focused on the reliability of automated data evaluation compared with manual extraction. The automated method of identifying VAE was more reliable than using a human abstractor. Both studies demonstrated patients with VAE had longer duration of mechanical ventilation, hospital LOS, and mortality compared with patients without VAE, and suggest in their discussions that the future performance improvement initiatives should be targeted on the prevention of VAE rather than VAP.[8]

One of the important selling points of the new VAE surveillance criteria is that it is based on objectivity and eliminates subjective criteria, thus reducing variability and increases validity of data and outcomes. Several recently published studies have argued that the nested definitions of possible-VAP and probable-VAP underperform, because they do not account for radiographic findings common in patients with VAP.[9,10] Lilly and colleagues[9] reviewed the charts of 8408 mechanically ventilated patients and identified a total of 83 incidences of clinical VAP. In this group, 27 patients met criteria for VAC, which means most patients (n = 56) that were diagnosed with clinical pneumonia in this study did not have any evidence of increased oxygen requirements. An even smaller number of patients in this cohort had either qualitative (possible-VAP, n = 18) or quantitative (probable-VAP, n = 4) microbiologic data supporting the VAP diagnosis. Another study by Chang and colleagues[10] demonstrated similar results; only one-third of the 165 episodes of clinically diagnosed VAP would have met VAC criteria with even fewer possible-VAP (12.1%) and probable-VAP (1.2%). Although this study demonstrated that patients with VAC had higher mortality than patients with clinical VAP, it is one of the few that demonstrates patients with possible- and probable-VAP have increased hospital mortality compared with the patients with clinical VAP.

Two studies published in 2015 attempted to better characterize VAC events. One study prospectively evaluated all patients admitted to an ICU and mechanically ventilated 2 or more days using the VAC surveillance criteria during a 12-month period from 2013 to 2014 in large teaching hospital. They identified 67 VACs in 1209 patients. They substantiated the finding that the mortality in patients with VAC was significantly higher than patients without VAC, and characterized the most common causes of VAC: IVAC (50.7%), ARDS (16.4%), pulmonary edema (14.9%), and atelectasis

(9.0%). Probable-VAP and possible-VAP accounted for 44.1% and 17.6% of the IVACs, whereas the remaining cases did not have microbiologic data to delineate the cause. This study also attempted to determine which cases of VAC were preventable. Two investigators reviewed each case and identified cases where medical error contributed to the respiratory complication or whether the VAC was a result of the patient's underlying disease process. They determined that 25 (37.3%) were potentially preventable events.[11] The other study was a large retrospective review of 16 years of data from a French national ICU database (OUTCOMEREA). This study evaluated the data for patients who were intubated a minimum of 5 consecutive days. They identified 3028 patients, 77% of them had VAC and 29% had IVAC. Patients with either possible-VAP or probable-VAP accounted for only 14.5% of VAC events and only 27.6% of the IVAC events. Other significant causes of VAC and IVAC were attributed to other nosocomial infections, failed extubation requiring reintubation, derecruitment during patient transport, and overresuscitation. The authors attribute the high rate of VAC to the study group; patients that require mechanical ventilation a minimum of 5 days are higher risk for adverse events. Both of these studies are important because they begin to characterize the frequent causes of respiratory deterioration in mechanically ventilated patients. By understanding how VACs occur clinicians can identify methods to prevent future events.[12]

These 15 studies discussed in this review are concisely summarized in Table 2. The studies are organized in alphabetical order by first author for each year published. The study design, patient population, and type of institution or database used and a succinct description of the each study findings are included. Additionally, the rates of the different categories of VAE identified for each study are presented. Four studies used the clinical definition of pneumonia to calculate their rate of VAP and are included in the table for comparison. The cumulative number of patients that were diagnosed with VAC, iVAC, possible- and probable-VAP from the studies that evaluated patients using the new NHSN VAE criteria is presented in Fig. 2. The sizes of the circles are proportional to the percentage of patients that meet the different categories of VAE. The total number of patients evaluated using VAE criteria was 33,276. VAC was diagnosed in 1808 (5.4%) of the patients and of these patients 738 (2.2%) met the iVAC criteria. The total number of patients with either possible- or probable-VAP was 458, representing 1.5% of all mechanically ventilated patients.

A recent report compared VAP rates by the NHSN and the Medicare Patient Safety Monitoring System (MPSMS).[13] Between 2006 and 2012, the rate of VAP per 1000 ventilator days reported by NHSN decreased from 3.1 to 0.9 (71% decline) in medical ICUs and 5.2 to 2.0 (62% decline) in surgical ICUs. In contrast, MPSMS VAP rates were stable over time: 10.8% during 2005 to 2006; 7.5% from 2007 to 2009; 10.4% from 2010 to 2011; and 10.2% from 2012 to 2013. This significant dichotomy between VAP rates reported to NHSN and measured in MPSMS is of significant concern, and is likely related to the different VAP definitions used by each group. Future studies must address this concern.

NEW DEFINITION, NEW FOCUS

Although the NHSN surveillance definition of VAE has been shown to be an effective method of characterizing respiratory deterioration, several areas may require further clarification. The current definition requires a 2-day period of stability with subsequent sustained increases in either PEEP or F_{IO_2}. This requirement necessarily eliminates any patient with a primary process that adversely affects the pulmonary status at the time of admission to the ICU. Stoeppel and colleagues[14] demonstrated a large number of surgery patients (77%) were excluded from meeting VAE criteria, because they never had a period of stability before their respiratory deterioration. In these patients, this deterioration was an evolution of their inciting process. Similarly, several studies have discussed that VAE criteria does not account for airway pressure release ventilation or similar modes that do not use PEEP, which results in underreporting the number of patients that would otherwise have VAE.[11,14,15] Potential solutions that would accommodate the use of these modes would be to include increasing requirements of mean airway pressure or potentially using changes in the P/ ratio. Although the goal of tracking VAE may be to track and trend preventable causes of respiratory failure; it is important for the surveillance criteria to have the broadest view including modes that directly affect the mean airway pressure so as to capture all events so that even these patterns of care may be analyzed for possible improvement.

Several studies in this article have criticized the new VAE surveillance definition for underidentifying clinical pneumonia. In these studies, the possible-VAP and probable-VAP identified using the VAE surveillance criteria were compared with clinical pneumonias. Frequently the clinical pneumonias were characterized using a hybrid of the objective probable-/possible-VAP criteria but allows the inclusion of the subjective radiographic criteria of PNU1. The comparisons have demonstrated that using the objective VAE surveillance criteria to identify pneumonia correlates poorly with the diagnosis of clinical pneumonia. Nearly all of the studies demonstrated that ventilator days, ICU LOS, and hospital LOS correlates more closely with VAC compared with clinical VAP. These findings support the decision of NHSN to place emphasis on identifying the broader range of VAEs even at the expense of missing some clinical VAPs.

As the focus of prevention shifts from VAP to VAC, more studies need to be designed to identify methods to reduce the duration of mechanical ventilation and subsequently the opportunity for VAC to occur. The Wake Up and Breathe Collaborative study evaluated how adherence to spontaneous awakening trials (SATs) and SBTs affects the incidence of VAE and VAP.[16] This collaborative was really an education initiative that prospectively tracked the incidence of daily SAT, SBT, and VAEs in participating ICUs over 2 years from 2011 to 2013. Each participating ICU designated a physician, nurse, and respiratory therapist to champion the education and data collection. The results of the study were impressive. Initial compliance with SAT and SBT in most centers was low but through the course of the study rates of daily SAT and SBT significantly improved while the rate of VAC and IVAC per episode of mechanical ventilation was significantly decreased. During the study, the duration of mechanical ventilation decreased by 2.4 days, ICU LOS by 3.0 days, and hospital LOS by 6.3 days. There were no changes in the rate of hospital morality or VAP. Not surprisingly, the rate of self-extubations per episode of mechanical ventilation increased but there was no change in the rate of reintubation within 24 hours. This paper brings to the forefront VAP is not an adequate surrogate for quality.

Dr Klompas, the architect of the new criteria, outlines future efforts directed at minimizing VAE in a recent review.[16] He summarizes several strategies to reduce or prevent VAEs. Intrinsic to the efforts are approaches that minimize the duration of mechanic ventilation and coincide with the Society of Critical Care Medicine's initiative Awakening, Breathing, Coordination, Delirium monitoring/management and Early exercise/mobility bundle. This bundle has been shown to improve patient outcomes by eliminating sedative and narcotic infusions, decreasing delirium, increasing patient participation in SATs and SBTs, and promoting early participation with occupational and physical therapy. All of these efforts, in turn, reduce duration of mechanical ventilation, and translate to decreased incidence of VAE.[16] Other efforts that may play a role in reducing VAE include using lung-protective ventilation and preventing overaggressive fluid or blood product resuscitation. Although there have not been any studies to date demonstrating the effects of these strategies on VAE, each has been shown to mitigate lung injury, which may lead to deterioration of pulmonary function in ventilated patients.

FUTURE DIRECTIONS

The application of NHSN Surveillance Definition of VAE to surgical patients has not been tested. Many of the publications reviewed in this article were performed in mixed populations and so how the criteria apply to surgical patients is unclear. Many surgical patients require mechanical ventilation secondary to another insult or injury and not from a primary pulmonary process as in many of the medicine patients. There is a bimodal distribution of pulmonary dysfunction in surgical patients. Some patients have early progressively worsening respiratory failure as a consequence of their initial injury or process and other patients develop late pulmonary dysfunction as a consequence of pneumonia or aggressive resuscitation secondary to the treatment of their primary event. The VAE criteria do not readily identify the first group because they never have a period of stability, but readily identify the other group. The appropriate resuscitation of a surgical patient with abdominal sepsis or the trauma patient with acute hemorrhage may secondarily exacerbate pulmonary dysfunction. Future studies that investigate VAE in these subsets of patients may help identify new end points for resuscitation that minimize pulmonary dysfunction while providing correction of acidosis and restoration of end-target organ perfusion.

SUMMARY

The new NHSN definition for VAE replaces the previous PNU1 definition of pneumonia. The VAE criteria stratify respiratory compromise of ventilated patient into a tiered system that includes VAC, iVAC, possible-VAP, and probable-VAP. Each classification has defined objective criteria that eliminate the subjectivity of previous PNU1 definition. The implementation of VAE criteria is intended to better characterize and quantitate the broader causes of respiratory deterioration in ventilated patients, and to shift the focus away from VAP as the only relevant ventilator-associated complication. This new definition eliminates radiographic finding as a component of the definition and, as a result, may underestimate the rate of clinical pneumonia. Instead these categories are intended to also capture all of the other noninfectious causes of respiratory compromise in ventilated patients. These objective criteria facilitate the automated collection of data from the EMR and reduce variability in reporting, which allows for easier comparison of data within institutions, between health care systems, and even across international borders. The current definition has been well studied in medicine patients but has not been well vetted in the surgical population. Additionally, these criteria may need to be amended to account for nonconventional modes of ventilation, such as airway pressure release ventilation. Using the new VAE surveillance definition serves as a quality indicator proxy. Adherence to the best practices standards of daily awakening and breathing trials and initiating early mobilization reduces the duration of ventilator dependence and the subsequent incidence of all classifications of VAE.

REFERENCES

1. Van Vught LA, Klowenberg PM, Spitoni C, et al, for the MARS Consortium. Incidence, risk factors, and attributable mortality of secondary infections in the intensive care unit after admission for sepsis. JAMA 2016;315(14):1469–79.

2. Magill SS, Klompas M, Balk R, et al. Developing a new, national approach to surveillance for ventilator-associated events. Am J Crit Care 2013;22(6):469–73.

3. Klompas M, Khan Y, Kleinman K, et al. Multicenter evaluation of a novel surveillance paradigm for complications of mechanical ventilation. PLoS One 2011;6: e18062.

4. Muscedere J, Sinuff T, Heyland DK, et al, on behalf of for the Canadian Critical Care Trials Group. The clinical impact and preventability of ventilator-associated conditions in critically ill patients who are mechanically ventilated. Chest 2013;144(5):1453–60.

5. Hayashi Y, Morisawa K, Klompas M, et al. Towards improved surveillance: the impact of ventilator-associated complications (VAC) on length of stay and antibiotic use in patients in intensive care units. Clin Infect Dis 2012;56(4):471–7.

6. Klouwenberg PM, van Mourik MS, Ong DS, et al. Electronic implementation of a novel surveillance paradigm for ventilator-associated events: feasibility and validation. Am J Respir Crit Care Med 2014;189(8):947–55.

7. Klompas M, Kleinman K, Murphy MV, for the CDC Prevention Epicenters Program. Descriptive epidemiology and attributable morbidity of ventilator-associated events. Infect Control Hosp Epidemiol 2014;35(5):502–10.

8. Stevens JP, Silva G, Gillis J, et al. Automated surveillance for ventilator-associated events. Chest 2014;146(6):1612–8.

9. Lilly CM, Landry KE, Sood RN, et al. Prevalence and test characteristics of national health safety network ventilator-associated events. Crit Care Med 2014; 42(9):2019–28.

10. Chang HC, Chen CM, Kung SC, et al. Differences between novel and conventional surveillance paradigms of ventilator-associated pneumonia. Am J Infect Control 2015;43(2):133–6.

11. Boyer AF, Schoenberg N, Babcock H, et al. A prospective evaluation of ventilator-associated conditions and infection-related ventilator-associated conditions. Chest 2015;147(1):68–81.

12. Boudma L, Sonneville R, Garrouste-Orgeas M, et al. Ventilator-associated events: prevalence, outcome, and relationship with ventilator-associated pneumonia. Crit Care Med 2015;43(9):1798–806.

13. Metersky ML, Wang Y, Klompas M, et al. Trend in ventilator-associated pneumonia rates between 2005 and 2013. JAMA 2016;316(22):2427–9.

14. Stoeppel CM, Eriksson EA, Hawkins K, et al. Applicability of the National Healthcare Safety Network's surveillance definition of ventilator-associated events in the surgical intensive care unit: a 1-year review. J Trauma Acute Care Surg 2014; 77(6):934–7.

15. McMullen KM, Boyer AF, Schoenberg N, et al. Surveillance versus clinical adjudication: differences persist with new ventilator-associated event definition. Am J Infect Control 2015;43(6):589–91.

16. Klompas M, Anderson D, Trick W, et al. The preventability of ventilator-associated events. The CDC prevention epicenters wake up and breathe collaborative. Am J Respir Crit Care Med 2015;191(3):292–301.

17. Lewis SC, Li L, Murphy MV, et al. Risk factors for ventilator-associated events: a case-control multivariable analysis. Crit Care Med 2014;42(8):1839–48.

18. Resetar E, McMullen KM, Russo AJ, et al. Development, implementation and use of electronic surveillance for ventilator-associated events (VAE) in adults. AMIA Annu Symp Proc 2014;2014:1010–7.

19. Nuckchady D, Heckman MG, Diehl NN, et al. Assessment of an automated surveillance system for detection of initial ventilator-associated events. Am J Infect Control 2015;43(10):1119–21.

20. Zhu S, Cai L, Ma C, et al. The clinical impact of ventilator-associated events: a prospective multi-center surveillance study. Infect Control Hosp Epidemiol 2015;36(12):1388–95.

21. Prospero E, Illuminati D, Marigliano A, et al. Learning from Galileo: ventilator-associated pneumonia surveillance. Am J Respir Crit Care Med 2012;186(12):1308–9.

22. Dessap AM, Katsahian S, Roche-Campo F, et al. Ventilator-associated pneumonia during weaning from mechanical ventilation: role of fluid management. Chest 2014;146(1):58–65.

Oxygen Therapeutics and Mechanical Ventilation Advances

Brian Weiss, MD[a], Lewis J. Kaplan, MD, FCCM, FCCP[a,b,c],*

KEYWORDS

- Oxygen • Intensive care unit • Ventilation • Therapeutics

KEY POINTS

- Advances in intensive care unit therapeutics are plentiful and rooted in technological enhancements as well as recognition of patient care priorities.
- A plethora of new devices and modes are available for use to enhance patient safety and support liberation from mechanical ventilation while preserving oxygenation and carbon dioxide clearance.
- Increased penetrance of closed loop systems is one means to reduce care variation in appropriate populations.
- Some therapeutics require additional evidence before routine use, or use only in specific patients.

INTRODUCTION

Recently, intensive care unit (ICU) admissions and use have come under intense scrutiny in large part related to high occupancy, emergency department to ICU admission delays, hospital readmission for sepsis,[1] sepsis and septic shock diagnosis,[2] ICU bed growth relative to specific patient populations,[3] as well as the diagnosis, interventions addressing, and prevention of both the post–intensive care syndrome (PICS)[4] and the persistent inflammation, infection, catabolism, syndrome.[5] Perhaps in part driven by the focused inquiry into each of these areas, several advances in critical care have directly and indirectly affected how critical care is practiced, and the outcomes from that practice.

Disclosures: None.
[a] Perelman School of Medicine, University of Pennsylvania, 51 North 39th Street, MOB 1, Philadelphia, PA 19104, USA; [b] Surgical Critical Care, Corporal Michael J Crescenz VA Medical Center, 3900 Woodland Avenue, Philadelphia, PA 19104, USA; [c] Division of Trauma, Surgical Critical Care and Emergency Surgery, Perelman School of Medicine, University of Pennsylvania, 51 North 39th Street, MOB 1, Philadelphia, PA 19104, USA
* Corresponding author. Division of Trauma, Surgical Critical Care and Emergency Surgery, Perelman School of Medicine, University of Pennsylvania, 51 North 39th Street, MOB 1, Philadelphia, PA 19104.
E-mail addresses: Lewis.Kaplan@uphs.upenn.edu; Lewis.Kaplan@va.gov

Crit Care Clin 33 (2017) 293–310
http://dx.doi.org/10.1016/j.ccc.2016.12.002
0749-0704/17/Published by Elsevier Inc.
criticalcare.theclinics.com

This article reviews key advances in critical care, addressing assessment of long-term outcomes of acute respiratory failure and mechanical ventilation, oxygen (O_2) therapeutics, premature device removal, oxygenation targets, noninvasive ventilation, modes of mechanical ventilation, ventilator weaning mechanisms and approaches, military relevant overlaps, and improvements in integrated ICU design.

OUTCOMES OF MECHANICAL VENTILATION

Understanding the implications of mechanical ventilation helps craft a natural history and target interventions to address undesirable outcomes. Although short-term mechanical ventilation has few negative outcomes associated with it in the confines of a modern ICU in a developed nation, long-term mechanical ventilation has a less salutary impact. A recent systematic review of long-term survival of patients with critical illness managed with long-term mechanical ventilation assessed outcomes at 1 year.[6] Documented mortality was 29% at discharge, and 62% at 1 year; only 19% were discharged home, with half ultimately being successfully liberated from ventilator support. Curiously, US-specific mortalities at hospital discharge (31% [confidence interval (CI), 26%–37%] vs 18% [CI, 14%–24%]) and at 1 year (73% [CI, 67%–78%] v 47% [CI, 29%–65%]) were worse than those documented abroad. Such data are informative because each patient who receives mechanical support is at risk for prolonged support. Recent preliminary data suggest that certain adjunctive modes (such as automatic tube compensation) may help with liberation by helping preserve normal neural conductive pathways, such as those of the dorsal phrenic nerve as evaluated using electrical impedance tomography.[7] Therefore, understanding the impact and outcome from mechanical ventilation is key.

Even more important may be understanding the setting in which mechanical ventilation is applied. A recent Cochrane analysis of automated versus nonautomated weaning found reduced weaning duration (30% shorter duration), use of prolonged mechanical ventilation (>21 days), and tracheostomy use with automated systems, but solely in medical and mixed populations; no benefit was noted in surgical populations.[8] No mortality or length-of-stay benefit was identified. Nonetheless, morbidity plays a significant role in shaping guidelines, protocols, and reporting requirements. It is plausible, and likely, that the blanket application of support techniques to everyone with an overarching diagnosis creates mismatch between the disease process, individual omics (gene, protein, metabolism), and leads to undesired outcomes. To address such potential mismatch, and to embed a precision medicine approach into ICU-relevant inquiry, a governing research agenda has been articulated for acute respiratory distress syndrome (ARDS), asking whether a therapy affords benefit, and, perhaps most importantly, for whom does the benefit accrue.[9] Mechanical ventilation in the ICU often begins via an urgently, emergently, or periprocedurally placed oral endotracheal tube whose management is designed to maintain it for an appropriate period of time while (seemingly paradoxically) also minimizing therapies focused on keeping the tube in place.

Intubation and Premature Removal of Device Events

Urgent or emergent intubation of the critically ill is often accompanied by hypoxemia, especially when performed using a rapid sequence technique such as bag-valve-mask ventilation is omitted to avoid gastric distension, regurgitation, and aspiration. Recognizing that there are a host of conditions whose outcomes may be negatively affected by episodes of hypoxia (eg, traumatic brain injury, stroke, acute myocardial infarction), a method of reducing hypoxemia may be beneficial. A recent trial of apneic oxygenation using 15 L/min high-flow nasal cannula O_2 (HF-NCo_2) compared with no O_2 for intubation of medical ICU patients failed to detect a difference in the lowest arterial O_2 saturation recorded.[10] The trial included only 150 patients, and was limited to medical patients who were intubated by critical care fellows, most importantly introducing a time bias (compared with anesthesiologists) with the mean time from induction to airway control in excess of 2 minutes; mean intubations per fellow was less than 70 over about a 2-year period of training. Also, given the medical patient population, preexisting pulmonary disease is highly prevalent, perhaps reducing oxygenation reserve. Other studies support the use of HF-NCo_2 in preserving oxygenation before intubation in a mixed medical-surgical unit compared with nonrebreather reservoir oxygenation before intubation.[11] One preliminary report in surgical patients supports the use of HF-NCo_2 before extubation to preserve oxygenation as well.[12] Many aspects of care may affect the maintenance of an oral endotracheal tube (OETT), including the competing interests of tube maintenance with sedation minimization, disordered sleep-wake cycles, and the desire to minimize polypharmacy. However, OETTs are occasionally removed before teams desire, with important impacts on care.

Often assumed to be fairly benign and an unavoidable consequence of minimizing mechanical ventilation, sedation, and the use of physical restraints, premature removal of device (PROD) events for endotracheal tubes bears a more ominous import. PROD-OETT occurred in a surgical ICU in 4% (39 of 939 patients) with 5.4% requiring reintubation.[13] Although that percentage is low, patients requiring OETT replacement had a higher likelihood of pulmonary infection, ventilator length of stay (LOS), tracheostomy use, and ICU as well as hospital LOS. A related study of 1775 intubated critically ill patients, using an unplanned extubation group (37 patients) and a control cohort (156 patients) matched for duration of mechanical ventilation identified risk factors for PROD-OETT.[14] Unsurprisingly, and seemingly intuitively, those with mild disease, higher Glasgow Coma Scale score, and more frequent restraint use all positively correlated with PROD-OETT as well as a lower ICU but not hospital mortality; disease severity instead correlated with hospital mortality. Therefore, it seems that successful self-extubation correlates with improved outcome, but failure carries with it undesirable outcomes. It is not clear whether the PROD triggers those outcomes, or whether they would have occurred as part of the index disease process requiring mechanical ventilation. Nonetheless, the support of patients who are either deliberately extubated by the critical care team or engage in self-extubation needs to be well coordinated to support CO_2 clearance as well as oxygenation.

Oxygenation Support

Several evidence-based O_2 support advances have emerged in the last decade (Box 1). In addition to mechanical processes such as head of bed elevation to reduce visceral weight and volume impedance of diaphragm excursion, supplemental, and generally humidified, O_2 is a staple. Most recently, oxygenation support using high-flow nasal cannula O_2 has been examined because it is increasingly commonly used both before and after liberation from mechanical ventilation. It is important to realize that the genesis of HF-NCo_2 systems lies in the entrainment of high volumes of low O_2 content room air when using traditional NCo_2 flows of 2 to 6 L/min. Moreover, because of the need for humidification, unheated bubble humidifiers are most commonly used but suffer from proportionate decreases in humidification efficacy as O_2 flows increase, especially in a room air temperature system. Realizing the care gap for patients who may not require noninvasive ventilation or reintubation,

---

Box 1
Evidence and opinion regarding oxygenation management advances in the intensive care unit

Clinical challenge: preintubation oxygenation support

Established evidence-based practice
1. HF-NCo$_2$ for hypoxemic rescue and support
2. Noninvasive ventilation for combined hypoxemic and hypercarbic failure

Author's opinion (more research required)
1. HF-NCo$_2$ for combined hypoxemic and hypercarbic failure in specific patient populations
2. Peri-intubation oxygenation maintenance including apneic oxygenation

Clinical challenge: postextubation oxygenation support

Established evidence-based practice
1. HF-NCo$_2$ for oxygenation support
2. Noninvasive ventilation for combined hypoxemic and hypercarbic failure

Author's opinion (more research required)
1. HF-NCo$_2$ for avoidance of reintubation

Clinical challenge: determining safe lower limits for oxygenation maintenance

Established evidence-based practice
1. Out of hospital O$_2$ tolerance limits in specific populations

Author's opinion (more research required)
1. Outcomes with reduced oxygenation targets in the critically ill

Clinical challenge: oxygenation support that improves ICU metrics

Established evidence-based practice
1. Noninvasive ventilation (NIV) as a rescue mode for hypoxemic failure, weaning facilitation, decreased ventilator-induced infection, decreased tracheostomy use, and decreased ICU LOS
2. Proportional Assist Ventilation (PAV) or neurally adjusted ventilatory assist (NAVA) support to improve patient comfort and improve patient-ventilator synchrony

Author's opinion (more research required)
1. Impact of HF-NCo$_2$ on outcomes
2. NIV to avoid reintubation after abdominal surgery
3. Optimal target population for PAV or NAVA
4. Impact of PAV or NAVA on sleep quality

Clinical challenge: improving extubation success

Established evidence-based practice
1. Spontaneous breathing trials to screen for liberation readiness
2. Weaning protocols to reduce ventilator LOS

Author's opinion (more research required)
1. Role of serum biomarkers such as β-natriuretic peptide in determining postextubation failure
2. Utility of derived indices such as the Timed Inspiratory Index in improving liberation success
3. Role and impact of ultrasonography as an evaluation tool for liberation appropriateness

Clinical challenge: enhancing ICU efficiency and integration

Established evidence-based practice
1. Planning for ICU design for technology integration and housing
2. Closed loop mechanical ventilation systems reduce the need for human input in management

Author's opinion (more research required)
1. Outcomes with closed loop mechanical ventilation for complex conditions

Clinical challenge: maintenance of diaphragm function or restoration of function after spinal cord injury (SCI)

Established evidence-based practice
1. Diaphragm exercise helps retard ventilator-induced diaphragm dysfunction
2. Phrenic nerve stimulation can improve diaphragm function in SCI

Author's opinion (more research required)
1. Optimal mode for preservation of diaphragm functional integrity
2. Outcomes using alternative functional electrical stimulation techniques to restore diaphragm function after SCI

---

but for whom oxygenation needs were inadequately supported by traditional NCO_2 systems, HF-NCO_2 systems were developed. Such systems outperform traditional NCO_2 delivery rates by an order of magnitude (60 L/min instead of 6 L/min).

The typical system comprises a heater humidifier coupled with a flow meter, an air-O_2 blending device, and a high flow rate–capable delivery tubing attachment (nasal prongs).[15] The rapid flow of heated humidified gas minimizes room air entrainment for nose breathers. Mouth breathers may entrain some gas, but substantially less so than with traditional NCO_2 flow rates. The rapid delivery of heated and humidified gas using HF-NCO_2 devices also aids in displacement of exhaled gas in the hypopharynx, further increasing the O_2 content of the next spontaneous breath. Furthermore, enriched O_2 priming of the pharynx and conducting upper airways effectively reduces dead space and reduces the patient's minute ventilation need; reduced work of breathing is an important corollary.

Additional device design advantages include avoiding a tight-fitting (often ill-fitting) nasal cannula or facemask, support of expectoration, and airway pressurization alveolar recruitment in a fashion akin to that of positive end-expiratory pressure (PEEP). One report documents an increase in measured hypopharynx pressure by 1 cm H_2O pressure for each 10 L/min flow increment as a reasonable metric and was accompanied by a lower respiratory rate and increased lung volumes.[16] The study was undertaken in post–cardiac surgical patients in whom extravascular lung water may be both more problematic as a result of cardiopulmonary bypass and more readily influenced by increased endotracheal pressure than in other clinical conditions, such as sepsis. Nonetheless, HF-NCO_2 seems to be a key tool competing for the same space occupied by noninvasive ventilation for those with oxygenation failure from a readily reversible cause but preserved CO_2 clearance and a patent airway. A variety of algorithms have been developed to guide the use of this specialized therapy. Underpinning the algorithms is the understanding that this therapy is generally not appropriate for general wards, but is instead most appropriately used in an intermediate-intensity or high-intensity care setting. Future applications that might be appropriate for all settings may include coupling therapeutic agent delivery via aerosolization using a high-flow setup with or without enriched O_2. Attractive targets for development include antibacterial and antiviral agents, but can readily include hypertonic saline for secretion clearance, as well as biofilm mitigation agents; these applications have yet to be developed.

Oxygenation Targets

Because O_2 saturation is so readily tracked using fixed, portable, as well as fingertip devices, a target safety range for general practice permeates alarm limits on ICU-relevant devices. Although there is a variety of data addressing the potential for O_2 toxicity on type II pneumocytes in particular, the safety of lower thresholds for oxygenation is less well studied. If a lower SpO_2 value were acceptable then the inspired O_2 concentration could, in theory, be decreased. Although there would be an impact on the Pao_2/fraction of inspired O_2 (Fio_2) ratio calculation for patients with ARDS, there might be no clinically relevant impact on outcome. This notion is buttressed by noting that military submarines generally operate with less than 21% Fio_2 (albeit for generally young and healthy sailors) without untoward effects. Additional support comes from the advanced chronic obstructive pulmonary disease (COPD) population whose baseline Spo_2 is less than 90% without a deleterious impact on cognition. These observations have led to increasing numbers of trials of conservative versus liberal O_2 targets in the critically ill requiring mechanical ventilation. One trial compared patients with mechanical ventilation for greater than 24 hours who were randomized to O_2 management targeting Spo_2 88% to 92% versus SpO_2 greater than or equal to 96%.[17] No relevant outcome differences were noted with regard to time spent with Sao_2 less than 88%, ICU LOS, or ICU or 90-day mortality. Note that this was a feasibility study with only 103 patients but its results justify a more robust investigation. A more recent trial used a before-and-after design spanning 2011 to 2014 in the Netherlands. A period of training was then followed by a computer decision-support system that was deployed to guide clinician order entry and target determination.[18] Hypoxic episodes were unchanged but hyperoxia (defined as Pao_2>85 torr and Sao_2>95%) was significantly reduced. If this approach is proved safe, significant changes are implied for weaning protocols, O_2 tolerances in ICUs, as well as potential revisions of ARDS definitions, and rapid response system triggers for O_2-related interventions.[19] Increasingly commonly, patients with hypoxemic respiratory failure are being managed with noninvasive ventilation on general wards as they transition to the ICU.

Noninvasive Ventilation

Because noninvasive ventilation (NIV) is not new, and detailed discussions of the mechanics, principles, and standard uses are available elsewhere, this article focuses on novel uses of the technique. Although NIV is commonly used as a rescue mode for hypoxemic as well as hypercarbic acute respiratory failure, as well as to help prevent reintubation in patients with a successful spontaneous breathing trial (SBT) but marginal mechanics after extubation (especially those with COPD or pulmonary edema), the use of NIV to facilitate weaning is uncommon. In this approach, patients who did poorly on an SBT, but for whom control of the primary process leading to intubation has been controlled, may benefit from extubation directly to an NIV modality with weaning of the NIV mode as the road to liberation from mechanical ventilation.[20] Both preliminary studies and randomized controlled trials support this approach with generally positive results in terms of time on mechanical ventilation, ICU LOS, ventilator-related infection, tracheostomy use, and survival (most profound impact in patients with underlying COPD).[21]

Although most trials of NIV include medical patients, one recent trial focused on the use of NIV to reduce tracheal reintubation in patients who have undergone abdominal surgery.[22] This multicenter trial evaluated patients randomized to NIV (n = 148) versus standard O_2 therapy (n = 145) for hypoxemic acute respiratory failure. The investigators noted reduced rates of reintubation in the NIV-supported group (33.1% vs 45.5%) within 7 days of randomization compared with those receiving standard O_2 therapy. NIV was associated with more ventilator-free days as well as reduced health care–associated infections. No intergroup differences were noted with regard to gas exchange or mortality at 90 days. The impact on infection is important and likely represents a salutary impact on pulmonary infection in particular (NIV pneumonia, 14.6% vs O_2 therapy pneumonia, 29.7%; P = .005). Therefore, there seems to be an important umbrella effect associated with NIV in patients with periprocedural hypoxemic acute respiratory failure, even after abdominal surgery. These data are even more important in light of the recent Cochrane Review that assessed the use of NIV after upper abdominal surgery, noting that although the approaches seemed to be safe, the data were of low or very low quality.[23]

Heated and Humidified High-flow Nasal Cannula

High-flow nasal cannula (HFNC) has emerged as a useful therapy in patients with respiratory failure, improving both oxygenation and patient comfort (Fig. 1).[24]

The FLORALI multicenter randomized trial enrolled 310 patients with acute hypoxemic respiratory failure without hypercapnia and Pao_2/Fio_2 ratio less than or equal to 300 mm Hg to HFNC, standard O_2 therapy delivered through a face mask, or NIV. No difference in the primary outcome measure of intubation rate was identified (38% HFNC, 47% standard O_2, 50% NIV, $P = .18$). However, in a post hoc adjusted analysis that included the 238 patients with severe initial hypoxemia ($Pao_2/Fio_2 \leq 200$ mm Hg), the intubation rate was significantly lower among patients who received HFNC than among the other 2 groups ($P = .009$). In the entire cohort, the number of ventilator-free days was significantly higher with HFNC (24 ± 8 days, vs 22 ± 10 days in the standard O_2 group and 19 ± 12 days in the NIV group; $P = .02$ for all comparisons). The hazard ratio for death at 90 days was 2.01 (95% CI, 1.01–3.99) with standard O_2 versus HFNC ($P = .046$) and 2.50 (95% CI, 1.31–4.78) with NIV versus HFNC ($P = .006$). Compared with the other strategies, HFNC was associated with less respiratory discomfort and a reduction in the severity of dyspnea, as measured by validated assessments of patient comfort.[25]

The accompanying editorial recommended "Although additional trials are needed, HFNC should be used for the treatment of patients without hypercapnia and with

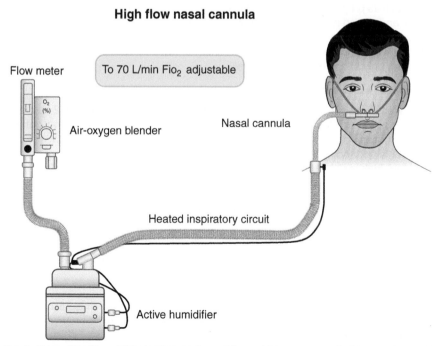

High flow nasal cannula

Flow meter

To 70 L/min Fio_2 adjustable

O_2 (%)

Air-oxygen blender

Nasal cannula

Heated inspiratory circuit

Active humidifier

Fig. 1. Heated and humidified HFNC. (*Adapted from* Nishimura M. High-flow nasal cannula oxygen therapy in adults. J Intensive Care 2015;3(1):15.)

acute severe hypoxemic respiratory failure in the emergency department, the ICU and hospital settings in which appropriate monitoring is available."[26]

A multicenter randomized noninferiority trial (BiPOP [Bilevel Positive Airway Pressure versus OPTIFLOW in Hypoxemic Patients After Cardiothroacic Surgery] Study) enrolled 830 patients after cardiothoracic surgery randomized to HFNC or NIV. The primary outcome (treatment failure defined as reintubation, switch to other study treatment, or premature treatment discontinuation) was not different (21.0% HFNC vs 21.9% NIV) with no differences in ICU mortality (6.8% HFNC vs 5.5% NIV).[27]

Since the publication of these trials, HFNC is increasingly being used. It is important to know the specifics regarding proper use of HFNC. The FLORALI trial used a gas flow rate of 50 L/min and an Fio_2 of 1.0 at initiation (Optiflow, Fisher and Paykel Healthcare). The fraction of O_2 in the gas flowing in the system was subsequently adjusted to maintain an Spo_2 of 92% or more. HFNC was applied for at least 2 calendar days; it could then be stopped and the patient switched to standard O_2 therapy. The high flow rates generate low levels of positive pressure in the upper airways, and the Fio_2 can be adjusted by changing the fraction of O_2 in the driving gas. The high flow rates may also decrease physiologic dead space by flushing expired carbon dioxide from the upper airway, a process that potentially explains the observed decrease in the work of breathing.

When HFNC or NIV fails to manage either hypoxic or hypercarbic (or both) acute respiratory failure, invasive mechanical ventilation is warranted.

INVASIVE MECHANICAL VENTILATION ADVANCES

Standard cyclic volume controlled ventilation as well as spontaneous breathing modes such as airway pressure release ventilation have been well reviewed elsewhere. Instead, this article focuses on novel approaches to invasive mechanical ventilation, such as proportional assist ventilation (PAV), neurally activated ventilator assist (NAVA), and closed loop mechanical ventilation. Assisted ventilation techniques seem focused on reducing patient-ventilator asynchrony, and seem poised to become preferred modes for likely longer-term weaning of patients, but offer advantages to those with only short-term needs as well.[28]

Proportional Assist Ventilation

PAV is a technique for mechanical ventilation that was described more than 2 decades ago by Younes.[29] PAV is designed to be applied to an actively breathing patient because it uses inspiratory flow to trigger the amount of support provided by the device; PAV is not appropriate for those requiring continuous heavy sedation or neuromuscular blockade. A byproduct of having the device respond to patient effort on a breath-by-breath basis is improved comfort and patient-ventilator synchrony, allowing amplification of the patient's own effort while allowing the patient to control the breathing pattern. The ability to rapidly and repeatedly measure pulmonary resistance and elastance underpins this mode's ability to adjust the proportion of the respiratory effort that is patient assisted compared with machine assisted, hence the designation of PAV. This relationship is described by the following equation of motion:

$$P_{musc} + P_{aw} = (flow \times R) + (V \times E) \text{ where}$$

P_{musc} = patient-generated airway pressure (derived from muscular effort); P_{aw} = machine-generated airway pressure; R = ventilator circuit resistant; V = volume; E = lung elastic recoil

Both flow and volume assistance adjustments are available on PAV-capable devices. The ability to rapidly determine R and E have defeated the major clinician impediment that previously hampered PAV deployment: the complex nature of making determinations and therefore ventilator adjustments. With PAV, flow, pressure, and the volume delivered and determined by patient effort to achieve a predetermined target of assistance[30] (Fig. 2). A variety of approaches have been described for how to initiate and manage PAV.[30] PAV has been associated with improved patient comfort, patient-ventilator synchrony,[31] as well as improved sleep quality.[32] Alternative studies support synchrony but do not link it with improved sleep quality.[33] It is likely that the differences between studies lies with patient selection (selected only from spontaneous effort vs targeting those with dyssynchrony), study design (only 1 mode vs switching back and forth between modes), and perhaps changes in sedative administration patterns over the past decade.

With technological advances in device application easing the use by bedside clinicians, rather than simply a percentage effort, clinicians may also determine a predefined range of respiratory effort that either enables or extinguishes support. One recent multicenter ICU study used PAV with load-adjustable gain factors to target a specific level of respiratory effort, in this case a peak respiratory muscle pressure between 5 and 10 cm H_2O.[34] Although the study was small (53 patients), it provided proof of concept for the 32 of 34 who tolerated it to liberation; 18 reverted to volume-cycled ventilation for continuous sedation and only 1 patient did not tolerate PAV. Issues surrounding the use of PAV in the ICU center not on whether the mode is feasible but whether it is ideal, especially because it is insensitive to the respiratory effort needed to overcome auto-PEEP in patients such as those with COPD; underestimation of machine assistance is the consequence. Moreover, the target patient population for the mode may be different from the population most commonly studied; those on a slow weaning program after critical illness recovery may benefit most, whereas those who can be rapidly extubated are often investigated.[35]

To that point, recent data were obtained in a mixed medical-surgical population of patients who received mechanical ventilation for 36 hours and were randomized to

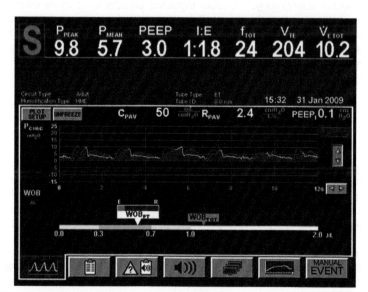

Fig. 2. PAV. (*Courtesy of* Medtronic, Proportional Assist and PAV are registered trademarks of The University of Manitoba, Canada; with permission.)

weaning using PAV versus pressure-support ventilation (PSV); weaning occurred by protocol in an unblended fashion.[36] The time from randomization to extubation was similar between groups, but ICU LOS (but not hospital LOS or mortality) was longer in the PSV group. Given the small number of subjects, the study was underpowered to assess clinical outcomes and instead serves as another feasibility study, suggesting that the appropriate target population has yet to be discovered for this mode. A related trial compared PAV with PSV and T tube for use as an SBT and noted no differences in clinically important outcomes such as reintubation, time to liberation from mechanical ventilation, or LOS.[37] The investigators concluded that PAV could instead serve as an alternative for the now well-ingrained SBT, for which PSV currently remains dominant.

A different approach was undertaken in a laboratory using test lungs and assessing the ability of PAV to provide resistive as well as elastic unloading.[38] Low and high compliance models were used to mimic infant respiratory distress syndrome compared with bronchopulmonary dysplasia. This study noted that elastic unloading in a low-compliance setting substantially reduced work of breathing; similar benefits were not noted for resistive unloading, suggesting that PAV would not be appropriate for that patient population. Although a pediatric-focused study, the methodology may be useful to better define appropriate adult patients for this mode. A related mode also uses a patient-derived variable to adjust machine effort NAVA.

Neurally Adjusted Ventilatory Assist

NAVA is a unique mode that adjusts the proportion of machine assistance to the electrical activity of the diaphragm (EAdi) and as such requires an esophageal catheter to record this variable (Fig. 3).[39] EAdi is taken to be the summed output of neural impulses transmitted to the diaphragm and is represented as a cyclic waveform of electrical energy. Similar to PAV, NAVA also improves patient-ventilator synchrony. In a sophisticated and elegant 3-way comparison of NAVA, PAV, and PSV, both PAV and NAVA avoided overdistension, improved neuromechanical coupling, restored variability in respiratory dynamics as assessed by breathing pattern, and reduced patient-ventilator asynchrony.[40] Double triggered breaths were more common with NAVA than with the other 2 modes. This study did not assess clinical outcomes because the study group was small (16 patients). Similar beneficial effects on tidal volume variability were noted for PAV and NAVA compared with PSV in an equally small study comparing the 3 modes.[41]

Data derived from the esophageal catheter have driven the incorporation of a new variable, neuroventilatory efficiency (NVE), into clinical parlance. NVE is defined as the ratio of tidal volume to EAdi (V_T/EAdi) and is purported to reflect the ability of the diaphragm to create inspiratory volume along a transpulmonary pressure gradient. Presumably, as patients successfully wean from mechanical support, NVE should also increase. The corollary is that decreases in NVE may be deleterious to the weaning process and ultimately liberation from ventilator support. One study explored the impact on NAVA as opposed to PSV on NVE during weaning.[42] Changing from NAVA to a PSV-driven SBT led to decreased NVE in both successful (−38%) and unsuccessful (−56%) SBTs compared with their NAVA NVE baseline. Furthermore, as NAVA decreased so too did NVE, corresponding with significant increases in EAdi and V_T; importantly, the NVE was then unchanged during SBT. These data suggest that NVE may be a useful variable in tracking the weaning progress. However, the major impediment seems to be the need for an esophageal monitoring catheter to determine EAdi, as well as an individual to interpret the data. Closed loop systems may be able to bridge the gap between data acquisition and decision determination to spur action.

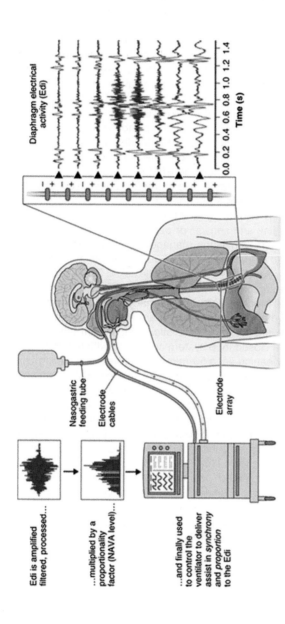

Fig. 3. NAVA ventilation. (*From* Brander L, Slutsky AS. Invasive mechanical ventilation. In: Spiro SG, Silvestri GA, Agusti A, editors. Clinical respiratory medicine. 4th edition. Philadelphia: Elsevier, Inc.; 2012; with permission.)

Closed Loop Mechanical Ventilation

Most commonly, mechanical ventilation prescriptive changes rest with a clinician. Many systems have evolved protocols (paper or electronic) that are to be followed, including ones that empower respiratory therapist independence with SBTs as a mechanism to support weaning assessment and progress toward liberation from mechanical ventilation. However, decisions regarding actionable data are generally routed back through a supervising clinician, creating an inherent time lag between data acquisition and action. Moreover, such protocols are not explicit and support interclinician variability in which the same data may lead to a different action.

In contrast, closed loop systems seek to eliminate the time delay by integrating patient information with ventilator data in a continuous fashion using predefined algorithms that are enacted under the supervision of a caregiver, but not at the discretion of the caregiver.[43] In this way, the protocols are explicit and reduce variability in decision making. Such a system is fundamentally different from computer decision-support tools commonly found in electronic health records because those tools still rely on the end user to decide what to do (by definition, an open system). Closed loop systems are already in use in the 2 modes discussed earlier (PAV and NAVA) using explicit protocols embedded in the ventilator programming. It is easy to envision closed loop O_2 management, or minute ventilation linked to $Paco_2$ with an indwelling arterial line and sensor, or perhaps using end-tidal CO_2 as was done for the negative pressure ventilation management of patients with polio more than 50 years ago.[44] Closed loop control of Fio_2 has been implemented after injury in a militarily relevant fashion as well as a civilian module called $CLiO_2$ from CareFusion (Yorba Linda, CA).[45] Two manufacturers offer a closed loop system on their devices: Smart-Care/PS from Drager Medical (Lubeck, Germany), and IntelliVent-ASV from Hamilton.[46] Both supportive and contrary studies are available spanning the last 10 years of investigation, including those with statistically significant but clinically insignificant differences between a closed loop system compared with respiratory therapy–based and protocol-driven weaning (ie, a 50-minute difference in weaning time favoring the respiratory therapy).[47] A recent Cochrane Review noted that automated systems reduced ventilation duration and ICU LOS as well as prolonged mechanical ventilation and tracheostomy use.[48] Even in patients with ARDS, closed loop system–based ventilation was assessed to be safe and to require fewer episodes of clinician input over a 48-hour period, perhaps supporting less clinician work, whereas the number of automated adjustments far outstripped the number of manual ventilator prescription adjustments (379 [range, 274–493] vs 17 [range, 10–27]).[49] It is perhaps the extreme number of automated adjustments that is most significant, raising the concern that there are opportunities for improvement on which bedside clinicians do not capitalize. The alternative, and intuitively attractive, view is that although many adjustments may be made, it is unclear whether all of them should be undertaken, especially because current weaning processes show reasonable success.

Weaning from Mechanical Ventilation

This process is well chronicled in many articles, chapters, and Web sites hailing the benefits of weaning protocols, sedation minimization, and early mobilization, leading instead to a focus on new additions to the weaning process. Recognizing that reductions in endoalveolar pressure during weaning may shift the pressure gradient toward fluid migration into the alveoli, it would be useful to be able to identify that event as the reason for weaning failure, as opposed to those related to infection, fatigue, and the like. In a trial of 21 patients who failed an initial SBT, and who were monitored using a pulmonary artery (PA) catheter, pressures, extravascular lung water, and plasma β-natriuretic peptide (BNP) level were measured along with plasma protein concentration and hemoglobin level during a second 60-minute T-tube trial.[50] For those with weaning-induced pulmonary edema (PA occlusion pressure >18 mm Hg), plasma protein, hemoglobin, and BNP levels were all increased. An increase in extravascular lung water of 14% (when indexed for body weight) correlated with weaning-induced pulmonary edema with a sensitivity of 67% and a specificity of 100%. Because few patients are monitored using a PA catheter at present, substituting changes in plasma protein, hemoglobin, and BNP concentrations seems to be potentially useful but would require planned resampling; an event that is unlikely to be cost-effective as a uniform event, but one that might be appropriate after an initially failed SBT.

Because SBTs are not universally predictive of weaning success, a search for an alternative index that may have greater fidelity would have utility. One such index is termed the timed inspiratory effort (TIE), whose derivation is based on the maximal inspiratory pressure (MIP) and the occlusion time required to achieve that pressure.[51] A study of 103 patients compared the TIE, the integrative weaning index (IWI), the Rapid Shallow Breathing Index (RSBI), as well as MIP and P0.1 indices and derivatives thereof for a total of 7 indices. Of all, the TIE generated the largest area under the receiver operating curve (0.9; RSBI area under the curve, = 0.8), and the TIE, IWI, and RSBI performed the best of the 7 indices assessed. Although the TIE may not be universally deployed, it does highlight that there are opportunities for further improvement in predicting liberation success.

One such opportunity may leverage the increased penetrance of ultrasonography in the ICU during the weaning process as well. Weaning readiness, in a fashion similar to weaning failure, is related to the interplay of both cardiac and pulmonary function leavened with renal competency, especially with regard to fluid balance. A recent review has parsed the potential contributions of ultrasonography with regard to weaning into 4 interwoven domains: (1) interrogation of cardiac function, (2) pulmonary function, (3) diaphragm function, and (4) presence of pleural fluid.[52] Included are indices that correspond with the likelihood of failing an SBT for each domain that is assessed. Note that not all of the indices are readily measured by typical intensivists, such as mitral diastolic inflow or thickening fraction of the diaphragm, requiring a dedicated ultrasonography evaluation that in many institutions might require 2 different operators; 1 from cardiology and 1 from radiology. Lung ultrasonography scoring focusing on the detection of aeration loss[53] as well as pleural effusion presence is more generally within the scope of practice for those using ultrasonography in the ICU. If clinicians were to identify correctable issues within each of the assessed domains, they might repair those before initiating an SBT, and thereby increase the likelihood of success when the SBT was undertaken. One specific instance of detected dysfunction is unable to be readily repaired without special intervention: diaphragmatic paralysis after spinal cord injury.

Diaphragm Paralysis and Dysfunction

Patients with high spinal cord injury may be committed to lifelong ventilator support because of diaphragm failure, whereas most others regain sufficient function to live without, or with only intermittent, support. Functional electrical stimulation describes the process of applying electrical stimulation in a pulsed fashion to a motor nerve, leading to induced muscular contraction. Such a technique has been applied to leg muscle groups of a small set of critically ill patients who then weaned at a faster rate than was anticipated.[54] When this technique is applied to the abdominal wall it is called abdominal functional electrical stimulation (AFES). In a small pilot study of

10 ventilator-dependent tetraplegic patients, AFES applied on a protocol led to improved VT (tidal volume) and VC (vital capacity) on and off stimulation as well as more rapid weaning compared with matched controls.[55] Previous attempts at diaphragm stimulation used individual phrenic nerve stimulation, as opposed to abdominal wall stimulation. Others investigators have more recently engaged in diaphragm stimulation using an intramuscular technique. This approach has been better studied than AFES and reports a success rate for liberation from mechanical ventilation of 40% to 72%, with earlier implantation seeming to increase liberation success.[56] These data suggest that diaphragm recruitment is feasible and may not only be a reasonable approach to diaphragm denervation from cervical injury but may also be anticipated to affect ventilator-induced diaphragm injury (VIDI).

VIDI may occur with as little as 1 day of mechanical support, is in part related to oxidative stress, and has been reviewed extensively.[57] Given that there is an association between oxidative stress and circulating angiotensin II (AT-II) levels in limb muscles that have undergone atrophy, it is plausible that blocking the generation or activity of AT-II would be protective against oxidative stress and diaphragm muscle atrophy. In a porcine model, angiotensin-converting enzyme inhibition did prevent the increase in AT-II level as predicted but failed to protect against diaphragm atrophy.[58] In contrast, an AT-II type 1 receptor antagonist reduced but did not abrogate oxidative stress and diaphragm weakness. These data may have implications for blood pressure control approaches for patients requiring mechanical ventilation if the preclinical data are proved in the clinical arena. The importance of these data lies in their cellular level approach to an organ-based issue.

Military Relevant Advances

Death from hemorrhage is a surrogate for O_2 delivery failure. In the quest for extending the envelope from which injured combatants who present in extremis are able to be salvaged, suspended animation techniques are central. One additional novel approach that has been articulated to support circulation and O_2 delivery is the use of an oxygenated micellar colloid. In a perimortem murine model of exsanguinating hemorrhage, oxygenated 20% intralipid was compared with lactated Ringer and albumin with efficacy determined for intravenous compared with intra-arterial infusion.[59] In addition, the value of infusion after apparent clinical death was assessed. Delayed resuscitation after clinical death with oxygenated 20% intralipid restored breathing and blood pressure and performed best when infused via the intra-arterial route. This approach to resuscitation offers promise for patients who would otherwise seem to be unsalvageable, including perhaps those with perioperative or periprocedural exsanguinating hemorrhage who require massive transfusion for rescue.

Intensive Care Unit Design

Advances in ICU design have been driven by the desire to manage environmental stimuli (or the lack thereof; especially natural light), incorporate family members into the space, accommodate more care devices, enable adaptive technology (including advanced informatics), as well as to incorporate education and administration into the space designed for care. A detailed breakdown of each aspect of the ICU from new design to renovation addressing patient room, central areas, and universal support services has been articulated.[60] It is essential to plan for where to house and deploy both invasive and noninvasive ventilator support devices, especially as the ICU grows in size. Many ICUs cohort respiratory therapy devices and supplies in a single location for ease of stocking and location, and use electronic tags to aid in equipment tracking and recovery. As the ICU footprint expands, a single location may be insufficient for rapid acquisition in case of emergency, and the new design or renovation should take these important considerations into account before plan finalization. Many designs may be successful, and ICU design may best parallel the move toward precision medicine in which 1 design fits no-one well, and individual customization is a necessity and no longer a luxury.

SUMMARY

Advances in ICU therapeutics are plentiful and rooted in technological enhancements as well as recognition of patient care priorities. A plethora of new devices and modes are available for use to enhance patient safety and support liberation from mechanical ventilation while preserving oxygenation and carbon dioxide clearance. Increased penetrance of closed loop systems is one means to reduce care variation in appropriate populations. Some therapeutics require additional evidence before routine use, or use only in specific patients. Regardless of which support devices or therapeutics are used by the bedside clinician, the intelligent design of the ICU space needs to be able to integrate the footprint of that device as well as the data streaming from it into a coherent whole that supports patient, family, and caregivers alike.

REFERENCES

1. Sun A, Netzer G, Small DS, et al. Association between index hospitalization and hospital readmission in sepsis survivors. Crit Care Med 2016;44(3):478–87.
2. Singer M, Deutschman CS, Seymour CW, et al. The Third International Consensus definitions for sepsis and septic shock (Sepsis-3). JAMA 2016;315(8):801–10.
3. Wallace DJ, Angus DC, Seymour CW, et al. Critical care bed growth in the United States. A comparison of regional and national trends. Am J Respir Crit Care Med 2015;191(4):410–6.
4. Harvey MA, Davidson JE. Postintensive care syndrome: right care, right now... and later. Crit Care Med 2016;44(2):381–5.
5. Vanzant EL, Lopez CM, Ozrazgat-Baslanti T, et al. Persistent inflammation, immunosuppression and catabolism syndrome after severe blunt trauma. J Trauma Acute Care Surg 2014;76(1):21–9.
6. Damuth E, Mitchell JA, Bartock JL, et al. Long-term survival of critically ill patients treated with prolonged mechanical ventilation: a systematic review and meta-analysis. Lancet Respir Med 2015;3(7):544–53.
7. Chang MY, Chang HT. Lung volume distribution in prolonged mechanical ventilation patients from assist control mode to spontaneous trial mode of automatic tube compensation in electrical impedance tomography. Intensive Care Med Exp 2015;3(Suppl 1):A666.
8. Rose L, Schultz MJ, Cardwell CR, et al. Automated versus non-automated weaning for reducing the duration of mechanical ventilation for critically ill adults and children (review). Cochrane Database Syst Rev 2014;(6):CD009235.
9. Beitler JR, Goligher EC, Schmidt M, et al. Personalized medicine for ARDS: the 2035 research agenda. Intensive Care Med 2016;42:756–67.
10. Semler MW, Janz DR, Lentz RJ, et al. Randomized trial of apneic oxygenation during endotracheal intubation of the critically ill. Am J Respir Crit Care Med 2016;193(3):273–80.
11. Miguel-Montanes R, Hajage D, Messike J, et al. Use of high-flow nasal cannula oxygen therapy to prevent desaturation during tracheal intubation of intensive care patients with mild-to-moderate hypoxemia. Crit Care Med 2015;43:574–83.

12. Ishii K, Morimatsu H, Ono K, et al. Early high flow nasal cannula before extubation can have predictable oxygenation. Crit Care Med 2015;43(12):189–90.

13. Fontenot AM, Malizia RA, Chopko MS, et al. Revisiting endotracheal self-extubation in the surgical and trauma intensive care unit: are they all fine? J Crit Care 2015;30:1222–6.

14. Chuang M-L, Lee C-Y, Huang S-F, et al. Revisiting unplanned endotracheal extubation and disease severity in intensive care units. PLoS One 2015;10(10): e0139864.

15. Levy SD, Allandina JW, Hibbert KA, et al. High-flow oxygen therapy and other inhaled therapies in intensive care units. Lancet Respir Med 2016;4:407–18.

16. Corley A, Caruana LR, Barnett AG, et al. Oxygen delivery through high-flow nasal cannulae increase end-expiratory lung volume and reduce respiratory rate in post-cardiac surgical patients. Br J Anaesth 2011;107:998–1004.

17. Panwar R, Hardie M, Bellomo R, et al. Conservative versus liberal oxygenation targets for mechanically ventilated patients. Am J Respir Crit Care Med 2016; 193(1):43–51.

18. Helmerhorst HJ, Schultz MJ, van der Voort PH, et al. Effectiveness and clinical outcomes of a two-step implementation of conservative oxygenation targets in critically ill patients: a before and after trial. Crit Care Med 2016;44(3):554–63.

19. Aneman A, Frost SA, Parr MJ, et al. Characteristics and outcomes of patients admitted to ICU following activation of the Medical Emergency Response Team: impact of introducing a two-tier response system. Crit Care Med 2015; 43(4):765–73.

20. Epstein SK. Use of noninvasive ventilation to facilitate weaning from mechanical ventilation. In: Esquinas AM, editor. Noninvasive mechanical ventilation and difficult weaning in critical care: key topics and practical approaches. Cham (Switzerland): Springer International Publishing; 2016. p. 165–71.

21. Burns KEA, Meade MO, Premji A, et al. Noninvasive ventilation as a weaning strategy for mechanical ventilation in adults with respiratory failure: a Cochrane systematic review. CMAJ 2014;186:E112–22.

22. Jaber S, Lescot T, Futier E, et al. Effect of noninvasive ventilation on tracheal re-intubation among patients with hypoxemic respiratory failure following abdominal surgery. A randomized clinical trial. JAMA 2016;315(13):1345–53.

23. Faria DA, da Silve EM, Atallah AN, et al. Noninvasive positive pressure ventilation for acute respiratory failure following upper abdominal surgery. Cochrane Database Syst Rev 2015;(10):CD009134.

24. Roca O, Hernández G, Díaz-Lobato S, et al, Spanish Multidisciplinary Group of High Flow Supportive Therapy in Adults (HiSpaFlow). Current evidence for the effectiveness of heated and humidified high flow nasal cannula supportive therapy in adult patients with respiratory failure. Crit Care 2016;20(1):109.

25. Frat JP, Thille AW, Mercat A, et al, FLORALI Study Group, REVA Network. High-flow oxygen through nasal cannula in acute hypoxemic respiratory failure. N Engl J Med 2015;372(23):2185–96.

26. Matthay MA. Saving lives with high-flow nasal oxygen. N Engl J Med 2015;372: 2225–6.

27. Stéphan F, Barrucand B, Petit P, et al, BiPOP Study Group. High-flow nasal oxygen vs noninvasive positive airway pressure in hypoxemic patients after cardiothoracic surgery: a randomized clinical trial. JAMA 2015;313(23):2331–9.

28. Kacmarek RM, Pirrone M, Berra L. Assisted mechanical ventilation: the future is now! BMC Anesthesiol 2015;15:110.

29. Younes M. Proportional assist ventilation, a new approach to ventilator support. Theory. Am Rev Respir Dis 1992;145:114–20.
30. Valdez C, Sarani B. Proportional assist ventilation. Curr Probl Surg 2013;50(10): 484–8.
31. Xirouchaki N, Kondili E, Vaporidi K, et al. Proportional assist with load adjustable gain factors in critically ill patients: comparison with pressure support. Intensive Care Med 2008;34:2026–34.
32. Bosma K, Ferreya G, Ambrogilo C, et al. Patient-ventilator interaction and sleep in mechanically ventilated patients: pressure support versus proportional assist ventilation. Crit Care Med 2007;35:1048–54.
33. Alexopoulou C, Kondili E, Palataki M, et al. Patient-ventilator synchrony and sleep quality with proportional assist ventilation and pressure support ventilation. Intensive Care Med 2013;39:1040–7.
34. Carteaux G, Mancebo J, Mercat A, et al. Bedside adjustment of proportional assist ventilation to target a predefined range of respiratory effort. Crit Care Med 2013;41(9):2125–32.
35. Manley C, Garpestad E, Hill NS. A new purpose for proportional assist ventilation? Crit Care Med 2013;41(9):2230–1.
36. Bosma KJ, Read BA, Bahrgard MJ, et al. A pilot randomized trial comparing weaning from mechanical ventilation on pressure support versus proportional assist ventilation. Crit Care Med 2016;44(6):1098–108.
37. Teixeira SN, Osaku EF, de Macedo Costa CRL, et al. Comparison of proportional assist ventilation plus, T-tube ventilation and pressure support ventilation as spontaneous breathing trials for extubation: a randomized study. Respir Care 2015;60(11):1527–35.
38. Chowdhury O, Bhat P, Rafferty G, et al. In vitro assessment of the effect of proportional assist ventilation on the work of breathing. Eur J Pediatr 2016;175: 639–43.
39. Sinderby C, Navaleski P, Beck J, et al. Neural control of mechanical ventilation in respiratory failure. Nat Med 1999;5:1433–6.
40. Schmidt M, Kindler F, Cecchini J, et al. Neurally adjusted ventilator assist and proportional assist ventilation both improve patient-ventilator interaction. Crit Care 2015;19:56.
41. Akoumianaki E, Pirinianakis G, Kondili E, et al. Physiologic comparison of neurally adjusted ventilator assist, proportional assist and pressure support ventilation in critically ill patients. Respir Physiol Neurobiol 2014;203:82–9.
42. Roze H, Repusseau B, Perrier V, et al. Neuro-ventilatory efficiency during weaning from mechanical ventilation using neutrally adjusted ventilator assist. Br J Anaesth 2013;111(6):955–60.
43. Wysocki M, Jouvet P, Jaber S. Closed loop mechanical ventilation. J Clin Monit Comput 2014;28:49–56.
44. Saxton GA, Myers G. A servomechanism for automatic regulation of pulmonary ventilation. J Appl Physiol 1957;11(2):326–8.
45. Johannigman JA, Branson RD, Edwards MG. Closed loop control of inspired oxygen concentration in trauma patients. J Am Coll Surg 2009;208(5):763–8.
46. Wallet F, Ledochoswski S, Bernet C, et al. Automated weaning modes. In: Esquinas AM, editor. Noninvasive ventilation and difficult weaning in critical care. Cham (Switzerland): Springer International Publishing; 2016. p. 21–8.
47. Taniguchi C, Victor ES, Pieri T, et al. Smart Care™ versus respiratory physiotherapy–driven manual weaning for critically ill adult patients: a randomized controlled trial. Crit Care 2015;19:246.

48. Rose L, Schultz MJ, Cardwell CR, et al. Automated versus non-automated weaning for reducing the duration of mechanical ventilation for critically ill adults and children: a Cochrane systematic review and meta-analysis. Crit Care 2015;19(1): 1.

49. Bialais E, Vignaux L, Wittebole X, et al. Comparison of an entirely automated ventilation mode, Intellivent-ASV, with conventional ventilation in ARDS patients: a 48-hour study. Crit Care 2013;17(2):1.

50. Dres M, Teboul J-L, Anguel N, et al. Extravascular lung water, B-type natriuretic peptide, and blood volume contraction enable diagnosis of weaning-induced pulmonary edema. Crit Care Med 2014;42:1882–9.

51. de Souza LC, Guimaraes FS, Lugon JR. Evaluation of a new index of mechanical ventilation weaning: the timed inspiratory index. J Intensive Care Med 2015;30(1): 37–43.

52. Mayo P, Volpocelli G, Lerolle N, et al. Ultrasonography evaluation during the weaning process: the heart, the diaphragm, the pleura and the lung. Intensive Care Med 2016;42:1107–17.

53. Soummer A, Perbet S, Brisson H, et al, The Lung Ultrasound Study Group. Ultrasound assessment of lung aeration loss during a successful weaning trial predicts postextubation distress. Crit Care Med 2012;40:2064–72.

54. Routsi C, Gerovasili V, Vasileiadis I, et al. Electrical muscle stimulation prevents critical illness polyneuromyopathy: a randomized parallel intervention trial. Crit Care 2010;14:R74.

55. McCaughey EJ, Berry HR, McLean AN, et al. Abdominal functional electrical stimulation to assist ventilator weaning in acute tetraplegia: a cohort study. PLoS One 2015;10(6):e0128589.

56. Garara B, Wood A, Marcus HJ, et al. Intramuscular diaphragm stimulation for patients with traumatic high cervical injuries and ventilator dependent respiratory failure: a systematic review of safety and effectiveness. Injury 2016;47(3):539–44.

57. Powers SK, Wiggs MP, Sollanek KJ, et al. Ventilator-induced diaphragm dysfunction: cause and effect. Am J Physiol Regul Integr Comp Physiol 2013;305: R464–77.

58. Kwon OS, Smuder AJ, Wiggs M, et al. AT_1 receptor blocker losartan protects against mechanical ventilation-induced diaphragmatic dysfunction. J Appl Physiol 2015;119(10):1033–41.

59. Simpkins C, Talluri K, Williams M. Intra-arterial perimortem resuscitation using a micellar colloid. Mil Med 2016;181(5):253–8.

60. Halpern NA. Innovative designs for the smart ICU. Chest 2014;145(3):646–58.

Tracheostomy Update
When and How

Bradley D. Freeman, MD

KEYWORDS

- Tracheostomy • Percutaneous dilational tracheostomy • Acute respiratory failure
- Intensive care units • Critical illness • Practice variation

KEY POINTS

- The presence of a tracheostomy identifies one of the most resource-intensive patient cohorts for which to provide care.
- Recent prospective trials have failed to demonstrate an effect of tracheostomy timing on outcomes, such as infectious complications, duration of mechanical ventilation, or intensive care unit (ICU) length of stay (LOS).
- Early tracheostomy is associated with greater patient comfort. Clinicians can defer tracheostomy placement for at least 2 weeks after the onset of acute respiratory failure to ensure need for ongoing ventilatory support.
- In appropriately selected patients, there are advantages of percutaneous dilational tracheostomy relative to surgical tracheostomy with respect to resource utilization and perioperative infection. These 2 techniques seem indistinguishable with respect to incidence of long-term complications (eg, tracheal stenosis).
- Tracheostomy practice varies substantially among disciplines, ICUs, and institutions. Use of protocols based on best evidence may be one strategy to lessen this variation.

INTRODUCTION

Tracheostomy is among the most commonly performed surgical procedures in patients with acute respiratory failure.[1–5] Although a minority of all individuals requiring respiratory support, tracheostomy patients place significant demands on ventilator, ICU, hospital, and posthospital discharge resources.[4,6–8] Financial expenditures to support the care of tracheostomy patients are among the highest of any diagnostic or procedural group.[9] Efforts to optimize tracheostomy practice may favorably affect both the quality of care provided this segment of the critically ill population and the resources expended delivering this care.[7,10]

The author has no conflicts of interest with any of the material presented.
Department of Surgery, Washington University School of Medicine, 660 South Euclid Avenue, Box 8109, St Louis, MO 63110, USA
E-mail address: freemanb@wustl.edu

Although a large body of literature exists regarding benefits, risks, and technical aspects of this procedure, little consensus exists as to what constitutes best tracheostomy practice in the setting of acute respiratory failure.[11] The intent of this article is to formulate recommendations based on contemporary evidence.

TRACHEOSTOMY INDICATIONS AND RATIONALE

A difficult airway in a patient requiring prolonged mechanical ventilation constitutes one of the few absolute indications for tracheostomy.[12] Difficult airway patients include those with conditions, such as significant maxillofacial trauma, angioedema, obstructing upper airway tumors, and other anatomic characteristics that render translaryngeal intubation difficult to perform in the event of airway loss.[12] Difficult airway patients constitute a small fraction of all individuals undergoing tracheostomy in most ICUs.[8] It is more often the case that patients requiring prolonged ventilatory support undergo tracheostomy to facilitate care.[11,13,14] In theory, there are several reasons why tracheostomy may be more advantageous than translaryngeal intubation in this context. The presence of a tracheostomy may promote oral hygiene and pulmonary toilet, enhance patient comfort, and allow oral nutrition and speech.[13–15] Because of greater airway security, patients with tracheostomy may be more practical to mobilize (such as transferring from bed to chair) and more likely to engage in physical therapy and conditioning regimens. Furthermore, the presence of a tracheostomy has been postulated to facilitate weaning from mechanical ventilation due to several factors.[16] Resistance to airflow in an artificial airway is proportional to air turbulence, tube diameter, and tube length.[13,17] Air turbulence is increased in the presence of extrinsic compression and inspissated secretions.[13,17] Because of its rigid design, shorter length, and – in some models – a removable inner cannula (to allow for evacuation of secretions), airflow resistance and associated work of breathing may be less with tracheostomies relative to endotracheal tubes.[13,17] Such effects, however, have not been consistently demonstrated in patients after tracheostomy.[18–20] Furthermore, the presence of a tracheostomy may allow clinicians to be more aggressive in weaning attempts.[12] Specifically, if a patient with a tracheostomy tube in place does not tolerate liberation from mechanical ventilation, he or she may be reconnected to the ventilator circuit. In contrast, if a patient who is maintained with translaryngeal intubation does not tolerate extubation, he or she must be sedated and reintubated. Concern about the development of respiratory failure when mechanical ventilation is withdrawn may represent a barrier to extubation in patients who are of marginal pulmonary status.[21] These and related benefits of tracheostomy relative to prolonged translaryngeal intubation are either unproved or subjective. As a consequence, widely accepted criteria to guide patient selection for tracheostomy are lacking.[11] The absence of such criteria may underlie the variability in tracheostomy that exists in clinical practice.[5,7,8,22–25]

TRACHEOSTOMY TIMING

One of the most debated aspects of tracheostomy practice concerns whether timing of this procedure affects clinically important outcomes.[26–36] Many studies addressing this question have produced conflicting findings owing to small sample sizes, heterogeneity in populations enrolled, variation in the quality of study design, inconsistencies as to the endpoints examined, and lack of protocols to direct care.[36] Three recent studies reported in this area merit comment.[37–39] In a large, multicenter investigation, Terragni and colleagues[39] randomized 419 patients to percutaneous tracheostomy after either 6 days to 8 days or 13 days to 15 days of mechanical ventilatory support. Tracheostomy timing had no effect on the primary outcome (ventilator-associated pneumonia). Although early tracheostomy was associated with significantly shorter duration of mechanical ventilation and ICU LOS, there were no differences in hospital LOS, 28-day mortality, or posthospital discharge destination (ie, proportion of patients requiring admission to a long-term care facility). In TracMan (Tracheostomy management in critical care), a large multi-center study conducted in the United Kingdom, 909 patients were randomized to undergo tracheostomy after either 1 day to 4 days versus greater than 10 days of ventilatory support.[37] Most tracheostomies (89%) were placed by percutaneous technique. Although tracheostomy timing produced no effect on the primary (mortality) or secondary (ICU or hospital LOS) endpoints, early tracheostomy was associated with less use of sedation.[37] In a study reported by Trouillet and colleagues,[38] patients requiring ventilatory support 5 days after cardiac surgery were randomized to percutaneous tracheostomy versus prolonged intubation. There was no effect of tracheostomy on the primary endpoints of duration of mechanical ventilation or mortality. Furthermore, treatment groups did not differ with respect to rates of ventilator-associated pneumonia, other infectious complications, ICU LOS, or hospital LOS. Patients undergoing tracheostomy experienced fewer unplanned extubations and required less sedative, analgesic, and antipsychotic use (for treatment of agitation and delirium) and were mobilized out of bed earlier in their ICU course. A minority of patients in the prolonged ventilation group (27%) underwent tracheostomy.

These studies had notable limitations. Terragni and colleagues[39] excluded patients with chronic obstructive pulmonary disease, anatomic deformity of the neck, history of prior tracheostomy, and active pneumonia. Such patients seem to constitute a large proportion of individuals who undergo tracheostomy in many ICUs.[7,8] TracMan investigators assigned patients in the early tracheostomy arm to undergo this procedure after 1 day to 4 days of mechanical ventilation.[37] Previous data suggest that a majority of patients maintained on mechanical ventilation during this time frame would be liberated from ventilatory support without need for tracheostomy.[8] Thus, it is unclear how the early intervention arm for TracMan would apply to most clinical settings.

These shortcomings notwithstanding, these trials provide useful information for guiding tracheostomy practice. First, these reports suggest that tracheostomy can be performed safely in critically ill patients. Although long-term follow-up is lacking, no deaths or serious short-term complications related to tracheostomy placement were reported in more than 1000 individuals undergoing this procedure.[37–39] Second, tracheostomy timing had no effect on mortality, incidence of ventilator-associated pneumonia, or LOS.[37–41] In contrast, the presence of a tracheostomy was associated with greater patient comfort, decreased sedative and antipsychotic drug administration, and lower incidence of unplanned extubation.[38] Finally, the challenge of predicting continued need for ventilatory support is evidenced by large numbers of patients randomized to late tracheostomy but who failed to undergo this procedure due to successful weaning from mechanical ventilation or death (ie, only 56.7% of patients in the study by Terragni and colleagues[39] and 45.5% of patients in TracMan randomized to late tracheostomy ultimately underwent this procedure).[37]

Based on the evidence provided by these 3 studies, clinicians should defer tracheostomy placement for at least 2 weeks after the onset of acute respiratory failure to insure need for ongoing ventilatory support.[37–39,42] This 2-week timing threshold corresponds to the control arm of the study reported by Terragni and colleagues.[39,41] Important caveats accompany this recommendation. Patients not addressed by studies to date include those with multiple failed extubations; those who require multiple general anesthetics whereby a surgical airway may be more safe, secure, and

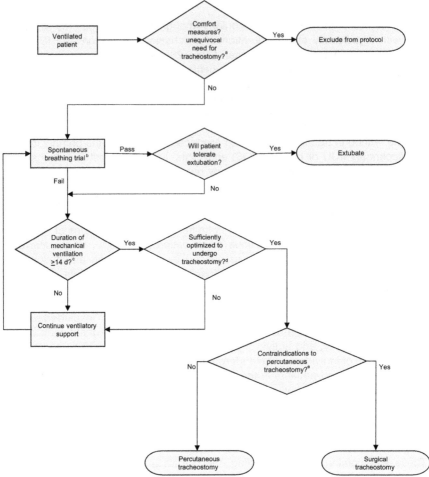

Fig. 1. Tracheostomy decision-making protocol. This algorithm is designed to guide tracheostomy decision making based on the best available evidence with respect to tracheostomy timing and technique. Such an approach is currently used in the surgical ICU of Barnes Jewish Hospital. [a] Ventilated patients are evaluated for their appropriateness for this protocol. Specifically, patients who have unequivocal need for tracheostomy (due to, for example, the presence of a difficult airway or a devastating intracranial injury) or who are managed with comfort measures only are excluded. [b] On a daily basis, patients undergo a spontaneous breathing trial, consistent with described methodology,[88] to determine their appropriateness for extubation. Those who successfully complete this evaluation typically proceed to extubation; those who fail this evaluation are maintained on ventilatory support. [c] Consistent with the evidence presented in the accompanying text, duration of mechanical ventilation is assessed, with those patients maintained on ventilatory support for at least 14 days considered candidates for tracheostomy. There are several clinical factors that may affect this timing threshold. For example, patients who have failed multiple extubation attempts may proceed to tracheostomy more quickly. [d] Patients deemed candidates for tracheostomy are evaluated to determine that they are sufficiently medically optimized to undergo this procedure (eg, coagulopathy corrected and level of ventilatory support appropriate). [e] Patients are assessed to determine the presence of contraindications to percutaneous tracheostomy (unstable cervical spine which may preclude optimal positioning, ambiguous surface anatomy, and so forth). If no such contraindications are present, this technique should be the preferred method of tracheostomy creation. Otherwise, surgical tracheostomy should be performed.

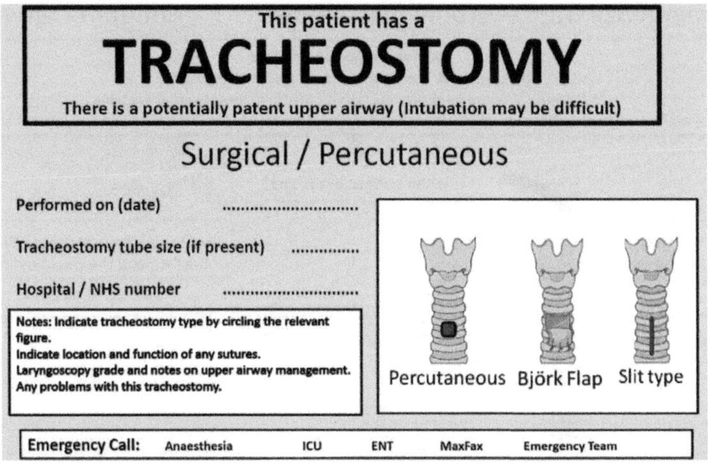

Fig. 2. Head-of-bed sign for tracheostomy. (*Reproduced from* McGrath BA, Bates L, Atkinson D, Moore JA. Multidisciplinary guidelines for the management of tracheostomy and laryngectomy airway emergencies. Anaesthesia. 2012 Jun 26. http://dx.doi.org/10.1111/j.1365-2044.2012.07217, with permission from the Association of Anaesthetists of Great Britain & Ireland/Blackwell Publishing Ltd.)

comfortable than repeated translaryngeal intubations; those with significant though potentially reversible cognitive impairment who are at risk of aspiration if extubated; and those with significant comorbidities.[37–39] These and other considerations will continue to factor prominently in decision for tracheostomy.

TRACHEOSTOMY TECHNIQUE

Traditionally, tracheostomies have been performed in the operating room according to standard surgical principles.[43] In 1985, Ciaglia and colleagues[44] described percutaneous dilational tracheostomy (PDT) in which tracheostomy is accomplished via modified Seldinger technique, typically with the aid of bronchoscopy. There have subsequently several technical modifications and refinements of this approach.[45] Several clinical studies and secondary data analyses have compared tracheostomy placed by these 2 approaches and suggest several advantages of PDT relative to surgically created tracheostomy.[46–65] PDT may be performed at the bedside, thus avoiding the inconvenience and risk associated with transporting a critically ill patient to the operating suite as well as the expense of these resources.[12,60,65,66] As a consequence, costs and charges associated with PDT are typically substantially less than those associated with surgical tracheostomy.[62–65] In addition, PDT is typically accomplished more quickly (reflecting the technical ease of this procedure) and is associated with less blood loss and lower rates of infectious complications (eg, peristomal infection and cellulitis) relative to surgically created tracheostomies.[48,55,58,60,61] These findings may reflect that there is minimal dead space separating the tracheostomy tube and adjacent pretracheal tissues after PDT, which may have a compressive effect on minor bleeding and serve as a barrier to infection.[60] Longitudinal follow-up suggests that incidence of delayed complications, such as clinically significant tracheal stenosis, are similar comparing these techniques.[45,52,53,67] Despite these potential advantages, PDT has been associated with a significant number of highly morbid complications,

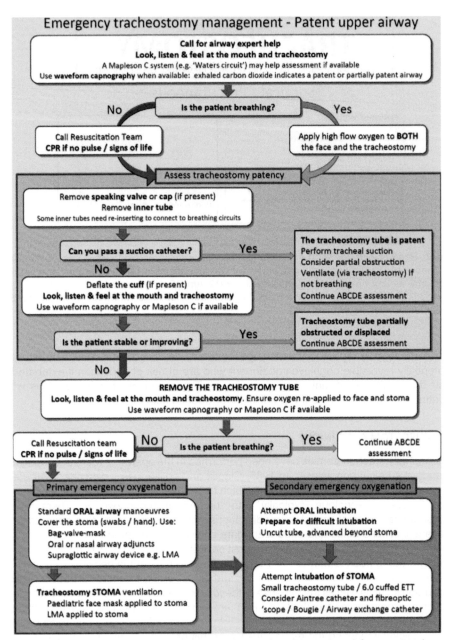

Fig. 3. Emergency tracheostomy management algorithm. (*Reproduced from* McGrath BA, Bates L, Atkinson D, Moore JA. Multidisciplinary guidelines for the management of tracheostomy and laryngectomy airway emergencies. Anaesthesia. 2012 Jun 26. http://dx.doi.org/10.1111/j.1365-2044.2012.07217, with permission from the Association of Anaesthetists of Great Britain & Ireland/Blackwell Publishing Ltd.)

many of which, such as tracheal laceration, aortic injury, and esophageal perforation, are unusual after surgical tracheostomies.[68–78]

Owing to these attributes as well as to the ease of this technique, which enables individuals who have not received in-depth surgical training to become facile in its use, PDT has gained wide acceptance and has become the predominate method of tracheostomy placement in many centers.[68,69,79–81] With notable caveats, PDT should be considered the preferred technique for tracheostomy creation.[82,83] Contraindications to PDT include ambiguous surface neck anatomy, which precludes identification of structural landmarks; clinical conditions resulting in a difficult airway (described previously); and the presence of an unstable cervical spine, which limits the ability to achieve optimal neck positioning.[10,66,84] Furthermore, PDT is an elective procedure and should not be used to establish an emergent airway.[11] Finally, although PDT is commonly performed competently by individuals not trained in surgical techniques, practitioners who are expert at surgical airway management should be immediately available in the event that complications arise.[12]

EVIDENCE-BASED APPROACH TO TRACHEOSTOMY PRACTICE

The manner in which this information might be integrated so as to guide practice is illustrated in Fig. 1.

TRACHEOSTOMY STANDARDIZED PROTOCOLS

Once a tracheostomy has been successfully performed, it is important to have standardized protocols for clinical care and for emergency airway management. These include hanging a sign above the head of the bed to provide essential details about the nature of the airway, tubes, and device; emergency contacts (Fig. 2); and emergency tracheostomy algorithm for patients who develop complications, such as hypoxemia, hypercarbia, or airway occlusion (Fig. 3). The National Tracheostomy Safety Project and the Global Tracheostomy Collaborative provide excellent resources for standardization of tracheostomy care for patients and families both in-hospital and at home.

SUMMARY

Although recent trials suggest that timing of tracheostomy does not influence ICU LOS and related endpoints of resource expenditure, there seems to be a beneficial effect of this intervention on sedation use, patient comfort, and mobility. Such patient-centric outcomes are difficult to quantify in the ICU setting, rendering it challenging to design and execute studies with these as primary endpoints. Nonetheless, the prevalence of tracheostomy use may be partly driven by the intrinsic value that clinicians assign to these attributes.[5,24,25] Future tracheostomy studies should incorporate methodologies that enable valuation of these and related variables. Furthermore, use of tracheostomy seems inextricably linked to many other facets of ICU care. Factors that are expected to influence duration of mechanical ventilation and ICU LOS — such as the primary disease process, acuity of illness, comorbid conditions, and use of and adherence to protocols directing weaning, sedation, and other aspects of care —also are expected to influence the frequency with which tracheostomy is used.[85–87] Although currently there are no benchmarks to define acceptable tracheostomy practice, use of this parameter can be envisioned as a surrogate for quality of care (eg, risk-adjusted comparison of rates of tracheostomy or in-hospital mortality of tracheostomy patients as an indicator for quality of care among institutions[7]). Given that variability in practice represents a potential opportunity for quality improvement, future research should assess the feasibility of establishing such benchmarks.[7,24,25] Finally, studies devoted to delineating optimal care after tracheostomy placement may enable more effective rehabilitation of patients recovering from prolonged periods of ventilatory support.[42]

REFERENCES

1. Cox CE, Carson SS, Holmes GM, et al. Increase in tracheostomy for prolonged mechanical ventilation in North Carolina, 1993-2002. Crit Care Med 2004; 32(11):2219–26.
2. Frutos-Vival F, Esteban A, Apezteguia C, et al. Outcome of mechanically ventilated patients who require a tracheostomy. Crit Care Med 2005;33:290–8.
3. Dewar DM, Kurek CJ, Lambrinos J, et al. Patterns in costs and outcomes for patients with prolonged mechanical ventilation undergoing tracheostomy: an analysis of discharges under diagnosis-related group 483 in New York state from 1992 to 1996. Crit Care Med 2003;27(12):2640–7.
4. Cox CE, Martinu T, Sathy S, et al. Expectations and outcomes of prolonged mechanical ventilation. Crit Care Med 2009;37(11):2888–94.
5. Mehta AB, Syeda SN, Bajpayee L, et al. Trends in tracheostomy for mechanically venitalated patients in the United States, 1993-2012. Am J Respir Crit Care Med 2015;192(4):446–54.
6. Kurek CJ, Cohen IL, Lambrinos J, et al. Clinical and economic outcome of patients undergoing tracheostomy for prolonged mechanical ventilation in New York state during 1993: analysis of 6,353 cases under diagnosis-related group 483. Crit Care Med 1997;25(6):983–8.
7. Freeman BD, Stwalley D, Lambert D, et al. High resource utilization does not affect mortality in acute respiratory failure patients managed with tracheostomy. Respir Care 2013;58(11):1863–72.
8. Freeman BD, Borecki IB, Coopersmith CM, et al. Relationship between tracheostomy timing and duration of mechanical ventilation in critically ill patients. Crit Care Med 2005;33:2513–20.
9. HCUP Fact Book #7: Procedures in U.S. Hospitals 2003. Available at: http://archive.ahrq.gov/data/hcup/factbk7/. Accessed December 29, 2016.
10. Freeman B, Kennedy C, Robertson TE, et al. Tracheostomy protocol: experience with development and potential utility. Crit Care Med 2008;36:1742–8.
11. Freeman BD, Morris PE. Concise defiinitive review: tracheostomy practice in adults with acute respiratory failure. Crit Care Med 2012;40:2890–6.
12. Freeman BD. Indications for and management of tracheostomy. In: Vincent JL, Abraham E, Moore FA, et al, editors. Textbook of critical care. 6th edition. Philadelphia: Elsevier/W. B. Saunders; 2011. p. 369–72.
13. Heffner JE, Hess D. Tracheostomy management in the chronically ventilated patient. Clin Chest Med 2001;22(1):55–69.
14. Plummer AL, Gracey DR. Consensus conference on artificial airways in patients receiving mechanical ventilation. Chest 1989;96(1):178–80.
15. Freeman-Sanderson AL, Togher L, Elkins MR, et al. Return of voice for ventilated tracheostomy patients in ICU: a randomized controlled trial of early-targeted intervention. Crit Care Med 2016;44(6):1075–81.
16. Heffner JE. The role of tracheotomy in weaning. Chest 2001;120(6):477S–81S.
17. Shah C, Kollef MH. Endotracheal tube intraluminal volume loss among mechanically ventilated patients. Crit Care Med 2004;32:120.

18. Lin MC, Huang CC, Yang CT, et al. Pulmonary mechanics in patients with prolonged mechanical ventilation requiring tracheostomy. Anaesth Intensive Care 1999;27(6):581–5.

19. Diehl JL, Atrous SE, Touchard D, et al. Changes in the work of breathing induced by tracheostomy in ventilator-dependent patients. Am J Respir Crit Care Med 2004;159:383–8.

20. Davis K Jr, Campbell RS, Johannigman JA, et al. Changes in respiratory mechanics after tracheostomy. Arch Surg 2004;134(1):59–62.

21. Thille AW, Harrois A, Schortgen F, et al. Outcomes of extubation failure in medical intensive care unit patients. Crit Care Med 2011;39(12):2612–8.

22. Nathens AB, Rivara FP, Mack CD, et al. Variations in the rates of trachestomy in the critically ill trauma patient. Crti Care Med 2006;34(12):2919–24.

23. Freeman BD, Kennedy C, Coopersmith CM, et al. Examination of non-clinical factors affecting tracheostomy practice in an academic surgical intensive care unit. Crit Care Med 2009;37:3070–8.

24. Mehta AB, Cooke CR, Wiener RS, et al. Hospital variation in early tracheostomy in the United States: a population-based study. Crit Care Med 2016;44(8):1506–14.

25. Freeman BD. Where the rubber meets the road. The discrepancy between evidence and reality for tracheostomy utilization in the setting of acute respiratory failure. Crit Care Med 2016;44(8):1610–1.

26. Blot F, Similowski T, Trouillet JL, et al. Early tracheostomy versus prolonged endotracheal intubation in unselected severely ill ICU patients. Intensive Care Med 2008;34:1779–87.

27. Rumbak MJ, Newton M, Truncale T, et al. A prospective randomized, study comparing early percutaneous dilational tracheotomy to prolonged translaryngeal intubation (delayed tracheotomy) in critically ill medical patients. Crit Care Med 2004;32:1689–94.

28. Griffiths J, Barber VS, Morgan L, et al. Systematic review and meta-analysis of studies of the timing of trachestomy in adult patients unergiong artifical ventilation. Br Med J 2005;330:1243–8.

29. Holevar M, Dunham M, Brautigan R, et al. Practice management guidelines for timing of tracheostomy: the EAST practice management guidelines work group. J Trauma 2009;67(4):870–4.

30. Dunham CM, LaMonica C. Prolonged tracheal intubation in the trauma patient. J Trauma 1984;24:120–4.

31. Maziak DE, Meade MO, Todd TRJ. The timing of tracheotomy - a systematic review. Chest 1998;114(2):605–9.

32. Blot F, Guiguet M, Antoun S, et al. Early tracheotomy in neutropenic, mechanically ventilated patients: rationale and results of a pilot study. Support Care Cancer 1995;3(5):291–6.

33. Brook AD, Sherman G, Malen J, et al. A comparison of early- vs. late-tracheostomy in patients requiring prolonged mechanical ventilation. Am J Crit Care 2000;9(5):352–9.

34. Lesnik I, Rappaport W, Fulginiti J, et al. The role of early tracheostomy in blunt, multiple organ trauma. Am Surg 1992;58(6):346–9.

35. Rodriguez JL, Steinberg SM, Luchetti FA, et al. Early tracheostomy for primary airway management in the surgical critical care setting. Surgery 1990;108:655–9.

36. Hosokawa K, Nishimura M, Vincent JL. Timing of tracheotomy in ICU patients: a systematic review of randomized controlled trials. Crit Care 2015;19:424.

37. Young D, Harrison DA, Cuthbertson BH, et al, TracMan Collaborators. Effect of early vs. late tracheostomy placement on survival in patients receiving mechanical ventilation: the TracMan randomized trial. JAMA 2013;309(20):2121–9.

38. Trouillet JL, Luyt CE, Guiguet M, et al. Early percutaneous tracheotomy versus prolonged intubation of mechanically ventilated patients after cardiac surgery. Ann Intern Med 2011;154:373–83.

39. Terragni PP, Antonelli M, Fumagalli R, et al. Early vs. late tracheotomy for prevention of pneumonia in mechanically ventilated adult ICU patients. JAMA 2010; 303(15):1483–9.

40. Paxtel SB, Kress JP. Early tracheostomy after cardiac surgery: not ready for prime time. Ann Intern Med 2011;154(6):434–5.

41. Scales DC, Ferguson ND. Early vs, late tracheotomy in ICU patients. JAMA 2010; 303(15):1537–8.

42. Combes A, Costa MA, Trouillet JL, et al. Morbidity, mortality, and quality-of-life outcomes of patinets requiring >14 days of mechanical ventilation. Crit Care Med 2003;31:1373–81.

43. Zollinger RM Jr, Zollinger RM. Atlas of surgical operations. 7th edition. New York: McGraw-Hill, Inc; 1993.

44. Ciaglia P, Firsching R, Syniec C. Elective percutaneous dilational tracheostomy. Chest 1985;87(6):715–9.

45. Dempsey GA, Morton B, Hammell C, et al. Long-term outcome following tracheostomy in critical care: a systematic review. Crit Care Med 2016;44(3):617–28.

46. Melloni G, Muttini S, Gallioli G, et al. Surgical tracheostomy versus percutaneous dilational tracheostomy - a prospective-randominzed study with long term follow-up. J Cardiovasc Surg 2002;43:113–21.

47. Higgins KM, Punthakee X. Meta-analysis comparison of open versus percutaneous tracheostomy. Laryngoscope 2007;117:447–54.

48. Delaney A, Bagshaw SM, Nalos M. Percutaneous dilatioinal tracheostomy versus surgical tracheostomy in critically ill patients: a systematic review and meta-analysis. Crit Care 2011;2006(10):R55.

49. Tabaee A, Geng E, Lin J, et al. Impact of neck length on the safety of percutaneous and surgicla tracheostomy: a prospective, randomized study. Laryngoscope 2005;115:1685–90.

50. Oliver ER, Gist A, Gillespie MB. Percutaneous versus surgical tracheostomy: an updated meta-analysis. Laryngoscope 2007;117:1570–5.

51. Massick DD, Yao S, Powell DM, et al. Bedside tracheostomy in the intensive care unit: a prospective randomized trial comparing open surgical tracheostomy with endoscopically guided percutaneous dilational tracheostomy. Laryngoscope 2001;111:494–500.

52. Silvester W, Goldsmith D, Uchino S, et al. Percutaneous versus surgical tracheostomy: a randomized controlled study with long-term follow-up. Crit Care Med 2006;34(8):2145–52.

53. Antonelli M, Michetti V, Di Palma A, et al. Percutaneous translaryngeal versus surgical tracheostomy: a randomized trial with 1-yr double-blind follow-up. Crit Care Med 2005;33(5):1015–20.

54. Porter JM, Ivatury RR. Preferred route of tracheostomy - percutaneous versus open at the bedside. Am Surg 1999;2:142–6.

55. Holdgaard HO, Pederson J, Jensen RH, et al. Percutaneous dilational tracheostomy versus conventional surgical tracheostomy. Acta Anaesthesiol Scand 1998; 42:545–50.

56. Hazard P, Jones C, Benitone J. Comparative clinical trial of standard operative tracheostomy with percutaneous tracheostomy. Crit Care Med 1991;19(8): 1018–24.
57. Gysin C, Dulguerov P, Guyot JP, et al. Percutaneous versus surgical tracheostomy - a doble-blind randomized trial. Ann Surg 1999;230(5):708–14.
58. Griggs WM, Myburgh JA, Worthley LIG. A prospective comparison of a percutaneous tracheostomy technique with standard tracheostomy. Intensive Care Med 1991;17:261–3.
59. Friedman Y, Fildes J, Mizock B, et al. Comparison of percutaneous and surgical tracheostomies. Chest 1996;110:480–5.
60. Freeman BD, Isabella K, Lin N, et al. A meta-analysis of prospective trials comparing percutaneous and surgical tracheostomy in critically ill patients. Chest 2000;118:1412–8.
61. Crofts SL, Alzeer A, McGuire GP, et al. A comparison of percutaneous and operative tracheostomies in intensive care patients. Can J Anaesth 1999;42(9):775–9.
62. Levin R, Trivikram L. Cost/Benefit analysis of open tracheotomy, in the OR and at the bedside, with percutaneous tracheotomy. Laryngoscope 2001;111:1169–73.
63. Heikkinen M, Pertti A, Hannukainen J. Percutaneous dilational tracheostomy or conventional surgical tracheostomy? Crit Care Med 2000;28(5):1399–402.
64. Fernandez L, Norwood S, Roettger R, et al. Bedside percutaneous tracheostomy with bronchoscopic guidance. Arch Surg 1996;131:129–32.
65. Freeman BD, Isabella K, Cobb JP, et al. A prospective, randomized study comparing percutaneous with surgical tracheostomy in critically ill patients. Crit Care Med 2001;29(5):926–30.
66. Freeman BD, Buchman TG. How does percutaneous tracheostomy compare with surgical tracheostomy? When is this alternate approach indicated? J Crit Illness 2002;17(9):329.
67. Freeman BD. Back to the present - does tracheostomy technique affect long-term complications? Crit Care Med 2016;44(3):648–9.
68. Petros S, Engelmann L. Percutaneous dilatational tracheostomy in the medical ICU. Intensive Care Med 1997;23:630–4.
69. Hill BB, Zweng TN, Maley RH, et al. Percutaneous dilatational tracheostomy: report of 356 cases. J Trauma 1996;40(8):238–44.
70. Pothman W, Tonner PH, Schulte am Esch J. Percutaneous dilatational tracheostomy: risks and benefits. Intensive Care Med 1997;23:610–2.
71. Klussman JP, Brochhagen HG, Sittel C, et al. Atresia of the trachea following repeated percutaneous dilational tracheostomy. Chest 2001;119(3):961–4.
72. Ayoub OM, Griffiths MV. Aortic arch laceration: a lethal complication after percutaneous tracheostomy. Laryngoscope 2007;117:176–8.
73. Malthaner RA, Telang H, Miller JD, et al. Percutaneous tracheostomy - is it really better? Chest 1998;144(6):1771–2.
74. Douglas WE, Flabouris A. Surgical emphysema following percutaneous tracheostomy. Anaesth Intensive Care 1999;27(1):69–72.
75. Alexander R, Pappachan J. Timing of surgical tracheostomy after failed percutaneous tracheostomy (letter). Anaesth Intensive Care 1997;25(1):91.
76. Kaloud H, Smolle-Juettner F, Prause G, et al. Iatrogenic rupture of the tracheobronchial tree. Chest 1997;112:774–8.
77. Briche T, Manach YL, Pats B. Complications of percutaneous tracheostomy. Chest 2001;119(4):1282–3.
78. Kaylie DM, Wax MK. Massive subcutaneous emphysema following percutaneous tracheostomy. Am J Otolaryngol 2002;23(5):300–2.

79. Durbin CG. Questions answered about tracheostomy timing. Crit Care Med 1999; 27(9):2024–5.
80. Kluge S, Baumann HJ, Maier C, et al. Tracheostomy in the intensive care unit: a nationwide survey. Anesth Analg 2008;107:1639–43.
81. Cooper RM. Use and safety of percutaneous tracheostomy in intensive care. Anaesthesia 1998;53:1209–27.
82. Muhammad JK, Major E, Patton DW. Evaluating the neck for percutaneous dilational tracheostomy. J Craniomaxillofac Surg 2000;28:336–42.
83. Mansharamani NG, Koziel H, Garland R, et al. Safety of bedside percutaneous dilational tracheostomy in obese patinets in the ICU. Chest 2000;117:1426–9.
84. Freeman BD. Should tracheostomy practice in the setting of trauma be standardized? Curr Opin Anesthesiol 2011;24:188–94.
85. Esteban A, Alia I, Tobin MJ, et al. Effect of spontaneous breathing trial duration on outcomes of attempts to discontinue mechanical ventilation. Am J Respir Crit Care Med 1999;159:512–9.
86. Ely EW, Meade MO, Haponik EF, et al. Mechanical ventilator weaning protocols driven by non-physician healthcare professionals: evidence-based clinical practice guidelines. Chest 2001;120(6 Suppl):454S–63S.
87. Girard TD, Kress JP, Thomason JWW, et al. Eficacy and safety of a paired sedation and ventilator weaning protocol for mechanically ventilated patients in intensive care (Awakening and Breating Controlled trial): a randomised controlled trial. Lancet 2008;371:126–34.
88. Esteban A, Frutos F, Tobin MJ, et al. A comparison of four methods of weaning patients from mechanical ventilation. N Engl J Med 1995;332(6):345–50.

Severe Sepsis and Septic Shock Trials (ProCESS, ARISE, ProMISe)

What is Optimal Resuscitation?

Tiffany M. Osborn, MD, MPH

KEYWORDS

- Severe sepsis • Septic shock • Resuscitation • Usual care • Lactate
- Hyperlactatemia • Sepsis

KEY POINTS

- Three large international randomized trials (Process, ARISE and Promise) confirmed that in the general population of patients with severe sepsis and septic shock, early goal-directed therapy did not confer a mortality benefit compared with usual resuscitation. The ability to generalize depends on the consistency of treatment provided as part of usual resuscitation in individual hospitals.
- All 3 trials used the established definitions for identifying septic patients. Until the SEPSIS-3 definitions are prospectively evaluated, their associated risks and benefits are unclear.
- Usual care in all 3 trials included early identification using standardized screening protocols, including lactate measurement, early intravascular fluid administration, and early antibiotics.
- Normotensive patients with lactate level greater than or equal to 4 mmol/L had a similar mortality to patients with refractory hypotension with a normal lactate level.

INTRODUCTION

Between 2014 and 2015, 3 independent, multicenter, government-funded, randomized controlled trials (RCTs) evaluating early goal-directed therapy (EGDT) were published. These trials were Protocolized Care for Early Septic Shock (ProCESS) from the United States,[1] Australasian Resuscitation in Sepsis Evaluation (ARISE),[2] and Protocolised Management in Sepsis (ProMISe)[3] in the United Kingdom.

The care of septic patients has progressed significantly over the years; mortality has significantly decreased but there is still much controversy and confusion. Which definition should be used to identify septic patients? Given that there was no survival

Section of Acute and Critical Care Surgery, Washington University School of Medicine, 4901 Forest Park Avenue, St. Louis, MO 63108, USA
E-mail address: osbornt@wustl.edu

Crit Care Clin 33 (2017) 323–344
http://dx.doi.org/10.1016/j.ccc.2016.12.004
0749-0704/17/© 2017 Elsevier Inc. All rights reserved.

criticalcare.theclinics.com

benefit of EGDT compared with usual resuscitation, how should usual resuscitation be defined in the context of the data? What interventions do clinicians need to provide and what is time dependent? This article reviews key findings of the 3 sepsis trials and reviews the following:

- Background on sepsis care before the original EGDT trial by Rivers and colleagues.[4]
- Key elements of ProCESS, ARISE, and ProMISe to assist comprehensive evaluation.
- Options for operationalization and future direction in the evolving care of septic patients.

Background

Death is not the enemy but occasionally needs help with timing.

—Peter Safar

Sepsis mortality before 2001 was traditionally high, with reports of mortality ranging between 30% and 60%.[5–9] There was no universal concept of urgency in the treatment of septic patients. Care was generally fractured, with little collaboration between the service line silos of the prehospital service, emergency department (ED), the intensive care unit (ICU), and the wards. Treatment might focus on using vasopressors to augment blood pressure with less emphasis on end-organ perfusion, resulting in ischemic limbs and colloquial names such as "leave 'em dead" for levophed.[10] In addition, universal use of ultrasonography in EDs or ICUs was nonexistent during this period.

After observing severe sepsis and septic shock mortality of 50% in local hospitals, an institutional quality improvement initiative led to a randomized controlled trial evaluating EGDT from 1997 to 2000.[4] In 2001, Rivers and colleagues[4] reported results of a new, protocolized resuscitation termed EGDT. EGDT was described as a structured treatment protocol that incorporated elements consistent with consensus guidelines.[11] EGDT is designed to optimize tissue oxygen transport through early identification and time-dependent hemodynamic optimization of oxygen delivery using continuous monitoring of prespecified physiologic targets.

- Preload: central venous pressure (CVP) was used as a surrogate target for intravascular volume.
- Afterload: mean arterial pressure (MAP) was targeted after volume repletion with vasoactive agents.
- Contractility and oxygen carrying capacity: central venous oxygen saturation ($ScvO_2$) guided delivery of inotropes and red blood cell transfusions.

At the time of publication, this protocol was novel because of the absolute mortality reduction, the time dependency element, and focus on the level of care rather than location of care. The absolute mortality benefit of 16% (46.5% to 30.5%) suggested that this was one of the most effective modalities to date.[12–14] Subsequent observational studies supported a mortality benefit of varying degrees.[15]

Although medicine traditionally functioned in silos, this study emphasized the level of care rather than location of care. During this period of time, central venous access, arterial access, and use of inotropes was generally reserved for the ICU. It was unique to provide several critical care modalities in locations outside of traditional critical care settings. Although novel in application, the idea was not a unique concept. Dr Peter Safar[16] described critical care as a continuum beginning prehospital, continuing with ED intervention, and culminating in ICU admission and management.

Also unique to the era, this study emphasized deliberate, time-dependent recognition and management of septic patients during the most proximal phase of hospital presentation in the ED. As part of the effort to reduce global mortality caused by severe sepsis and septic shock, EGDT was incorporated into the first iterations of the international management guidelines of the Surviving Sepsis Campaign (SSC).[12–14,17] Given that half of the estimated cases of severe sepsis and septic shock originally present to the ED,[18] the American College of Emergency Physicians representative worked on the guidelines writing committee, endorsed all iterations of the guidelines, and actively supported their distribution and implementation.[19]

Despite incorporation into the SSC guidelines and nonrandomized trials reporting benefit, adoption was not universal.[20,21] Concerns regarding universal adoptions centered on the ability to generalize, protocol complexity, high control arm mortality, and financial and infrastructure implications.

To address these concerns, ProCESS, ARISE, and ProMISe, three international, independent, multicentered, government-funded trials were undertaken. Principal investigators decided before enrollment to reconcile key protocol design and operational elements to facilitate combining data on completion for a patient-level meta-analysis and further evaluation of specific components that would not be possible based on single trials alone.[22]

Shock is a rude unhinging of the machinery of life.
—Samuel D. Gross (A System of Surgery)[23]

PATIENT EVALUATION OVERVIEW
Identification/Inclusion Criteria

Identification is inherently linked to how the patient population is defined (Table 1). All 3 trials used the same established definitions,[24] in combination with lactate level (≥4 mmol/L) as did the original EGDT trial to identify adult ED patients with severe sepsis or septic shock (Fig. 1).

Fluid Refractory Hypotension

Fluid refractory hypotension was originally defined in ProCESS as low blood pressure after a 30-mL/kg fluid bolus, which was later changed to the same threshold, a 1-L fluid challenge, used by both ProMISe and ARISE. The time of fluid bolus administration was more than 30 minutes in ProCESS and 60 minutes in ARISE and ProMISe (see Table 1).

Increased Lactate level

Increased lactate level (>2 mmol/L) is an established indicator of critical illness and predictor of decreased survival.[25–31] Mortality reportedly increases with increasing hyperlactatemia similar to a dose-response relationship.[31] Further, normotensive patients with a lactate level greater than or equal to 4 mmol/L have a similar mortality to hypotensive patients who are not hyperlactemic.[3,25,26,32,33] Lactate screening was a component of the protocol in all 3 trials. For consistency with the original EGDT trial, ProMISe, ProCESS, and ARISE used lactate level greater than 4 mmol/L as an independent inclusion criterion. Lactate level greater than 4 mmol/L was the sole identifier in almost half of the recruited patients (Table 2).

When comparing sole hyperlactatemia (lactate level >4 mmol/L in normotensive patients), sole refractory hypotension (hypotension with normal lactate), and the two combined, the inclusion criteria met most often in ProCESS and ProMISe was

Table 1
Inclusion criteria across trials

	ProCESS	ARISE	ProMISe	EGDT
Age >18 y	✔	✔	✔	✔
Infection: Suspected, presumed, or known	✔	✔	✔	✔
Serum lactate screening required[a]	✔	✔	✔	✔
Serum lactate >4 mmol/L	✔	✔	✔	✔
Refractory hypotension	✔	✔	✔	✔
Fluid requirement	✔	✔	✔	✔
Fluid amount[b]	20 cc/kg changed to 1 liter	1 liter	1 liter	20 – 30 cc/kg
SBP <90 mm Hg[c]	✔	✔	✔	✔
MAP <65 mm Hg	✗	✔	✔	✗
Antibiotics required prior to randomization[d]	✗	✔	✔	✗

[a] EDGT lactate screening for enrolment.
[b] Amount of fluid required to meet study definition of refractor hypotension.
[c] Blood pressure parameter required for inclusion (either SBP or MAP in ProMISe/ARISE).
[d] Antibiotics encouraged within 6 hours (ProCESS), no universally accepted standard for timing at time of EGDT – timing per clinical determination.

hyperlactatemia followed by refractory hypotension. The most common criterion in ARISE was sole refractory hypotension followed by sole hyperlactatemia. In all 3 trials, the least common criterion was patients with both refractory hypotension and hyperlactatemia (see Table 1).

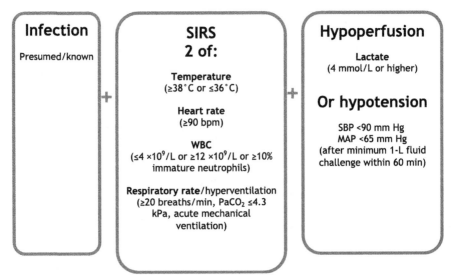

Fig. 1. Severe sepsis and septic shock definitions were the inclusion criteria. All 3 trials used the established definitions for inclusion criteria. WBC, white blood cell count.

Table 2
ProCESS/ARISE/ProMISe prevalence of hyperlactatemia versus hypotension in the usual resuscitation group

	ProCESS Lactate >4 mmol/L	ARISE Lactate >4 mmol/L	ProMISe Lactate >4 mmol/L	SEPSIS-3* Lactate >4 mmol/L
Hyperlactatemia Only[a] (%)	46.7	30.2	44.4	9.9
Refractory Hypotension Only[b] (%)	39.3	53.5	36.3	22.0
Both Refractory Hypotension and Hyperlactatemia[c] (%)	14.0	16.3	19.3	23.6
Any Lactate >4 mmol/L (%)	60.7	46.5	63.7	9.9

[a] Normotension and hyperlactatemia (lactate level >4 mmol/L).
[b] Refractory hypotension after a 1-L fluid challenge without hyperlactatemia.
[c] Concurrent refractory hypotension and hyperlactatemia.
   Data from Mouncey PR, Osborn TM, Power GS, et al. Trial of early, goal-directed resuscitation for septic shock. N Engl J Med 2015;372(14):1301–11 [supplemental material] and Shankar-Hari M, Phillips GS, Levy ML, et al. Developing a new definition and assessing new clinical criteria for septic shock: for the third international consensus definitions for sepsis and septic shock (Sepsis-3). JAMA 2016;315(8):775–87.

Antibiotic

Antibiotic delivery time is associated with survival in both severe sepsis[34] and septic shock.[34,35] Antibiotic initiation was required before randomization in ProMISe and ARISE (Fig. 2). ProCESS encouraged early antibiotic delivery and, during the era of the original EGDT trial, there was no universally agreed-on time frame of antibiotic delivery except that it be as soon as possible as established by the clinician (see Table 1).

Time Requirements

Time requirements were substantial for all the trials. In the original EGDT trial, ProMISe and ARISE patients had to meet inclusion criteria within 6 hours of presentation to the

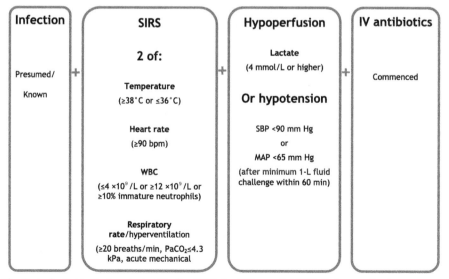

Fig. 2. Inclusion criteria required in ProCESS, ProMISe, and ARISE. Before patients were randomized in all 3 trials, identification criteria had to be met (requiring early identification/fluid administration) and antibiotics initiated.

ED. In ProCESS, patients had to meet inclusion criteria within 12 hours of ED presentation. Once inclusion criteria were met, all trials had up to 2 hours to obtain consent and enroll the patient (Fig. 3).

Thus, before being randomized into the treatment or usual-resuscitation arms, the patients required early identification, including either refractory hypotension or hypoperfusion (lactate level >4 mmol/L), and early intravenous fluid administration and early antibiotics (ARISE, ProMISe).

TREATMENT OPTIONS

ProMISe and ARISE had 2 arms to which patients were randomized, consisting of treatment and usual resuscitation. ProCESS randomized to 1 of 3 arms: treatment, usual resuscitation, and a protocolized standard therapy arm. The treatment arms consisted of similar processes to those described in the 2001 EGDT articles (Fig. 4), which entailed continuous monitoring of prespecified physiologic targets, including CVP, MAP, and central venous oxygen saturation (Scvo$_2$), to guide delivery of intravenous fluids, vasoactive drugs, and packed red blood cell transfusions.

The ProCESS protocolized standard care arm was a 6-hour protocol that consisted of ensuring venous access (peripheral or central) and administration of fluid and vasoactive agents to a shock index goal and hourly clinical assessment of fluid status and hypoperfusion (Fig. 5).

How the protocols were delivered and monitored was similar between trials. ARISE and ProMISe delivered the protocols within existing resources and required each hospital to have a plan for delivery. ProCESS required a designated team outside of the ED work flow to deliver protocolized care in the two treatment arms.

ProCESS patients had higher acute physiology and chronic health evaluation (APACHE) II scores, whereas ProMISe had the higher lactate values, followed by ARISE. ProMISe had the greatest percentage of patients with lactate levels greater than 4 mmol/L, and all 3 trial had baseline Scvo$_2$ greater than or equal to 70% (Table 3). All 3 trials had greater fluid, vasopressor, red cell, and dobutamine administration in the EGDT group compared with usual resuscitation. Central venous catheters and arterial catheters were placed in 50% to 60% and 60% to 75% of usual resuscitation patients respectively.

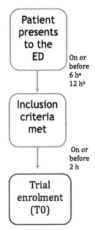

Fig. 3. Timeline overview. [a] ProMISe and ARISE required inclusion criteria to be met on or before 6 hours. [b] ProCESS required inclusion criteria to be met on or before 12 hours. All 3 trials required randomization within 2 hours of meeting inclusion criteria.

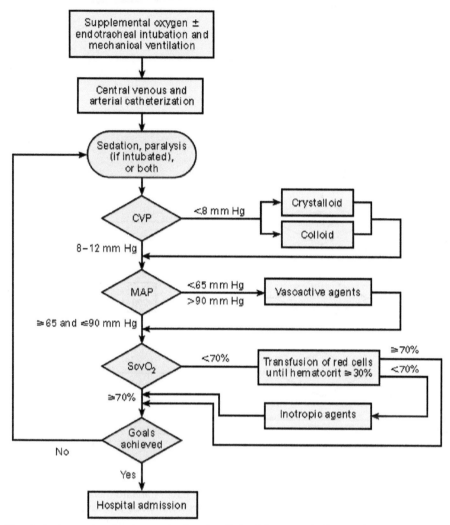

Fig. 4. Early, protocolized resuscitation in all 3 trials were similar to the original EGDT protocol. (*From* Rivers E, Nguyen B, Havstad S, et al. Early goal-directed therapy in the treatment of severe sepsis and septic shock. N Engl J Med 2001;345(19):1368–77; with permission.)

Vasopressors, red cell transfusions, and dobutamine were administered in approximately half, less than 7%, and less than 4% respectively (Table 4).

The good physician treats the disease; the great physician treats the patient who has the disease.

—*William Osler*

EVALUATION OF OUTCOME

In the evaluation of adults with early signs of septic shock who presented to the ED, ProCESS, ARISE, and ProMISe reported no significant difference in hospital or 90-day mortality among patients receiving 6 hours of EGDT and those receiving usual

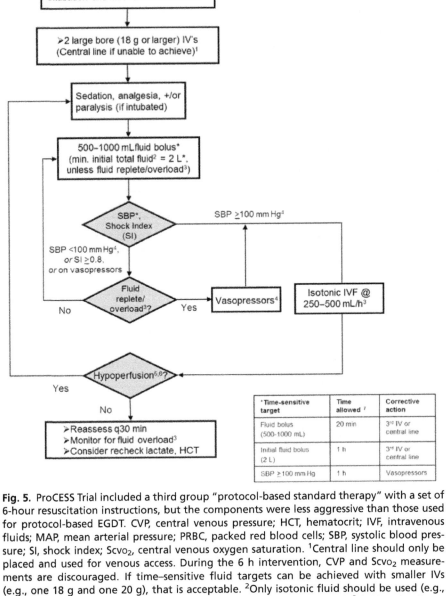

Fig. 5. ProCESS Trial included a third group "protocol-based standard therapy" with a set of 6-hour resuscitation instructions, but the components were less aggressive than those used for protocol-based EGDT. CVP, central venous pressure; HCT, hematocrit; IVF, intravenous fluids; MAP, mean arterial pressure; PRBC, packed red blood cells; SBP, systolic blood pressure; SI, shock index; Scvo$_2$, central venous oxygen saturation. [1]Central line should only be placed and used for venous access. During the 6 h intervention, CVP and Scvo$_2$ measurements are discouraged. If time–sensitive fluid targets can be achieved with smaller IVs (e.g., one 18 g and one 20 g), that is acceptable. [2]Only isotonic fluid should be used (e.g., saline, lactated Ringer's). Colloids are neither encouraged nor excluded. [3]Fluid replete/overload is defined here as a clinical diagnosis by the treating ProCESS Investigator. Signs and symptoms of overload include jugular venous distention, rales, and decreased pulse oximetry readings. Discontinue all IVF (boluses, background rate) once this occurs, until no longer deemed fluid replete/overload. [4]If patient's SBP is within 10% of known baseline SBP, AND patient is not deemed to be clinically hypoperfused, the SBP >100 mmHg target can be deemed fulfilled. Arterial lines allowed if deemed necessary, but not mandatory. Shock index = heart rate/systolic blood pressure. [5]Hypoperfusion is defined here as a clinical diagnosis by the treating ProCESS Investigator. Signs and symptoms include, but are not limited to, MAP <65 despite SBP >100, arterial lactate >4, mottled skin, oliguria, and altered sensorium. [6]Transfuse PRBCs for Hgb <7.5 g/dL. [7]From time of prompt by protocol (i.e., not from time of physician order, or from when intravenous fluid bag hung). (*From* Process Investigators, Yealy DM, Kellum JA, et al. A randomized trial of protocol-based care for early septic shock. N Engl J Med. 2014;370(18):1683–93; with permission.)

Table 3
Baseline values versus resuscitation end points

	ProCESS		ARISE		ProMISe		EGDT	
	EGDT	UR	EGDT	UR	EGDT	UR	EGDT	UR
APACHE II[a]	20.8	20.7	15.4	15.8	18	17	21.4	20.4
SOFA[a]	—	—	—	—	4	4	—	—
SBP (mm Hg)	100.2	99.9	78.8	79.6	77.7	78.4	106	109
SBP, 6 h (mm Hg)	—	—	—	—	113.1	110.7	—	—
Lactate (mM/L)	4.8	4.9	6.7	6.6	7.0	6.8	7.7	6.9
Lactate, 6 h (mm Hg)	—	—	2.8	2.9	—	—	—	—
Lactate >4 mM/L (%)	59	60	46.0	46.5	65.4	63.7	79[b]	
CVP	—	—	—	—	—	—	—	—
CVP, 6 h (mm Hg)	—	—	11.4	11.9	11.2	11.7	13.8	11.8
Scvo$_2$%	71	—	72.7	—	70.1	—	48.6	49.2
Scvo$_2$% (6 h)	—	—	75.9	—	74.2	—	77.3	66.0

Abbreviations: UR, usual resuscitation; HR, heart rate; CVP, central venous pressure; Scvo$_2$%, central venous oxygen saturation (%).
[a] Median (interquartile range [IQR]).
[b] Value found in Table 3 from Nguyen Crit Care (2016).[51]

resuscitation (Table 5). In all 3 evaluations, the overall rate of death was lower than anticipated. ARISE and ProMISe evaluated ED length of stay (LOS) and reported significantly higher LOS in the usual-resuscitation groups. However, the maximum median time of 2 hours from ED presentation is significantly lower than the 6-hour national average of ED LOS for critically ill patients in the United States.[36] None of the 3 trials showed a significant difference in hospital LOS. ProMISe reported an increased ICU LOS in the EGDT group with ProCESS and ARISE reporting no difference. ProMISe was the only trial of the three to evaluate quality of life and resource consumption. Quality of life of patients with severe sepsis and septic shock (0.60) was substantially lower than that of age-matched and gender-matched people in the general population (0.80). ProMISe also reported a low probability that EGDT was cost-effective because of increased treatment intensity in the EGDT groups and no difference in outcomes.

The benefits of EGDT treatment in the original trial were substantial. Why would 3 trials now show such divergent results? Possibilities include:

- The benefits derived in the original single-center RCT might not have been generalizable, and the multiple observational, before/after, historical control studies were compromised by bias, confounding, sample size, or chance.
- Recruitment time could have encompassed practice changes within the institutions that could have modified the effect benefit.
- The intervention (EGDT) was not blinded in ProCESS, ARISE, or ProMISe. However, the risk of bias was minimized through central randomization and the use of a primary outcome not subject to observer bias. In the original EGDT RCT, the ED, where the treatment was administered, was not blinded. However, the ICU practitioners were blinded to who received EGDT in the ED.
- Change of care over the 15 years between trials may have affected the results. The mortality in the 3 recent trials was substantially reduced compared with those reported by Rivers and colleagues[4] (see Table 5). In addition, severity of illness

Table 4
Interventions delivered during a 6-hour period

	ProCESS		ARISE		ProMISe		EGDT	
	EGDT	UR	EGDT	UR	EGDT	UR	EGDT	UR
Arterial Catheter Insertion (%)[a]	Required	—	91.4	76.3	74.2	62.2	Required	Required
CVC Insertion (%)[a,b]	93.6	57.9	90	61.9	92.1	50.9	Required	Required
Any IV Fluid (mL)[a]	2805 (±1957)	2279 (±1881)	1964 (±1415)	1713 (±1404)	2226 (±1443)	2022 (±1271)	4981 (±2984)	3499 (±2438)
Vasopressor (%)[a]	54.9	44.1	66.6	57.8	53.3	46.6	27.4	30.3
Red Cell Transfusion (%)[a]	14.4	7.5	13.6	7.0	8.8	3.8	64.1	18.5
Dobutamine (%)[a]	8	0.9	15.4	2.6	18.1	3.8	13.7	.8

Abbreviations: CVC, central venous catheter; IV, intravenous.

[a] Significant difference (P<.001).

[b] CVC: ProMISe and ProCESS, any CVC placement; ARISE CVC, EGDT is $Scvo_2$, UR is non-$Scvo_2$.

Table 5
Outcomes

	ProCESS		ARISE		ProMISe		EGDT	
	EGDT	UR	EGDT	UR	EGDT	UR	EGDT	UR
Hospital Death (%)	21	18.9	14.5	15.7	25.6	24.6	30.5	46.5[a]
Death by 60 d (%)	—	—	—	—	—	—	33.3	49.2[a]
Death by 90 d (%)	31.9	33.7	18.6	18.8	29.5	29.2	—	—
Median ED LOS (IQR)[a]	—	—	1.4 (0.5–2.7)	2.0 (1.0–3.8)	1.5 (0.4–3.1)	1.3 (0.4–2.9)	—	—
Median ICU LOS (IQR)	5.1 (±6.3)	4.7 (±5.8)	2.8 (1.4–5.1)	2.8 (1.5–5.7)	2.6 (1.0–5.8)	2.2[a] (0–5.3)	—	—
HLOS[b]	11.1 (±10)	11.3 (±10.9)	8.2 (4.9–16.7)	8.5 (4.9–16.5)	9 (4–21)	9 (4–18)	—	—

ProCESS used combined in hospital death or death by 60 days.

± denotes mean with standard deviation.

Abbreviations: HLOS, hospital length of stay; LOS, length of stay.

[a] Significant difference (*P*<.01).

[b] Unless otherwise noted, median (IQR).

seemed greater in the Rivers and colleagues[4] trial. The ProMISe and ARISE trial patients had lower APACHE II scores, and all 3 trials had lower lactate levels and higher $Scvo_2$ (see Table 3). Patients from all 3 trials received antibiotics very quickly. Receiving antibiotics before randomization was an inclusion criterion for ProMISe and ARISE, and ProCESS encouraged rapid administration (Fig. 6, Table 6). Other care elements, such as lung-protective ventilation, that would now most likely be part of general practice would not have been in 1997 to 2000.

For the general population of patients with severe sepsis and septic shock, rigid protocols requiring universal application of central venous catheters, red cell transfusion, and inotropes was not effective. Given that the 3 trials had baseline $Scvo_2$ greater than 70%, it is unclear whether there may be a subset of this patient population that could benefit from normalizing an abnormally low $Scvo_2$. Important to ensuring individual intuitional replication of these results is a clear understanding of what usual resuscitation entailed in ProCESS, ARISE, and ProMISe.

What Was Usual Care?

Often the question arises, "How did all that treatment equate to no care?" The answer is that usual care, in this case usual resuscitation, did not equate to no care. Usual care equated to a standardized protocol requiring early identification (including lactate screening), early intravenous fluids, and early antibiotics (see Fig. 6, Table 6). The hospital mortality in the usual-care groups of ProCESS, ARISE, and ProMISe were 18.9%, 15.7%, and 24.6% respectively (see Table 5). Before translating these results to individual institutions, specific parameters for quality improvement projects should consider the current hospital mortality and the following specific parameters. It is unclear that individual institutions would have the same results without similar quality maintenance processes in place (see Table 6).

- Early identification
  - ○ Definition: the foundation of how septic patients are identified centers on how the disorder is defined. As with most major sepsis evaluations to date, the definition used in all 3 of these large, prospective RCTs and the original EGDT RCT

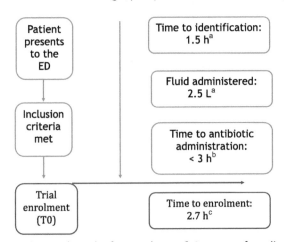

Fig. 6. Timeline overview and results for usual care. [a] Average of median values from all 3 trials. [b] Antibiotic administration was required before randomization. Longest time to randomization of usual care was 3 hours (±1.6 hours). [c] Average time to enrollment of all 3 trials was 2.7 hours.

Table 6
Early treatment in usual resuscitation patients

	PROCESS	ARISE	ProMISe
Hours to Identification	1.5 (+/−0.75)	1.3[a] (0.5–2.4)	1.7 (+/−1.4)
Identification by lactate alone[b]	45%	30%	45%
Hours to antibiotic[a] administration	76.1% less than 3 hours[c]	1.12 (.63–1.8)	1.3 α (0.6–2.4)
Fluids prior to randomization (liters)	2.1 (+/−1.4)	2.6 (+/−1.3)	2.0 (+/−1.1)
Hours to randomization[a]	3.0 (+/−1.6)	2.7 (2.0–3.9)	2.5 (1.8–3.5)
Fluids 0–6 h (liters)[a]	2.8	1.7	2.0
Central venous catheter	58%	62%	51%
Vasopressor use	48%	58%	47%
ED LOS[a] (h)	NR	2.0 (1.0–3.8)	1.3 (.4–2.9)

(+/−) denote means with standard deviation; α point at which all inclusion criteria met in ProMISe include antibiotic initiation.
Abbreviation: NR, Not Reported.
[a] Median (IQR) unless otherwise noted.
[b] Percent of normotensive, usual resuscitation patients identified by lactate ≥4 mmol/l alone.
[c] Related to randomization time.

was based on the established definition of severe sepsis and septic shock[24] and lactate screening.

- o Structured screening protocol: all 3 trials had structured screening of ED patients on arrival and during the ED stay with a standardized tool. Screening tools allowed consistency among providers.
- o Lactate screening: using lactate as a component of sepsis screening was essential. Sole hyperlactatemia (lactate level >4 mmol/L) identified up to half of the eligible patients. In addition, point-of-care lactate measurement was found to be effective in further reducing time to identification.
- o Time to identification: the median or mean time to identification from ED presentation was less than 2 hours in all 3 trials (see Fig. 6, Table 6).
- Treatments provided to patients before randomization:
- o Early intravenous antibiotics: antibiotics administration before randomization was required in ARISE and ProMISe and was encouraged in ProCESS. The median time to antibiotic administration was 1 to 2 hours from ED presentation in ARISE and ProMISe and less than 3 hours in all 3 trials.
- o Early fluid administration: before randomization, usual-care patients received 2 to 3 L of fluid between the 3 trials.
- Treatments provided to usual resuscitation patients after randomization:
- o In all 3 trials, usual resuscitation patients received monitoring, investigations, and treatment, considered appropriate by the treating clinicians.
- o ED LOS: median ED LOS was 1 hour (ProMISe) to 2 hours (ARISE) before admission (see Table 5).

PATIENT IDENTIFICATION: WHAT DEFINITION SHOULD BE USED?

Representatives from 2 critical care organizations (Society of Critical Care Medicine and the European Society of Intensive Care Medicine) recently formed a task force to derive new sepsis definitions for screening and identification.[32,37,38] After completing their work, the definitions were sent to other organizations for review and endorsement. The organizations should be commended for their efforts to devise definitions that incorporate large data evaluation in conjunction with expert opinion. This set of sepsis definitions was the first to include rigorous evaluations resulting in derivation and validation of new sepsis definitions and supporting documents.[32] However, the proposed definitions have not been universally accepted.[39–41] The guidelines were not endorsed by the American College of Chest Physicians, the Infectious Disease Society of America, the American College of Emergency Physicians, or the Latin American Sepsis Institute, among others. The concerns can be categorized into 2 areas: clinical and operational.

CLINICAL
Screening

Its authors propose Quick Sequential Organ Failure Assessment (qSOFA) as a tool to screen infected patients for severe sepsis or septic shock. Infected patients with 2 or more criteria of hypotension, altered mental status, and increased respiratory rate were found to be at risk for the primary outcome of death and the secondary outcome of death with or without ICU stay of 3 days or more (Table 7).

The traditional paradigm has been to treat the sick but cast a wide net, screening for patients who may deteriorate and treat to arrest progression.[1–3,42–47] Many clinicians consider infected patients with hypotension and/or altered mental status to no longer be at risk of decline but within an active deterioration phase of organ system dysfunction and/or failure.[42,43,48,49] In the ICU, the higher level of specificity compared with sensitivity is understood. If a patient at risk for deterioration is missed, the person is still within a monitored hospital setting and ICU resources can be managed. However, misidentifying a patient at risk of decline on the floor or in the ED can result in a different outcome. The investigators show eloquently that qSOFA is associated with high risk for poor outcomes.[38] However, as its authors state, the applicability as a screening tool remains a question for prospective evaluation and further

Table 7
Comparisons of established, SEPSIS-3 definitions and SSC Guidelines application

	Established Definition (Used by CMS)	Sepsis - 3 Definition
Sepsis	Presumed/known infection + ≥2 SIRS	≥2 SOFA criteria (present or increased) Includes: hypotension + normal lactate (shock)
Severe Sepsis	Sepsis + End organ dysfunction, Lactate >4 mmol/L	Not a category
Septic shock	Sepsis + Refractory hypotension (+/− lactate)	Vasopressors AND lactate >2 mmol/L
Mortality Ratio = $\frac{\text{Observed Mortality}}{\text{Expected mortality}}$ Example	Sepsis = low acuity Observed mortality low / Expected mortality low	Sepsis = higher acuity Observed mortality higher / Expected mortality low

Mortality ratio, national quality metrics based on established definitions (expected mortality). When clinicians apply a low acuity diagnosis (sepsis) to a higher acuity patient (SEPSIS-3 definition of sepsis), the observed mortality will be higher than expected. Results in similar care appearing worse based on different definitions applied to the same patients.

discrimination of patients who currently are identified and treated who are not considered within this paradigm.

Application: Screening and Identification of Sepsis and Septic Shock

The SEPSIS-3 definitions categorize sepsis as infected patients with an increase of greater than or equal to 2 Sequential Organ Failure Assessment (SOFA) points from baseline in the ICU (area under the curve, 0.79). Outside of the ICU, it is recommended that clinicians obtain information for SOFA calculations if 2 qSOFA criteria are attained.[37] Both systems were validated in secondary databases (Table 8).

The new definitions categorize septic shock as hypotension requiring vasopressors and increased lactate level (>2 mmol/L). This combination was highly predictive of poor outcomes with an estimated mortality of 42%[32,37] (Table 9). There is concern that use of the SEPSIS-3 definitions may foster under-recognition of partially compensated septic shock phenotypes. Cryptic shock, as shown by increased lactate level alone, is a phenotype that portends a worse outcome rather than simply a bad infection. Some clinicians are concerned about patients who may be missed, especially in the early phases of care when durable long-term improvements are most possible.

It is unclear why lactate, an established indicator of critical illness,[25–31] was not retained in the qSOFA screening criteria. It is possible that hyperlactatemia is not as good an indicator of decline in septic patients as was previously considered. As its authors point out, it is also possible that the infrequent lactate evaluations may have contributed. Only 9% of infected patients from the derivation set and validation set had lactate evaluation on the day of admission. A post-hoc evaluation of qSOFA and lactate levels was done in the Kaiser Permanente Northern California health system data set, in which 57% of patients with suspected infection had lactate levels measured on the day of admission; however, only 20% had lactate level increases greater than or equal to 2 mmol/L.[38]

In ProCESS, ARISE, and ProMISe, in which lactate measurement was one of the inclusion criteria, lactate level greater than 4 mmol/L was the sole identifier in 30% to 45% of patients (see Table 6). Further, when evaluating patients across 240 ICUs across the United Kingdom, the prevalence of lactate level greater than 4 mmol/L in normotensive infected patients presenting to the ICU was 44.5%. This finding is consistent with ProCESS, ARISE, and ProMISe.

The mortality of normotensive hyperlactemic patients in the ARISE data set was 26% and in the Sepsis-3 article the prevalence for lactate level greater than 4 mmol/L was 9.9%; however, the mortality was 29.9%. The mortality for hyperlactatemia (29.9%) is equivalent to the mortality of hypotensive patients (29.7%); however, hypotension is part of the definition but lactate level is not a component until the patient has concurrent hypotension (see Table 9).

For example, consider a 55-year-old woman, absent preexisting organ dysfunction (baseline SOFA 0), who is infected from a urinary source. Initially she is normotensive and her lactate level is 5 mmol/L. She would not fit the proposed definition paradigm offered by Sepsis-3. In addition, she might not have lactate level evaluated because it is only considered in the proposed Sepsis-3 definitions if the patient is hypotensive.

If this same woman presents with hypotension (MAP of 60 mm Hg) after receiving fluids (SOFA 1), she may not be considered septic until vasopressors are initiated and not considered in septic shock until her lactate result is known, if it is increased. This patient's classification depends on clinical decisions or processes rather than clinical presentation and progression.

Table 8
Sequential [Sepsis-Related] Organ Failure Assessment Score

System	Score				
	0	1	2	3	4
Respiration					
Pao₂/Fio₂, mm Hg (kPa)	$\geq$400 (53.3)	<400 (53.3)	<300 (40)	<200 (26.7) with respiratory support	<100 (13.3) with respiratory support
Coagulation					
Platelets, × 10³/μL	$\geq$150	<150	<100	<50	<20
Liver					
Bilirubin, mg/dL (μmol/L)	<1.2 (20)	1.2–1.9 (20–32)	2.0–5.9 (33–101)	6.0–11.9 (102–204)	>12.0 (204)
Cardiovascular	MAP $\geq$70 mm Hg	MAP <70 mm Hg	Dopamine <5 or dobutamine (any dose)[a]	Dopamine 5.1–15 or epinephrine $\leq$0.1 or norepinephrine $\leq$0.1[a]	Dopamine >15 or epinephrine >0.1 or norepinephrine >0.1[a]
Central nervous system					
Glasgow Coma Scale score[b]	15	13–14	10–12	6–9	<6
Renal					
Creatinine, mg/dL (μmol/L)	<1.2 (110)	1.2–1.9 (110-170)	2.0–3.4 (171–299)	3.5–4.9 (300–440)	>5.0 (440)
Urine output, mL/d	—	—	—	<500	<200

Abbreviations: Fio₂, fraction of inspired oxygen; MAP, mean arterial pressure; Pao₂, partial pressure of oxygen.
[a] Catecholamine doses are given as μg/kg/min for at least 1 hour.
[b] Glasgow Coma Scale scores range from 3–15; higher score indicates better neurological function.
Adapted from Singer M, Deutschman CS, Seymour CW, et al. The third international consensus definitions for sepsis and septic shock (Sepsis-3). JAMA 2016;315(8):801–10.

Table 9
Hyperlactatemia and refractory hypotension: prevalence and mortality

N = 18,840	Sepsis-3 Definition Refractory Hypotension Only	Sepsis-3 Definition Lactate >2–4 mmol/L	Sepsis-3 Definition Lactate >4 mmol/L	ICNARC Lactate >4 mmol/L N = 12,004
Hyperlactatemia Only N (% total)	—	4106 out of 18,840[a] (21)	1856 out of 18,840 (9.9)	5339 out of 12,004 (44.5)
Hyperlactatemia Only Mortality N (%)	—	1086 out of 4108[a] (26.4)	555 out of 1856 (29.9)	1397 out of 5339 (26.2)
Refractory Hypotension Only[b] N (%)	4135 out of 18,840 (22.0)	—	—	2186 out of 12,004 (18.2)
Refractory Hypotension Only[b] Mortality N (%)	1226 out of 4135 (29.7)	—	—	1397 out of 5339 (26.2)
Both Refractory Hypotension and Hyperlactatemia[c] N (%)		4295 out of 18,840 (22.8)	4448 out of 18,840 (23.6)	4479 out of 12,004 (37.3)
Both Refractory Hypotension and Hyperlactatemia[c] Mortality N (%)		1498 out of 4295 (34.2)	2198 out of 4448 (49.4)	2485 out of 4479 (55.5)

Authors; ARISE data adapted from Table S22 (Mouncey et al,[3] 2015).

[a] Combined groups 4 and 5.
[b] Combined groups 2 and 6.
[c] Combined groups 1 and 3.

Adapted from Table 3 in Shankar-Hari M, Phillips GS, Levy ML, et al. Developing a new definition and assessing new clinical criteria for septic shock: for the Third International Consensus Definitions for Sepsis and Septic Shock (Sepsis-3). JAMA 2016;315(8):775–87.

If lactate assessment is only considered proposed in the Sepsis-3 definitions when combined with hypotension, will some clinicians, especially in resource-limited areas, stop looking for it before hypotension? It was reported[32,37] that hyperlactatemia in normotensive patients occurred more often than refractory hypotension alone. However, given that mortality for both was high (see Table 9), which care opportunities will be missed and how would they be affected?

Operationalization and the Law of Unintended Consequence

Clinicians using the new Sepsis-3 definition will seem to provide worse care for patients with sepsis than clinicians using the established definition. This difference may occur in any country or environment where a mortality index is used to assist with monitoring value-based care or care quality. This difference may exist despite the quality of care provided.

One method of national quality and value monitoring is the mortality index. The mortality index (MI) is the ratio of observed deaths to expected deaths.

$$MI = \frac{\text{Observed deaths}}{\text{Expected deaths}}$$

There has been no decision to date that third parties will change from using the established definitions. Centers for Medicare & Medicaid Services stated at the time of the SEP-3 definition articles release[32,37] that they had no current plans to change the definitions they were currently using. Because the established definition of sepsis has a low mortality, the expected deaths are low. In the proposed definition, patients who would normally be classified as having septic shock (hypotension plus normal or no lactate measurement) would now be classified as having sepsis. Although the observed deaths would be higher, the expected deaths (based on the established, older sepsis definition) would remain low.

For example:

$$MI = \frac{\text{Observed deaths}}{\text{Expected deaths}}$$

$$MI = \frac{\text{Infection hypotension+no/normal lactate}}{\text{Above patient "Septic shock" diagnosis}} = \frac{\text{Observed Mortality}}{\text{Expected Death 30\%+}}$$

$$MI = \frac{\text{Infection hypotension+no/normal lactate}}{\text{Above patient "Sepsis" diagnosis}} = \frac{\text{Observed Mortality}}{\text{Expected Death 15\%+}}$$

Percentages presented with the plus symbol (+) are estimates for example purposes only. Septic shock mortality is based on SSC database. Expected mortality for sepsis is based on 2016 global report.[50]

REVISED SEPSIS BUNDLE

With the publication of 3 sepsis RCTs that do not show superiority of EGDT in patients with sepsis who have received timely antibiotics and fluid resuscitation compared with controls, the Surviving Sepsis Campaign guidelines revised the sepsis bundles to the following (http://www.survivingsepsis.org/SiteCollectionDocuments/SSC_Bundle.pdf):

To be completed within 3 hours of time of presentation[a]:

1. Measure lactate level.
2. Obtain blood cultures before administration of antibiotics.
3. Administer broad-spectrum antibiotics.
4. Administer 30 mL/kg crystalloid for hypotension or lactate level greater than or equal to 4 mmol/L.

To be completed within 6 hours of time of presentation:

5. Apply vasopressors (for hypotension that does not respond to initial fluid resuscitation) to maintain an MAP greater than or equal to 65 mm Hg.
6. In the event of persistent hypotension after initial fluid administration (MAP <65 mm Hg) or if initial lactate level was greater than or equal to 4 mmol/L, reassess volume status and tissue perfusion and document findings according to Table 1.
7. Remeasure lactate if initial lactate level is increased.

Document reassessment of volume status and tissue perfusion with:

Either:

- Repeat focused examination (after initial fluid resuscitation) by licensed independent practitioner, including vital signs and cardiopulmonary, capillary refill, pulse, and skin findings.

Or 2 of the following:

- Measure CVP
- Measure $Scvo_2$
- Bedside cardiovascular ultrasonography
- Dynamic assessment of fluid responsiveness with passive leg raise or fluid challenge

[a] Time of presentation is defined as the time of triage in the ED or, if presenting from another care venue, from the earliest chart annotation consistent with all elements of severe sepsis or septic shock ascertained through chart review.

LONG-TERM RECOMMENDATIONS

1. Identification: it is suggested that it may be prudent to wait for prospective validation of the proposed Sepsis-3 definitions before universally implementing them clinically and use the established definitions currently. If clinicians or hospitals think that using the proposed definitions will facilitate patient care, they should consider using them.
2. Usual care in ProCESS, ProMISe, and ARISE for patients with severe sepsis and septic shock entailed early identification with standardized screening protocols, including lactate measurement, early fluid administration for hypotensive patients, and early antibiotic administration within 3 hours.
3. Data measurement: there should be some form of data collection and monitoring for on-going quality-assessment purposes.

SUMMARY

Usual resuscitation may have evolved over the last 15 years since the original EGDT trial. In-hospital and 90-day survival of patients receiving usual resuscitation were similar to those achieved with EGDT when they were identified early through a screening program including lactate measurement and received early intravenous fluids and antibiotics. The addition of continuous $Scvo_2$ monitoring and strict protocolization did not improve outcomes. It is unclear whether there are subpopulations that might benefit from additional treatment.

REFERENCES

1. Process Investigators, Yealy DM, Kellum JA, et al. A randomized trial of protocol-based care for early septic shock. N Engl J Med 2014;370(18):1683–93.
2. ARISE Investigators, Anzics Clinical Trials Group, Peake SL, et al. Goal-directed resuscitation for patients with early septic shock. N Engl J Med 2014;371(16): 1496–506.
3. Mouncey PR, Osborn TM, Power GS, et al. Trial of early, goal-directed resuscitation for septic shock. N Engl J Med 2015;372(14):1301–11.
4. Rivers E, Nguyen B, Havstad S, et al. Early goal-directed therapy in the treatment of severe sepsis and septic shock. N Engl J Med 2001;345(19):1368–77.
5. Salvo I, de Cian W, Musicco M, et al. The Italian SEPSIS study: preliminary results on the incidence and evolution of SIRS, sepsis, severe sepsis and septic shock. Intensive Care Med 1995;21(Suppl 2):S244–9.
6. Brun-Buisson C, Doyon F, Carlet J, et al. Incidence, risk factors, and outcome of severe sepsis and septic shock in adults. A multicenter prospective study in intensive care units. French ICU Group for Severe Sepsis. JAMA 1995;274(12):968–74.
7. Zeni F, Freeman B, Natanson C. Anti-inflammatory therapies to treat sepsis and septic shock: a reassessment. Crit Care Med 1997;25(7):1095–100.
8. Sands KE, Bates DW, Lanken PN, et al. Epidemiology of sepsis syndrome in 8 academic medical centers. JAMA 1997;278(3):234–40.
9. Angus DC, Linde-Zwirble WT, Lidicker J, et al. Epidemiology of severe sepsis in the United States: analysis of incidence, outcome, and associated costs of care. Crit Care Med 2001;29(7):1303–10.
10. Nasraway SA. Norepinephrine: no more "leave 'em dead"? Crit Care Med 2000; 28(8):3096–8.
11. Practice parameters for hemodynamic support of sepsis in adult patients in sepsis. Task force of the American College of critical care medicine, Society of critical care medicine. Crit Care Med 1999;27(3):639–60.
12. Dellinger RP, Carlet JM, Masur H, et al. Surviving Sepsis Campaign guidelines for management of severe sepsis and septic shock. Intensive Care Med 2004;30(4): 536–55.
13. Dellinger RP, Levy MM, Carlet JM, et al. Surviving Sepsis Campaign: international guidelines for management of severe sepsis and septic shock: 2008. Crit Care Med 2008;36(1):296–327.
14. Dellinger RP, Levy MM, Rhodes A, et al. Surviving Sepsis Campaign: international guidelines for management of severe sepsis and septic shock, 2012. Intensive Care Med 2013;39(2):165–228.
15. Otero RM, Nguyen HB, Huang DT, et al. Early goal-directed therapy in severe sepsis and septic shock revisited: concepts, controversies, and contemporary findings. Chest 2006;130(5):1579–95.
16. Safar P. Critical care medicine–quo vadis? Crit Care Med 1974;2(1):1–5.
17. Huang DT, Osborn TM, Gunnerson KJ, et al. Critical care medicine training and certification for emergency physicians. Ann Emerg Med 2005;46(3):217–23.
18. Wang HE, Shapiro NI, Angus DC, et al. National estimates of severe sepsis in United States emergency departments. Crit Care Med 2007;35(8):1928–36.
19. Osborn TM, Nguyen HB, Rivers EP. Emergency medicine and the Surviving Sepsis Campaign: an international approach to managing severe sepsis and septic shock. Ann Emerg Med 2005;46(3):228–31.

20. McIntyre LA, Hebert PC, Fergusson D, et al, Canadian Critical Care Trials Group. A survey of Canadian intensivists' resuscitation practices in early septic shock. Crit Care 2007;11(4):R74.

21. Sivayoham N. Management of severe sepsis and septic shock in the emergency department: a survey of current practice in emergency departments in England. Emerg Med J 2007;24(6):422.

22. ProCESS/ARISE/ProMISe Methodology Writing Committee, Huang DT, Angus DC, Barnato A, et al. Harmonizing international trials of early goal-directed resuscitation for severe sepsis and septic shock: methodology of ProCESS, ARISE, and ProMISe. Intensive Care Med 2013;39(10):1760–75.

23. Gross SD. A system of surgery. Philadelphia: 1872.

24. Bone RC, Balk RA, Cerra FB, et al. Definitions for sepsis and organ failure and guidelines for the use of innovative therapies in sepsis. The ACCP/SCCM consensus conference committee. American College of Chest Physicians/Society of Critical Care Medicine. Chest 1992;101(6):1644–55.

25. Ranzani OT, Monteiro MB, Ferreira EM, et al. Reclassifying the spectrum of septic patients using lactate: severe sepsis, cryptic shock, vasoplegic shock and dysoxic shock. Rev Bras Ter Intensiva 2013;25(4):270–8.

26. Puskarich MA, Trzeciak S, Shapiro NI, et al. Outcomes of patients undergoing early sepsis resuscitation for cryptic shock compared with overt shock. Resuscitation 2011;82(10):1289–93.

27. Singer AJ, Taylor M, Domingo A, et al. Diagnostic characteristics of a clinical screening tool in combination with measuring bedside lactate level in emergency department patients with suspected sepsis. Acad Emerg Med 2014;21(8):853–7.

28. Puskarich MA, Trzeciak S, Shapiro NI, et al. Whole blood lactate kinetics in patients undergoing quantitative resuscitation for severe sepsis and septic shock. Chest 2013;143(6):1548–53.

29. Arnold RC, Shapiro NI, Jones AE, et al. Multicenter study of early lactate clearance as a determinant of survival in patients with presumed sepsis. Shock 2009;32(1):35–9.

30. Shapiro NI, Fisher C, Donnino M, et al. The feasibility and accuracy of point-of-care lactate measurement in emergency department patients with suspected infection. J Emerg Med 2010;39(1):89–94.

31. Shapiro NI, Howell MD, Talmor D, et al. Serum lactate as a predictor of mortality in emergency department patients with infection. Ann Emerg Med 2005;45(5):524–8.

32. Shankar-Hari M, Phillips GS, Levy ML, et al. Developing a new definition and assessing new clinical criteria for septic shock: for the third international consensus definitions for sepsis and septic shock (Sepsis-3). JAMA 2016;315(8):775–87.

33. Levy MM, Dellinger RP, Townsend SR, et al. The Surviving Sepsis Campaign: results of an international guideline-based performance improvement program targeting severe sepsis. Intensive Care Med 2010;36(2):222–31.

34. Ferrer R, Martin-Loeches I, Phillips G, et al. Empiric antibiotic treatment reduces mortality in severe sepsis and septic shock from the first hour: results from a guideline-based performance improvement program. Crit Care Med 2014;42(8):1749–55.

35. Kumar A, Roberts D, Wood KE, et al. Duration of hypotension before initiation of effective antimicrobial therapy is the critical determinant of survival in human septic shock. Crit Care Med 2006;34(6):1589–96.

36. McCaig LF, Nawar EW. National hospital ambulatory medical care survey: 2004 emergency department summary. Adv Data 2006;(372):1–29.

37. Singer M, Deutschman CS, Seymour CW, et al. The third international consensus definitions for sepsis and septic shock (Sepsis-3). JAMA 2016;315(8):801–10.

38. Seymour CW, Liu VX, Iwashyna TJ, et al. Assessment of clinical criteria for sepsis: for the third international consensus definitions for sepsis and septic shock (Sepsis-3). JAMA 2016;315(8):762–74.

39. Vincent JL, Martin GS, Levy MM. qSOFA does not replace SIRS in the definition of sepsis. Crit Care 2016;20(1):210.

40. Machado FR, Salomao R, Pontes de Acevedo LC, et al. Latin American Sepsis Institute (LASI). Why LASI did not endorse the new definitions of sepsis published today in JAMA 2016. Available at: http://ilas.org.br/assets/arquivos/upload/declaracao%20sepse%203.0%20ILAS%20-%20English%20version.pdf. Accessed October 10, 2016.

41. Simpson SQ. New sepsis criteria: a change we should not make. Chest 2016; 149(5):1117–8.

42. Levy MM, Rhodes A, Phillips GS, et al. Surviving Sepsis Campaign: association between performance metrics and outcomes in a 7.5-year study. Crit Care Med 2015;43(1):3–12.

43. Dellinger RP, Levy MM, Rhodes A, et al. Surviving Sepsis Campaign: international guidelines for management of severe sepsis and septic shock: 2012. Crit Care Med 2013;41(2):580–637.

44. Levy MM, Artigas A, Phillips GS, et al. Outcomes of the Surviving Sepsis Campaign in intensive care units in the USA and Europe: a prospective cohort study. Lancet Infect Dis 2012;12(12):919–24.

45. Levy MM, Dellinger RP, Townsend SR, et al. The Surviving Sepsis Campaign: results of an international guideline-based performance improvement program targeting severe sepsis. Crit Care Med 2010;38(2):367–74.

46. Dellinger RP, Levy MM, Carlet JM, et al. Surviving Sepsis Campaign: international guidelines for management of severe sepsis and septic shock: 2008. Intensive Care Med 2008;34(1):17–60.

47. Dellinger RP, Carlet JM, Masur H, et al. Surviving Sepsis Campaign guidelines for management of severe sepsis and septic shock. Crit Care Med 2004;32(3): 858–73.

48. Osborn TM, Phillips G, Lemeshow S, et al. Sepsis severity score: an internationally derived scoring system from the Surviving Sepsis Campaign database*. Crit Care Med 2014;42(9):1969–76.

49. Marshall JC, Cook DJ, Christou NV, et al. Multiple organ dysfunction score: a reliable descriptor of a complex clinical outcome. Crit Care Med 1995;23(10): 1638–52.

50. Fleischmann C, Scherag A, Adhikari NK, et al. Assessment of global incidence and mortality of hospital-treated sepsis. Current estimates and limitations. Am J Respir Crit Care Med 2016;193(3):259–72.

51. Nguyen HB, Jaehne AK, Jayaprakash N, et al. Early goal-directed therapy in severe sepsis and septic shock: insights and comparisons to ProCESS, ProMISe, and ARISE. Crit Care 2016;20(1):160.

Anemia and Red Blood Cell Transfusion

Advances in Critical Care

Lena M. Napolitano, MD, FCCP, MCCM

KEYWORDS

- Anemia • Red blood cell transfusion • Transfusion • Blood transfusion • Hemoglobin
- Critical care • Critically ill

KEY POINTS

- Anemia is common in all critically ill patients and is due to anemia of inflammation (high hepcidin levels resulting in iron-restricted erythropoiesis) and low erythropoietin (EPO) levels.
- A new hormone (erythroferrone) has been identified, which mediates hepcidin suppression to allow increased iron absorption and mobilization from iron stores.
- In general, in critically ill patients and those with severe sepsis and septic shock, a restrictive strategy (consider red blood cell [RBC] transfusion when hemoglobin [Hb] ≤7 g/dL) is recommended; in patients with acute coronary syndrome, consider RBC transfusion when Hb ≤8 g/dL.
- The decision to transfuse RBCs should not be solely based on the hemoglobin level and should include clinical factors and patient preferences with use of a Patient Blood Management approach.
- All strategies to prevent anemia in the intensive care unit (decreased phlebotomy, low volume sampling tubes, medical treatment of anemia) should be implemented.

INTRODUCTION

Anemia is common in the intensive care unit (ICU), resulting in frequent administration of red blood cell (RBC) transfusions. Significant advances have been made in understanding the pathophysiology of anemia in the ICU that will be reviewed. Most studies document that approximately 30% to 50% of patients receive RBC transfusions while in the ICU with an average of 5 units transfused during their ICU stay.[1–9] Higher RBC transfusion rates are reported in burn patients.[10] RBC transfusions are most commonly administered to ICU patients with anemia, and not bleeding. Several recent

Disclosure: The author has nothing to disclose; no conflicts of interest.

Division of Acute Care Surgery [Trauma, Burns, Critical Care, Emergency Surgery], Department of Surgery, University of Michigan Health System, University Hospital, Room 1C340-UH, 1500 East Medical Drive, SPC 5033, Ann Arbor, MI 48109-5033, USA

E-mail address: lenan@umich.edu

randomized controlled trials (RCTs) have providing increased evidence regarding the safety of restrictive RBC transfusion strategies in ICU patients, and this review summarizes the findings of these important studies. ICUs with evidence-based restrictive transfusion protocols significantly reduced the risk of transfusion in ICU patients controlling for patient and ICU factors, confirming the effectiveness of restrictive transfusion protocols.[11]

Anemia in the Intensive Care Unit: Pathophysiology

The pathophysiology of anemia in critical illness is consistent with an "anemia of chronic disease" and "anemia of inflammation."[12] Anemia in ICU patients is the result of 3 main abnormalities related to the host inflammatory response: (1) dysregulation of iron homeostasis due to increased hepcidin concentrations; (2) impaired proliferation of erythroid progenitor cells; and (3) blunted erythropoietin response. Hepcidin is the master regulator of iron homeostasis. Increased hepcidin concentrations reduce iron availability via 2 mechanisms: (1) internalization and destruction of the iron-exporting protein ferroportin, which in turn leads to an inability to export iron out cells, locking iron primarily in macrophages of the reticuloendothelial system (RES); and (2) decreased absorption of iron through the gastrointestinal tract (**Fig. 1**).[13] High hepcidin concentrations result in a state of functional iron deficiency.[14]

Reduced production of erythropoietin and a blunted response of the bone marrow to erythropoietin further contribute to anemia in critically ill patients (**Fig. 2**). A new hormone (erythroferrone, ERFE) has been identified, which mediates hepcidin suppression to allow increased iron absorption and mobilization from iron stores.

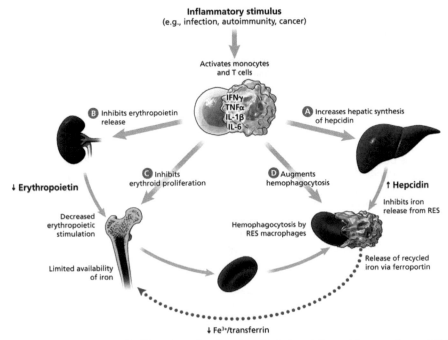

Fig. 1. Anemia in critically ill patients is related to high hepcidin and low erythropoietin levels. IFNγ, interferon γ; IL-1β, interleukin-1β; IL-6, interleukin-6; TNFα, tumor necrosis factor α. (*From* Zarychanski R, Houston DS. Anemia of chronic disease: a harmful disorder or an adaptive, beneficial response? CMAJ 2008;179;333–7.)

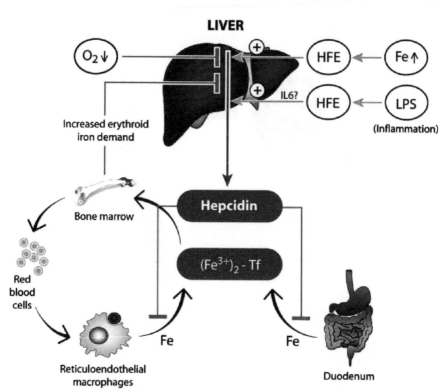

Fig. 2. Increased hepcidin serum concentrations are responsible for anemia in the ICU, resulting in iron-restricted erythropoiesis by blocking iron absorption from the gastrointestinal tract, and blocking iron release from the reticuloendothelial system. HFE protein, human hemochromatosis protein; LPS, lipopolysaccharide.

ERFE is produced by erythroblasts in response to erythropoiesis-stimulating agent (ESA) treatment and is responsible in part for decreased hepcidin expression (Fig. 3).[15]

Both anemia and RBC transfusion are associated with risk in critically ill patients.[16] However, it is not clear that RBC transfusion mitigates the risk of anemia in critically ill patients. Furthermore, ICU patients are heterogenous and may respond differently to both anemia and RBC transfusion.[17] Finally, the efficacy of RBC transfusion in the critically ill is in question, particularly whether oxygen delivery will be improved by RBC transfusion.[18–20]

Prevention of Anemia in the Intensive Care Unit

Multiple strategies can be implemented to prevent anemia in the ICU, most related to blood conservation.[21] Given the significant risks associated with RBC transfusion treatment of anemia, all of the following strategies should be implemented in ICU patients to prevent anemia in the ICU.

- Reduction in phlebotomy for diagnostic laboratory testing, which can account for 40% of RBC transfusion requirements[22,23]
- Use of pediatric or low-volume adult blood sampling tubes instead of conventional tubes[24,25]

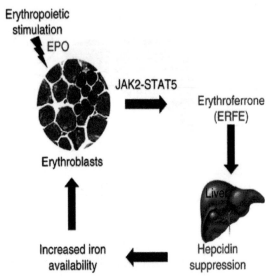

Fig. 3. ERFE is a new hormone and erythroid regulator that has been identified. ERFE suppresses the hepatic synthesis of the principal iron-regulatory protein hepcidin, resulting in increased iron uptake. ERFE production by erythroblasts is greatly increased when RBC synthesis is stimulated, such as after bleeding, or in response to anemia. In normal volunteers, erythropoietin administration was sufficient to profoundly lower serum hepcidin levels in less than a day without any significant changes in serum iron concentrations, and its action was presumed to be mediated via ERFE. (*Reprinted by permission from* Macmillan Publishers Ltd: Kautz L, Jung G, Valore EV, et al. Identification of erythroferrone as an erythroid regulator of iron metabolism. Nat Genet 2014;46(7):678–84. Copyright © 2014.)

- Use of in-line closed blood conservation devices on arterial and central lines for reinfusion of waste blood, which was associated with reduced blood loss, reduced RBC transfusions, and even decreased mortality[26–29]
- Cell salvage during surgical procedures, which is effective in reducing RBC transfusion requirements (21% absolute risk reduction) in adult elective cardiac and orthopedic surgery[30]

Anemia Treatment in the Intensive Care Unit

Erythropoiesis-stimulating agents

ESAs are indicated for treatment of critically ill patients with chronic kidney disease.[31] However, ESAs are not currently recommended for treatment of anemia in critically ill patients because multiple RCTs did not confirm a reduction in RBC transfusions.[32–36] However, only one study administered intravenous (IV) iron in association with ESA, so treatment failure may have been related to inadequate iron supplementation in these studies.

In contrast to general critical care patients, ESA use in trauma critically ill patients was associated with significantly increased survival in 2 large RCTs.[37] A recent meta-analysis and systematic review documented that the administration of ESAs to critically ill trauma patients was associated with a significant improvement in mortality without an increase in the rate of lower limb proximal deep venous thrombosis.[38] Additional clinical trials are warranted to confirm these important findings.[39]

Iron supplementation

A recent meta-analysis of 5 RCTs of iron supplementation (4 IV iron, 1 oral [PO] iron) in adult critical care with 665 patients found no difference in RBC transfusion rates or hemoglobin (Hb). There was also no difference in secondary outcomes of mortality, in-hospital infection, or length of stay. However, there is considerable heterogeneity between trials in study design, interventions, and outcomes.[40]

Additional studies demonstrate conflicting results. A study of 200 anemic surgical ICU patients compared PO iron to placebo and confirmed less RBC transfusions in the iron group, and no difference in infection rates.[41] A double-blind RCT of 150 anemic trauma patients compared IV iron sucrose (100 mg 3 times per week) to placebo and confirmed 40% of patients had iron-deficient erythropoiesis. However, there was no impact of iron therapy on hemoglobin, RBC transfusion rate, or infection.[42]

Most recently, the IRONMAN trial compared IV iron (500 mg ferric carboxymaltose, FCM) to placebo in 140 critically ill patients (86% surgical ICU patients). Patients received up to 4 doses if Hb was less than 10 g/dL, ferritin was less than 1200 ng/mL, and TSAT was less than 50%, but in the study, only 15 patients received 2 doses, and only 2 patients received 3 doses. The iron group received less RBC units (97 versus 136; 95% confidence interval, CI [0.43–1.18], $P = .19$), but was not statistically significant. Median Hb at hospital discharge was significantly higher in the IV iron group (10.7 vs 10.0 g/dL, $P = .02$). There was no significant difference between the groups in any safety outcome.[43]

However, it should be noted that the IV iron FCM dose in the IRONMAN trial (and in all prior iron ICU anemia trials) was substantially lower than in the REPAIR-IDA trial of IV iron to treat iron-deficiency anemia in non–dialysis-dependent chronic kidney disease. In the REPAIR-IDA study, 1500 mg of FCM was compared with 1000 mg of iron sucrose, and the mean hemoglobin increase was higher with FCM (1.13 g/dL in FCM group vs 0.92 g/dL in the iron sucrose group; 95% CI, 0.13–0.28).[44]

Additional well-designed trials are needed to investigate the optimal iron-dosing regimens in ICU patients and strategies to identify which patients are most likely to benefit from iron, together with patient-focused outcomes.

Nutritional and vitamin supplementation

Nutritional and vitamin deficiency as a cause of anemia in the ICU is uncommon. In one study, only 2% of ICU patients had vitamin B12 deficiency and another 2% had folate deficiency.[45] These deficiencies should be evaluated as a cause of anemia in ICU patients, and appropriately treated if identified.

Antihepcidin strategies

Erythropoietin stimulation via ESA treatment results in decreased hepcidin expression.[39,46] Additional antihepcidin strategies are now being studied in clinical trials for anemia treatment and are an exciting potential for the treatment of anemia in ICU patients.[47,48]

Patient Blood Management in the Intensive Care Unit

Patient blood management (PBM) is defined as "the timely application of evidence-based medical and surgical concepts designed to maintain hemoglobin concentration, optimize hemostasis and minimize blood loss in an effort to improve patient outcome."[49] PBM is a comprehensive concept that seeks to optimize the utilization of blood components to improve patient safety and outcome.

There is robust scientific evidence for PBM with a focus on the increasing evidence for restrictive rather than liberal transfusion practice and the use of electronic blood ordering and decision support to facilitate its implementation.[50] PBM includes 3 strategies: (1) anemia management; (2) blood conservation; and (3) appropriate blood use through implementation of evidence-based transfusion guidelines. PBM programs have achieved significant reductions in RBC utilization with associated improved patient outcomes.[51–57] The PBM Guidelines for Critical Care established in Australia are an excellent evidence-based resource.[58]

The Joint Commission Blood Management Performance Measures

From 2007 to 2010, The Joint Commission developed a set of Blood Management Performance Measures. They are currently developing a new set of PBM performance measures that update the previous measure set and are derived exclusively from electronic health records (ePBM).[59] At present, there is a set of 5 draft candidate performance measures that are being tested by volunteer hospitals, with one related to PBM:

- ePBM-01: Preoperative Anemia Screening, Selected Elective Surgical Patients
- ePBM-02: Preoperative Hemoglobin Level, Selected Elective Surgical Patients
- ePBM-03: Preoperative Type and Crossmatch, Type and Screen, Selected Elective Surgical Patients
- ePBM-04: Initial Transfusion Threshold
- ePBM-05: Outcome of Patient Blood Management, Selected Elective Surgical Patients

Red Blood Cell Transfusion Risks

Increasing high-quality evidence is now available linking increased risk of nosocomial infection with RBC transfusions. A systematic review and meta-analysis of 18 RCTs with 7593 patients with restrictive versus liberal RBC transfusion strategies were examined to evaluate whether RBC transfusion thresholds are associated with the risk of health care–associated infection (pneumonia, mediastinitis, wound infection, and sepsis) and whether risk was independent of leukocyte reduction.[60]

The pooled risk of all serious infections was 11.8% (95% CI, 7.0%-16.7%) in the restrictive group and 16.9% (95% CI, 8.9%-25.4%) in the liberal group. The number needed to treat with restrictive strategies to prevent serious infection was 38 (95% CI, 24–122). Implementing restrictive RBC transfusion strategies in the ICU therefore has the potential to lower the incidence of health care-associated infection.

Red Blood Cell Transfusion Thresholds

Clinical practice guidelines recommend a restrictive RBC transfusion practice (consider RBC transfusion if Hb <7 g/dL) in the ICU, with the goal of minimizing exposure to allogeneic blood.[61,62] There is current evidence supporting a higher hemoglobin trigger (consider RBC transfusion if Hb <8 g/dL) for some specific patient populations (Fig. 4).

General critically ill patient

There is increasing level 1 evidence from prospective randomized trials that restrictive blood transfusion strategies are associated with decreased mortality and improved outcomes in general critically ill patients. A recent systematic review and meta-analysis included pooled results from 3 trials (1966–2013) with 2364 participants.[63] They reported that a restrictive Hb transfusion trigger of less than 7 g/dL resulted in significantly improved outcomes compared with a more liberal strategy (Table 1). The number needed to treat with a restrictive strategy to prevent 1 death was 33. Pooled data from randomized trials with less restrictive transfusion strategies (Hb >7 g/dL) showed no significant effect on outcomes. They concluded that in

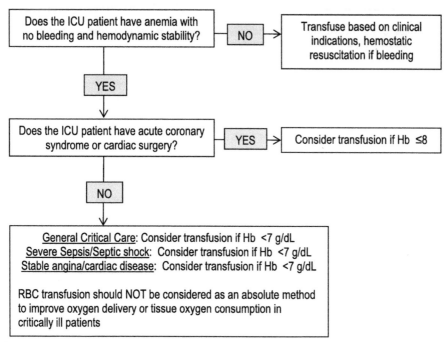

Fig. 4. RBC transfusion management of ICU patients with anemia.

patients with critical illness or bleed, restricting blood transfusions by using an Hb trigger of less than 7 g/dL significantly reduced cardiac events, rebleeding, bacterial infections, and total mortality.

A *Cochrane Database Systematic Review* compared clinical outcomes with restrictive versus liberal transfusion thresholds (triggers) in 19 trials with 6264 randomized patients.[64] Restrictive transfusion strategies reduced the risk of receiving an RBC transfusion by 39% (risk ratio [RR] 0.61, 95% CI 0.52–0.72), which equated to an average absolute risk reduction of 34% (95% CI 24% to 45%). The volume of RBCs transfused was reduced on average by 1.19 units (95% CI 0.53–1.85 units). However, heterogeneity between trials was statistically significant ($P<.00001$; $I^{(2)} \geq 93\%$) for these outcomes. Restrictive transfusion strategies did not appear to impact the rate of adverse events compared with liberal transfusion strategies (ie, mortality, cardiac events, myocardial infarction, stroke, pneumonia, and thromboembolism). Restrictive transfusion strategies were associated with a statistically significant reduction in hospital mortality (RR 0.77, 95% CI 0.62–0.95) but not 30-day mortality (RR 0.85, 95% CI 0.70–1.03). The use of restrictive transfusion strategies did not reduce functional recovery, hospital, or intensive care length of stay. The existing evidence supports the use of restrictive transfusion triggers in most patients, including those with pre-existing cardiovascular disease.[65]

An updated systematic review with trial sequential analysis included 31 trials that compared restrictive versus liberal transfusion strategy in adults or children and included 9813 randomized patients.[66] Restrictive transfusion strategies were associated with a reduced RBC unit transfused and number of patients transfused, but mortality, overall morbidity, and myocardial infarction were unaltered (**Figs. 5** and **6**). Similarly, a review of 7 RCTs with 5,566 high-risk patients compared restrictive versus liberal transfusion strategy, confirming noninferiority, safety, and a significant reduction

Table 1
Outcomes for Restrictive Transfusion Strategy (hemoglobin transfusion trigger <7 g/dL), compared with Liberal Transfusion Strategy

Outcome	Trials	Patients	RR or MD	RD	No. Needed to Treat
Mortality					
Hospital mortality	2	1727	RR, 0.74 (CI, 0.60–0.92)	RD, −0.04 (CI, −0.04 to −0.00)	25
30-d mortality	3	2364	RR, 0.81 (CI, 0.61–0.96)	RD, −0.02 (CI, −0.04 to −0.00)	50
Total mortality	3	2364	RR, 0.80 (CI, 0.65–0.98)	RD, −0.03 (CI, −0.05 to −0.00)	33
Cardiac events					
Acute coronary syndrome	2	1727	RR, 0.44 (CI, 0.22–0.89)	RD, −0.02 (CI, −0.03 to −0.00)	50
Pulmonary edema	3	2364	RR, 0.48 (CI, 0.33–0.73)	RD, −0.03 (CI, −0.05 to −0.01)	33
Other outcomes					
Rebleeding	1	889	RR, 0.64 (CI, 0.45–0.90)	RD, −0.06 (CI, −0.10 to −0.01)	17
Bacterial infections	3	2364	RR, 0.86 (CI, 0.73–1.00)	RD, −0.03 (CI, −0.06 to −0.00)	33
Blood transfusions					
Patients exposed to blood	3	2364	RR, 0.57 (CI, 0.46–0.70)	RD, −0.41 (CI, −0.52 to −0.29)	2
Units transfused per patient	3	2364	MD −1.98 (CI, −3.22 to −0.74)	—	—

Abbreviations: MD, mean difference; RD, risk difference.
From Salpeter SR, Buckley JS, Chatterjee S. Impact of more restrictive blood transfusion strategies on clinical outcomes: a meta-analysis and systematic review. Am J Med 2014;127:124–31.

in RBC transfusions in the restrictive group.[67] Restrictive transfusion strategies were safe and liberal transfusion strategies were not shown to convey any benefit to patients.

Trauma critically ill patient

The resuscitation of patients with traumatic hemorrhagic shock requires the use of damage control resuscitation with minimization of crystalloid, permissive hypotension, transfusion of a balanced ratio of blood products, and goal-directed correction of coagulopathy, covered in detail in a recent publication.[68] Once blood product resuscitation for hemorrhagic shock is complete and hemorrhage control is achieved, then all current data support a restrictive RBC transfusion strategy.[69] This restrictive RBC transfusion strategy was used as the clinical standard operating procedure to guide RBC transfusion after the immediate resuscitation phase (acute hemorrhage has been controlled, initial resuscitation is complete, patient is stable in ICU without ongoing bleeding) and to minimize the adverse consequences of potentially unnecessary RBC transfusions.[70]

Severe sepsis and septic shock

RBC transfusions are frequently administered to patients with severe sepsis and septic shock related to previous guideline recommendations to transfuse for Hb <10 g/dL

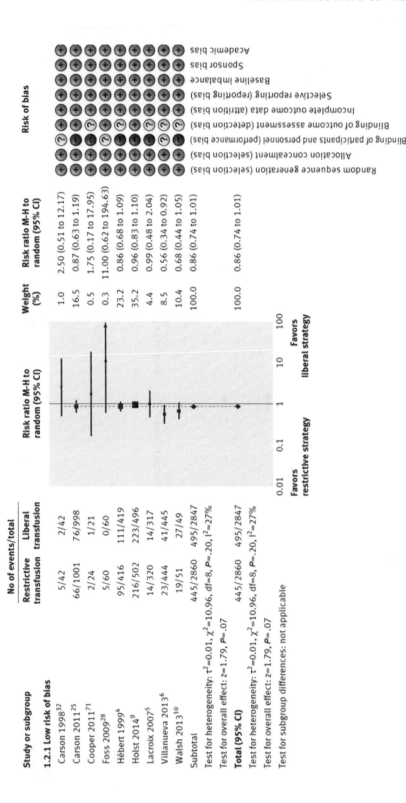

	Risk of bias								
Academic bias	+	+	+	+	+	+	+	+	+
Sponsor bias	+	+	+	+	+	+	+	+	+
Baseline imbalance	+	+	+	+	+	+	+	+	+
Selective reporting (reporting bias)	+	+	+	+	+	+	+	+	+
Incomplete outcome data (attrition bias)	+	+	+	+	+	+	+	+	+
Blinding of outcome assessment (detection bias)	+	+	?	+	?	+	?	?	?
Blinding of participants and personnel (performance bias)	?	●	●	?	●	●	●	?	●
Allocation concealment (selection bias)	+	+	+	+	+	+	+	+	+
Random sequence generation (selection bias)	+	+	+	+	+	+	+	+	+

Study or subgroup	No of events/total		Risk ratio M-H to random (95% CI)	Weight (%)	Risk ratio M-H to random (95% CI)
	Restrictive transfusion	Liberal transfusion			
1.2.1 Low risk of bias					
Carson 1998[32]	5/42	2/42		1.0	2.50 (0.51 to 12.17)
Carson 2011[25]	66/1001	76/998		16.5	0.87 (0.63 to 1.19)
Cooper 2011[71]	2/24	1/21		0.5	1.75 (0.17 to 17.95)
Foss 2009[28]	5/60	0/60		0.3	11.00 (0.62 to 194.63)
Hébert 1999[4]	95/416	111/419		23.2	0.86 (0.68 to 1.09)
Holst 2014[9]	216/502	223/496		35.2	0.96 (0.83 to 1.10)
Lacroix 2007[5]	14/320	14/317		4.4	0.99 (0.48 to 2.04)
Villanueva 2013[6]	23/444	41/445		8.5	0.56 (0.34 to 0.92)
Walsh 2013[10]	19/51	27/49		10.4	0.68 (0.44 to 1.05)
Subtotal	445/2860	495/2847		100.0	0.86 (0.74 to 1.01)
Test for heterogeneity: τ^2=0.01, χ^2=10.96, df=8, P=.20, I^2=27%					
Test for overall effect: z=1.79, P=.07					
Total (95% CI)	445/2860	495/2847		100.0	0.86 (0.74 to 1.01)
Test for heterogeneity: τ^2=0.01, χ^2=10.96, df=8, P=.20, I^2=27%					
Test for overall effect: z=1.79, P=.07					
Test for subgroup differences: not applicable					

Fig. 5. Forest plot of mortality in lower risk of bias trials. Size of squares for risk ratio reflects weight of trial in pooled analysis. Horizontal bars represent 95% CIs. M-H, mantel haenszel. (*From* Holst LB, Petersen MW, Haase N, et al. Restrictive versus liberal transfusion strategy for red blood cell transfusion: systematic review of randomised trials with meta-analysis and trial sequential analysis. BMJ 2015;350:h1354; with permission.)

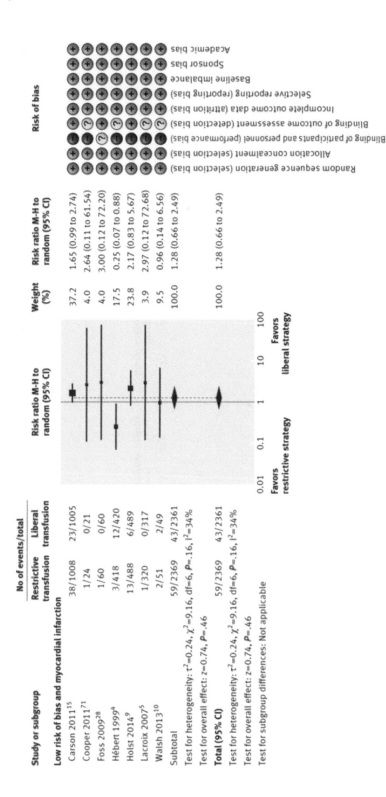

Fig. 6. Forest plot of myocardial infarctions in lower risk of bias trials. Size of squares for risk ratio reflects weight of trial in pooled analysis. Horizontal bars represent 95% CIs. (*From* Holst LB, Petersen MW, Haase N, et al. Restrictive versus liberal transfusion strategy for red blood cell transfusion: systematic review of randomised trials with meta-analysis and trial sequential analysis. BMJ 2015;350:h1354; with permission.)

in the early goal-directed therapy (EGDT) algorithm.[71] However, studies have documented that RBC transfusions may not be associated with improved cellular oxygenation or improved central venous oxygen saturation.[72-76]

The recent Transfusion Requirements in Septic Shock (TRISS) trial (n = 998) randomized ICU septic shock patients with an Hb of 9 g/dL or less to receive 1 unit of leukoreduced RBCs when the Hb level was 7 g/dL or less (lower threshold) or 9 g/dL (higher threshold) during the ICU stay. In the ICU, the lower-threshold group received a median of 1 unit of blood (interquartile range [IQR], 0–3) and the higher-threshold group received a median of 4 units (IQR, 2–7). No differences in 90-day mortality (43.0% vs 45.0%, RR 0.94; 95% CI 0.78–1.09; $P = .44$), or secondary outcomes (ischemic events, life support use), were identified in septic shock patients randomized to receive transfusion if Hb was less than 7 or 9 g/dL.[77] Subgroup analyses also confirmed no survival benefit in any subgroup with a hemoglobin threshold of 9 g/dL.[78] Long-term mortalities and health-related quality of life also did not differ between the 2 study cohorts.[79]

Three additional large multicenter RCTs documented no outcome benefit to higher RBC transfusion threshold in management of severe sepsis and septic shock patients (ProCESS, ARISE, and ProMISe) as part of EGDT, protocol-based care, or usual care.

In the *ProCESS* study (n = 1341), 3 different therapeutic strategies (EGDT [Hb trigger10 g/dL] versus protocol-based therapy [Hb trigger 8 g/dL] versus usual care) were compared, and no difference in the primary end point (60-day mortality) was found. Significantly more patients in the EGDT group than in the protocol-based or the usual-care group received RBC transfusions (14.4% vs 8.3% and 7.5%, respectively; $P = .001$) with no improvement in outcomes.[80]

The ARISE trial (n = 1600) randomized patients to EGDT (Hb trigger 10 g/dL) or usual care. No mortality or outcome differences were identified. Significantly more patients received RBC transfusions in the EGDT group compared with usual care (13.6% vs 7.0%, $P<.001$).[81]

The ProMISe trial (n = 1260) included randomized patients to EGDT (Hb trigger 10 g/dL) or usual care. No mortality or outcome differences were identified. Higher rates of RBC transfusions were confirmed in the EGDT group (8.8% of patients in EGDT vs 3.8% in usual care). However, interestingly, lower median volume of RBC transfusion was noted in the EGDT group (309, IQR 285–577 EGDT vs 535, IQR 305–607 in usual care group).[82]

These 3 studies are limited in that the specific indication for RBC transfusion was not identified. In contrast, the TRISS trial specifically compared lower versus higher RBC transfusion triggers in severe sepsis and septic shock.

Acute respiratory failure requiring mechanical ventilation
RBC transfusion practices are widely variable in patients receiving mechanical ventilation.[83] No studies to date have reported that increased RBC transfusion is associated with improved outcomes in mechanically ventilated patients. A post hoc subgroup analysis of the TRICC trial did not demonstrate differences in mortality for patients who required mechanical ventilation.[84]

The RELIEVE (Restrictive vs liberal transfusion strategies for older mechanically ventilated critically ill patients) trial compared restrictive or liberal blood transfusion strategies used to treat anemic (Hb ≤9 g/dL) critically ill patients of age 55 years and older requiring 4 days or more of mechanical ventilation in ICU. This parallel-group multicenter RCT enrolled patients (n = 100) in 6 ICUs in the United Kingdom (8/2009 to 12/2010) and randomized to a restrictive (Hb trigger, 7 g/dL; target,

7–9 g/dL) or liberal (9 g/dL; target, 9–11 g/dL) transfusion strategy for 14 days or the remainder of ICU stay, whichever was longest.

Mortality at 180 days was higher in the liberal (55%) than in the restrictive group (37%): RR 0.68 (95% CI, 0.44–1.05; $P = .073$). This trend remained in a survival model adjusted for age, gender, ischemic heart disease, Acute Physiology and Chronic Health Evaluation II score, and total nonneurologic Sequential Organ Failure Assessment score at baseline (hazard ratio, 0.54 [95% CI, 0.28–1.03]; $P = .061$).

The RELIEVE trial demonstrated an unexpectedly large difference in mortality at 180 days favoring the restrictive transfusion strategy.[85] These data support the importance of the need for a large RCT to further clarify the risk versus benefit of RBC transfusions in older mechanically ventilated critically ill patients.

Acute coronary syndrome

Anemia is common during acute myocardial infarction, persists after discharge, and is associated with higher in-hospital and long-term mortality.[86–89] Observational studies have explored the clinical consequences of anemia and RBC transfusion in patients with acute coronary syndromes or acute myocardial infarction with diverse findings.[90–95]

A meta-analysis of 10 studies (203,665 participants) confirmed that RBC transfusion was associated with increased all-cause mortality (RR 2.91; 95% CI, 2.46–3.44) and increased risk of subsequent myocardial infarction (RR 2.04; 95% CI, 1.06–3.93).[96] Multivariate metaregression confirmed that the mortality increase was independent of baseline Hb, nadir Hb, or change in Hb level during the hospital stay. The accompanying editorial and additional publications review the significant limitations in interpreting these observational studies.[97,98]

Two small pilot RCTs compared liberal versus restrictive transfusion strategies in patients with acute myocardial infarction or symptomatic cardiac disease. The CRIT randomized pilot study compared a liberal (hematocrit <30%) or restrictive RBC transfusion strategy (hematocrit <24%) in 45 patients with acute myocardial infarction and anemia (hematocrit ≤30%) and reported worse clinical outcomes (in-hospital death, recurrent myocardial infarction, or new/worsening congestive heart failure) with the liberal strategy (38% vs 13%, $P = .046$).[99]

The Myocardial Ischemia and Transfusion pilot trial enrolled 110 patients with acute coronary syndrome or stable angina undergoing cardiac catheterization and anemia (Hb <10 g/dL) and compared a transfusion threshold of less than 10 g/dL versus 8 g/dL. The predefined primary outcome was the composite of death, myocardial infarction, or unscheduled revascularization 30 days after randomization. The primary outcome occurred in 6 patients (10.9%) in the liberal group and 14 patients (25.5%) in the restrictive group (risk difference 15.0%; 95% CI 0.7%–29.3%; $P = .054$ and adjusted for age $P = .076$).[100]

A definitive trial of RBC transfusion in patients with acute coronary syndromes is needed to establish the optimal transfusion threshold. At this point, based on the data available, an Hb threshold less than 8.0 g/dL is likely safe for patients with acute coronary syndrome or acute myocardial infarction, although transfusion decisions should be individualized.

Cardiovascular disease

In a subgroup analysis of 357 critically patients with cardiovascular disease from the TRICC trial, overall mortality was comparable in the liberal transfusion group (Hb threshold 10 g/dL) and the restrictive transfusion group (Hb threshold 7.0 g/dL).[101] Changes in multiple organ dysfunction from baseline scores were significantly less in the restrictive transfusion group overall (0.2 ± 4.2 vs 1.3 ± 4.4; P = .02). In 257 patients with severe ischemic heart disease, there were no statistically significant differences in all survival measures, but this was the only subgroup wherein the restrictive group had lower but nonsignificant absolute survival rates.

The Transfusion Trigger Trial for Functional Outcomes in Cardiovascular Patients Undergoing Surgical Hip Fracture Repair (FOCUS) trial compared a liberal (Hb <10 g/dL) with a restrictive transfusion strategy (Hb <8 g/dL or symptoms) in 2016 patients more than 50 years of age with a history or risk factors for cardiovascular disease undergoing hip fracture repair.[102] No differences were identified between the 2 groups for measures of functional outcome (ability to walk independently at 60 days; 35.2% liberal vs 34.7% restrictive), in-hospital acute coronary syndrome or death (4.3% liberal vs 5.2% restrictive), or 60-day mortality (7.6% liberal vs 6.6% restrictive). In a subsequent study of long-term outcome (median 3.1 years) of the FOCUS participants, long-term mortality did not differ between the groups (43.2% liberal vs 40.8% restrictive; hazard ratio 1.09 [95% CI 0.95–1.25]; P = .21) nor were there any differences in cause of death.[103] These study results confirm that patients with stable cardiac disease can tolerate Hb levels between 7 and 8 g/dL.

Cardiac surgery

There are 2 recent large RCTs in cardiac surgery. The Transfusion Requirements After Cardiac Surgery (TRACS) study compared a liberal (hematocrit ≥30%) versus restrictive strategy (hematocrit ≥24%) in patients (n = 502) undergoing elective cardiac surgery.[104] There was no difference in the restrictive (11%) versus liberal (10%) strategy for the composite end point of 30-day all-cause mortality and severe morbidity (cardiogenic shock, acute respiratory distress syndrome, or acute renal injury requiring dialysis or hemofiltration) occurring during the hospital stay. The mean Hb concentration was 10.5 g/dL in the liberal group and 9.1 g/dL in the restrictive group.

A substudy of the TRACS trial compared outcomes based on age (≥60 vs <60 years). No outcome differences were identified in older patients (11.9% liberal vs 16.8% restrictive; P = .254) or patients less than 60 years (6.8% liberal vs 5.6% restrictive; P = .714). In older patients, cardiogenic shock was more frequent in the restrictive group (12.8% vs 5.2%, P = .31), but 30-day mortality, acute respiratory distress syndrome, and acute renal injury were no different in both age groups.[105]

The largest cardiac surgery trial is the TITRe 2 Trial (n = 2007).[106] This multicenter RCT compared a liberal (Hb <9.0 g/dL) versus restrictive transfusion threshold (Hb <7.5 g/dL). The primary outcome was serious infection (sepsis or wound infection) or ischemic event (stroke, myocardial infarction, gut infarct, acute kidney injury). There was no difference between the restrictive and liberal groups in the primary outcome, 35.1% versus 33% (OR 1.11, 95% CI, 0.91–1.34, P = .30). However, there were more deaths in the restrictive group at 90 days (4.2% vs 2.6%, hazard ratio 1.64, 95% CI, 1.00–2.67, P = .045), which was a secondary outcome. Independent of transfusion strategy, the number of transfused RBC units was an independent risk factor for clinical complications or death at 30 days (hazard ratio for each additional unit transfused, 1.2 [95% CI, 1.1–1.4]; P = .002).

These data support the use of a restrictive threshold (Hb <8.0 g/dL) for elective cardiac surgery patients. The Transfusion Requirements in Cardiac Surgery III (NCT02042898) trial, an international multicenter open-label RCT comparing liberal (Hb <9.5 g/dL) and restrictive (Hb <7.5 g/dL) transfusion strategies in high-risk patients having cardiac surgery, is recruiting patients. The primary outcome measure is a composite score of (1) all-cause mortality; (2) myocardial infarction; (3) new renal failure requiring dialysis; or (4) new focal neurologic deficit. The results of this clinical trial should be able to address the concerns raised by the secondary analysis in TITRe 2.

REFERENCES

1. Vincent JL, Baron JF, Reinhart K, et al, ABC (Anemia and Blood Transfusion in Critical Care) Investigators. Anemia and blood transfusion in critically ill patients. JAMA 2002;288:1499–507.
2. Vincent JL, Sakr Y, Sprung C, et al. Are blood transfusion associated with greater mortality rates? Results of the sepsis occurrence in acutely ill patients (SOAP) study. Anesthesiology 2008;108:31–9.
3. Corwin HL, Gettinger A, Pearl RG, et al. The CRIT Study: anemia and blood transfusion in the critically ill—current clinical practice in the United States. Crit Care Med 2004;32:39–52.
4. Shapiro MJ, Gettinger A, Corwin H, et al. Anemia and blood transfusion in trauma patients admitted to the intensive care unit. J Trauma 2003;55:269–74.
5. Hebert PC, Wells G, Blajchman MA, et al. A multicenter, randomized, controlled clinical trial of transfusion requirements in critical care. Transfusion Requirements in Critical Care investigators, Canadian Critical Care Trials Group. N Engl J Med 1999;340:409–17.
6. Rao MP, Boralessa H, Morgan C, et al. Blood component use in critically ill patients. Anaesthesia 2002;57:530–4.
7. Walsh TS, Garrioch M, Maciver C, et al, Audit of Transfusion in Intensive Care in Scotland Study Group. Red cell requirements for intensive care units adhering to evidence-based transfusion guidelines. Transfusion 2004;44:1405–11.
8. Walsh TS, McClelland DB, Lee RJ, et al. Prevalence of ischemic heart disease at admission to intensive care and its influence on red cell transfusion thresholds: multicenter Scottish Study. Br J Anaesth 2005;94:445–52.
9. Shehata N, Forster A, Lawrence N, et al. Changing trends in blood transfusion: an analysis of 244,013 hospitalizations. Transfusion 2014;54(10 Pt 2): 2631–9.
10. Palmieri TL, Caruso DM, Foster KN, et al. Effect of blood transfusion on outcome after major burn injury: a multicenter study. Crit Care Med 2006;34:1602–7.
11. Seitz KP, Sevransky JE, Martin GS, et al. Evaluation of RBC transfusion practice in adult ICUs and the effect of restrictive transfusion protocols on routine care. Crit Care Med 2016. [Epub ahead of print].
12. Hayden SJ, Albert TJ, Watkins TR, et al. Anemia in critical illness: insights into etiology, consequences, and management. Am J Respir Crit Care Med 2012; 185(10):1049–57.
13. Sihler KC, Raghavendran K, Westerman M, et al. Hepcidin in trauma: linking injury, inflammation, and anemia. J Trauma 2010;69:831–7.
14. Girelli D, Nemeth E, Swinkels DW. Hepcidin in the diagnosis of iron disorders. Blood 2016;127(23):2809–13.
15. Kautz L, Jung G, Valore EV, et al. Identification of erythroferrone as an erythroid regulator of iron metabolism. Nat Genet 2014;46(7):678–84.
16. Vincent JL. Which carries the biggest risk: anaemia or blood transfusion? Transfus Clin Biol 2015;22(3):148–50.
17. Mirski MA, Frank SM, Kor DJ, et al. Restrictive and liberal red cell transfusion strategies in adult patients: reconciling clinical data with best practice. Crit Care 2015;19:202.

18. Napolitano LM, Corwin HL. Efficacy of red blood cell transfusion in the critically ill [review]. Crit Care Clin 2004;20(2):255–68.

19. Josephson CD, Glynn SA, Kleinman SH, et al, State-of-the Science Symposium Transfusion Medicine Committee. A multidisciplinary "think tank": the top 10 clinical trial opportunities in transfusion medicine from the National Heart, Lung, and Blood Institute-sponsored 2009 state-of-the-science symposium. Transfusion 2011;51(4):828–41.

20. Blajchman MA, Glynn SA, Josephson CD, et al, State-of-the Science Symposium Transfusion Medicine Committee. Clinical trial opportunities in transfusion medicine: proceedings of a National Heart, Lung, and Blood Institute state-of-the-science symposium. Transfus Med Rev 2010;24(4):259–85.

21. Fowler RA, Berenson M. Blood conservation in the intensive care unit. Crit Care Med 2003;31:653–7.

22. Chant C, Wilson G, Friedrich JO. Anemia, transfusion, and phlebotomy practices in critically ill patients with prolonged ICU length of stay: a cohort study. Crit Care 2006;10:R140.

23. Shaffer C. Diagnostic blood loss in mechanically ventilated patients. Heart Lung 2007;36:217–22.

24. Smoller BR, Kruskall MS, Horowitz GL. Reducing adult phlebotomy blood loss with the use of pediatric-sized blood collection tubes. Am J Clin Pathol 1989; 91:701–3.

25. Dolman HS, Evans K, Zimmerman LH, et al. Impact of minimizing diagnostic blood loss in the critically ill. Surgery 2015;158(4):1083–7.

26. Page C, Retter A, Wyncoll D. Blood conservation devices in critical care: a narrative review. Ann Intensive Care 2013;3:14.

27. Mukhopadhyay A, Yip HS, Prabhuswamy D, et al. The use of a blood conservation device to reduce red blood cell transfusion requirements: a before and after study. Crit Care 2010;14(1):R7.

28. MacIsaac CM, Presneill JJ, Boyce CA, et al. The influence of a blood conserving device on anaemia in intensive care patients. Anaesth Intensive Care 2003; 31(6):653–7.

29. Peruzzi WT, Parker MA, Lichtenthal PR, et al. A clinical evaluation of a blood conservation device in medical intensive care unit patients. Crit Care Med 1993;21: 501–6.

30. Carless PA, Henry DA, Moxey AJ, et al. Cell salvage for minimising perioperative allogeneic blood transfusion. Cochrane Database Syst Rev 2010;(4):CD001888.

31. KDIGO anemia work group. KDIGO clinical practice guideline for anemia in chronic kidney disease. Kidney Int Suppl 2012;2(4):279–335.

32. Corwin HL, Gettinger A, Rodriguez RM, et al. Efficacy of recombinant human erythropoietin in the critically ill patient: a randomized, double-blind, placebo-controlled trial. Crit Care Med 1999;27:2346–50.

33. Corwin HL, Gettinger A, Pearl RG, et al. Efficacy of recombinant human erythropoietin in critically ill patients: a randomized controlled trial. JAMA 2002;288: 2827–35.

34. Corwin HL, Gettinger A, Fabian TC, et al. Efficacy and safety of epoetin alfa in critically ill patients. N Engl J Med 2007;357:965–76.

35. Silver M, Corwin MJ, Bazan A, et al. Efficacy of recombinant human erythropoietin in critically ill patients admitted to a long-term acute care facility: a randomized, double-blind, placebo-controlled trial. Crit Care Med 2006;34:2310–6.

36. Zarychanski R, Turgeon AF, McIntyre L, et al. Erythropoietin-receptor agonists in critically ill patients: a meta-analysis of randomized controlled trials. CMAJ 2007; 177:725–34.

37. Napolitano LM, Fabian TC, Kelly KM, et al. Improved survival of critically ill trauma patients treated with recombinant human erythropoietin. J Trauma 2008;65(2):285–97 [discussion: 297–9].

38. French CJ, Glassford NJ, Gantner D, et al. Erythropoiesis-stimulating agents in critically ill trauma patients: a systematic review and meta-analysis. Ann Surg 2017;265(1):54–62.

39. Corwin HL, Napolitano LM. Erythropoietin for critically ill trauma patients: a missed opportunity? J Trauma Acute Care Surg 2014;77(5):774–9.

40. Shah A, Roy NB, McKechnie S, et al. Iron supplementation to treat anaemia in adult critical care patients: a systematic review and meta-analysis. Crit Care 2016;20(1):306.

41. Pieracci FM, Henderson P, Rodney JR, et al. Randomized, double-blind, placebo-controlled trial of effects of enteral iron supplementation on anemia and risk of infection during surgical critical illness. Surg Infect (Larchmt) 2009; 10(1):9–19.

42. Pieracci FM, Stovall RT, Jaouen B, et al. A multicenter, randomized clinical trial of IV iron supplementation for anemia of traumatic critical illness. Crit Care Med 2014;42(9):2048–57.

43. IRONMAN Investigators, Litton E, Baker S, et al, Australian and New Zealand Intensive Care Society Clinical Trials Group. Intravenous iron or placebo for anaemia in intensive care: the IRONMAN multicentre randomized blinded trial: a randomized trial of IV iron in critical illness. Intensive Care Med 2016; 42(11):1715–22.

44. Onken JE, Bregman DB, Harrington RA, et al. Ferric carboxymaltose in patients with iron-deficiency anemia and impaired renal function: the REPAIR-IDA trial. Nephrol Dial Transplant 2014;29(4):833–42.

45. Rodriguez RM, Corwin HL, Gettinger A, et al. Nutritional deficiencies and blunted erythropoietin response as causes of the anemia of critical illness. J Crit Care 2001;16:36–41.

46. Sasaki Y, Noguchi-Sasaki M, Yasuno H, et al. Erythropoietin stimulation decreases hepcidin expression through hematopoietic activity on bone marrow cells in mice. Int J Hematol 2012;96(6):692–700.

47. Corwin HL, Napolitano LM. Anemia in the critically ill: do we need to live with it? Crit Care Med 2014;42(9):2140–1.

48. Ruchala P, Nemeth E. The pathophysiology and pharmacology of hepcidin. Trends Pharmacol Sci 2014;35(3):155–61.

49. Available at: http://www.sabm.org/. Accessed October 2, 2015.

50. Murphy MF, Goodnough LT. The scientific basis for patient blood management. Transfus Clin Biol 2015;22(3):90–6.

51. Oliver JC, Griffin RL, Hannon T, et al. The success of our patient blood management program depended on an institution-wide change in transfusion practices. Transfusion 2014;54(10 Pt 2):2617–24.

52. Leahy MF, Roberts H, Mukhtar SA, et al, Western Australian Patient Blood Management Program. A pragmatic approach to embedding patient blood management in a tertiary hospital. Transfusion 2014;54(4):1133–45.

53. Mehra T, Seifert B, Bravo-Reiter S, et al. Implementation of a patient blood management monitoring and feedback program significantly reduces transfusions and costs. Transfusion 2015;55(12):2807–15.

54. Gross I, Seifert B, Hofmann A, et al. Patient blood management in cardiac sur-gery results in fewer transfusions and better outcome. Transfusion 2015;55(5): 1075–81.

55. Theusinger OM, Kind SL, Seifert B, et al. Patient blood management in ortho-paedic surgery: a four-year follow-up of transfusion requirements and blood loss from 2008 to 2011 at the Balgrist University Hospital in Zurich, Switzerland. Blood Transfus 2014;12(2):195–203.

56. Goodnough LT, Maggio P, Hadhazy E, et al. Restrictive blood transfusion prac-tices are associated with improved patient outcomes. Transfusion 2014;54(10 Pt 2):2753–9.

57. Roubinian NH, Escobar GJ, Liu V, et al, NHLBI Recipient Epidemiology and Donor Evaluation Study (REDS-III). Trends in red blood cell transfusion and 30-day mortality among hospitalized patients. Transfusion 2014;54(10 Pt 2): 2678–86.

58. Available at: https://www.blood.gov.au/system/files/documents/pbm-module-4.pdf. Accessed October 2, 2015.

59. Available at: http://www.jointcommission.org/electronic_clinical_quality_measures_for_patient_blood_management/. Accessed October 2, 2015.

60. Rohde JM, Dimcheff DE, Blumberg N, et al. Health care-associated infection af-ter red blood cell transfusion: a systematic review and meta-analysis. JAMA 2014;311(13):1317–26.

61. Napolitano LM, Kurek S, Luchette FA, et al. Clinical practice guideline: red blood cell transfusion in adult trauma and critical care. Crit Care Med 2009;37: 3124–57.

62. Carson JL, Guyatt G, Heddle NM, et al. Clinical practice guidelines from the AABB: red blood cell transfusion thresholds and storage. JAMA 2016;316(19): 2025–35.

63. Salpeter SR, Buckley JS, Chatterjee S. Impact of more restrictive blood transfu-sion strategies on clinical outcomes: a meta-analysis and systematic review. Am J Med 2014;127:124–31.

64. Carson JL, Carless PA, Hebert PC. Transfusion thresholds and other strategies for guiding allogeneic red blood cell transfusion. Cochrane Database Syst Rev 2012;(4):CD002042.

65. Roubinian NH, Carson JL. Restrictive red blood cell transfusion strategies appear safe in most clinical settings. Evid Based Med 2015;20(5):170.

66. Holst LB, Petersen MW, Haase N, et al. Restrictive versus liberal transfusion strategy for red blood cell transfusion: systematic review of randomised trials with meta-analysis and trial sequential analysis. BMJ 2015;350:h1354.

67. Spahn DR, Spahn GH, Stein P. Evidence base for restrictive transfusion triggers in high-risk patients. Transfus Med Hemother 2015;42(2):110–4.

68. Chang R, Holcomb JB. Optimal fluid therapy for traumatic hemorrhagic shock. Crit Care Clin 2017;33(1):15–36.

69. McIntyre L, Hebert PC, Wells G, et al, Canadian Critical Care Trials Group. Is a restrictive transfusion strategy safe for resuscitated and critically ill trauma pa-tients? J Trauma 2004;57(3):563–8 [discussion: 568].

70. West MA, Shapiro MB, Nathens AB, et al, Inflammation and the Host Response to Injury Collaborative Research Program. Inflammation and the host response to injury, a large-scale collaborative project: patient-oriented research core-standard operating procedures for clinical care. IV. Guidelines for transfusion in the trauma patient. J Trauma 2006;61(2):436–9.

71. Rivers E, Nguyen B, Havstad S, et al, Early Goal-Directed Therapy Collaborative Group. Early goal-directed therapy in the treatment of severe sepsis and septic shock. N Engl J Med 2001;345(19):1368–77.

72. Fuller BM, Gajera M, Schorr C, et al. Transfusion of packed red blood cells is not associated with improved central venous oxygen saturation or organ function in patients with septic shock. J Emerg Med 2012;43(4):593–8.

73. Marik PE, Sibbald WJ. Effect of stored-blood transfusion on oxygen delivery in patients with sepsis. JAMA 1993;269:3024–30.

74. Dietrich KA, Conrad SA, Hebert CA, et al. Cardiovascular and metabolic response to red blood cell transfusion in critically ill volume-resuscitated nonsurgical patients. Crit Care Med 1990;18:940–4.

75. Conrad SA, Dietrich KA, Hebert CA, et al. Effect of red cell transfusion on oxygen consumption following fluid resuscitation in septic shock. Circ Shock 1990; 31:419–29.

76. Mazza BF, Machado FR, Mazza DD, et al. Evaluation of blood transfusion effects on mixed venous oxygen saturation and lactate levels in patients with SIRS/sepsis. Clinics (Sao Paulo) 2005;60:311–6.

77. Holst LB, Haase N, Wetterslev J, for the TRISS Trial Group and the Scandinavian Critical Care Trials Group. Lower versus higher hemoglobin threshold for transfusion in septic shock. N Engl J Med 2014;371:1381–91.

78. Rygård SL, Holst LB, Wetterslev J, et al, TRISS Trial Group; Scandinavian Critical Care Trials Group. Higher vs. lower haemoglobin threshold for transfusion in septic shock: subgroup analyses of the TRISS trial. Acta Anaesthesiol Scand 2017;61(2):166–75.

79. Rygård SL, Holst LB, Wetterslev J, et al, TRISS Trial Group; Scandinavian Critical Care Trials Group. Long-term outcomes in patients with septic shock transfused at a lower versus a higher haemoglobin threshold: the TRISS randomised, multicentre clinical trial. Intensive Care Med 2016;42(11):1685–94.

80. Angus DC, Yealy DM, Kellum JA, ProCESS Investigators. Protocol-based care for early septic shock. N Engl J Med 2014;371(4):386.

81. ARISE Investigators; ANZICS Clinical Trials Group, Peake SL, Delaney A, Bailey M, et al. Goal-directed resuscitation for patients with early septic shock. N Engl J Med 2014;371(16):1496–506.

82. Mouncey PR, Osborn TM, Power GS, et al, ProMISe Trial Investigators. Trial of early, goal-directed resuscitation for septic shock. N Engl J Med 2015; 372(14):1301–11.

83. Levy MM, Abraham E, Zilberberg M, et al. A descriptive evaluation of transfusion practices in patients receiving mechanical ventilation. Chest 2005;127: 928–35.

84. Hébert PC, Blajchman MA, Cook DJ, et al. Transfusion requirements in critical care investigators for the Canadian critical care trials group: do blood transfusions improve outcomes related to mechanical ventilation? Chest 2001;119: 1850–7.

85. Walsh TS, Boyd JA, Watson D, et al, RELIEVE Investigators. Restrictive versus liberal transfusion strategies for older mechanically ventilated critically ill patients: a randomized pilot trial. Crit Care Med 2013;41(10):2354–63.

86. Salisbury AC, Amin AP, Reid KJ, et al. Hospital-acquired anemia and in-hospital mortality in patients with acute myocardial infarction. Am Heart J 2011;162(2): 300–9.

87. Salisbury AC, Kosiborod M, Amin AP, et al. Recovery from hospital-acquired anemia after acute myocardial infarction and effect on outcomes. Am J Cardiol 2011;108(7):949–54.
88. Salisbury AC, Reid KJ, Amin AP, et al. Variation in the incidence of hospital-acquired anemia during hospitalization with acute myocardial infarction (data from 57 US hospitals). Am J Cardiol 2014;113(7):1130–6.
89. Hanna EB, Alexander KP, Chen AY, et al. Characteristics and in-hospital outcomes of patients with non-ST-segment elevation myocardial infarction undergoing an invasive strategy according to hemoglobin levels. Am J Cardiol 2013;111(8):1099–103.
90. Wu WC, Rathore SS, Wang Y, et al. Blood transfusion in elderly patients with acute myocardial infarction [comment]. N Engl J Med 2001;345(17):1230–6.
91. Hebert PC, Fergusson DA. Do transfusions get to the heart of the matter? JAMA 2004;292:1610–2.
92. KP1 Alexander, Chen AY, Wang TY, et al. Transfusion practice and outcomes in non-ST-segment elevation acute coronary syndromes. Am Heart J 2008;155(6):1047–53.
93. Salisbury AC, Reid KJ, Marso SP, et al. Blood transfusion during acute myocardial infarction: association with mortality and variability across hospitals. J Am Coll Cardiol 2014;64(8):811–9.
94. Rao SV, Jollis JG, Harrington RA, et al. Relationship of blood transfusion and clinical outcomes in patients with acute coronary syndromes [see comment]. JAMA 2004;292(13):1555–62.
95. Shishehbor MH, Madhwal S, Rajagopal V, et al. Impact of blood transfusion on short- and long-term mortality in patients with ST-segment elevation myocardial infarction. JACC Cardiovasc Interv 2009;2(1):46–53.
96. Chatterjee S, Wetterslev J, Sharma A, et al. Association of blood transfusion with increased mortality in myocardial infarction: a meta-analysis and diversity-adjusted study sequential analysis. JAMA Intern Med 2013;173:132–9.
97. Carson JL, Hebert PC. Here we go again—blood transfusion kills patients? JAMA Intern Med 2013;173:139–40.
98. Gerber DR. Transfusion of packed red blood cells in patients with ischemic heart disease. Crit Care Med 2008;36(4):1068–74.
99. Cooper HA, Rao SV, Greenberg MD, et al. Conservative versus liberal red cell transfusion in acute myocardial infarction (the CRIT Randomized Pilot Study). Am J Cardiol 2011;108(8):1108–11.
100. Carson JL, Brooks MM, Abbott JD, et al. Liberal versus restrictive transfusion thresholds for patients with symptomatic coronary artery disease. Am Heart J 2013;165(6):964–71.
101. Hébert PC, Yetisir E, Martin C, et al, Transfusion Requirements in Critical Care Investigators for the Canadian Critical Care Trials Group. Is a low transfusion threshold safe in critically ill patients with cardiovascular diseases? Crit Care Med 2001;29(2):227–34.
102. Carson JL, Terrin ML, Noveck H, et al, FOCUS Investigators. Liberal or restrictive transfusion in high-risk patients after hip surgery. N Engl J Med 2011;365(26):2453–62.
103. Carson JL, Sieber F, Cook DR, et al. Liberal versus restrictive blood transfusion strategy: 3-year survival and cause of death results from the FOCUS randomised controlled trial. Lancet 2015;385:1183–9.
104. Hajjar LA, Vincent JL, Galas FR, et al. Transfusion requirements after cardiac surgery: the TRACS randomized controlled trial. JAMA 2010;304:1559–67.

105. Nakamura RE, Vincent JL, Fukushima JT, et al. A liberal strategy of red blood cell transfusion reduces cardiogenic shock in elderly patients undergoing cardiac surgery. J Thorac Cardiovasc Surg 2015;150(5):1314–20.

106. Murphy GJ, Pike K, Rogers CA, et al, TITRe2 Investigators. Liberal or restrictive transfusion after cardiac surgery. N Engl J Med 2015;372:9971008.

Renal Replacement Therapy in Acute Kidney Injury: Controversies and Consensus

 CrossMark

Michael Heung, MD, MS*, Lenar Yessayan, MD, MS

KEYWORDS

- Acute kidney injury • Dialysis • Continuous renal replacement therapy

KEY POINTS

- Acute kidney injury (AKI) occurs commonly among intensive care unit (ICU) patients, and about 5% of ICU patients require renal replacement therapy (RRT).
- There are several different modalities of RRT, and each has potential advantages and disadvantages depending on the clinical situation. In hemodynamically unstable patients, continuous RRT (CRRT) has become the standard of care.
- The established target dose for CRRT is a delivered effluent rate of 20 to 25 mL/kg/h. To achieve this, a prescribed dose of 25 to 30 mL/kg/h may be required.
- Regional citrate anticoagulation has emerged as a first-line form of anticoagulation to maintain CRRT circuit patency.
- Despite recent advances, there remain many gaps in the evidence basis, and therefore physicians must understand basic principles and use appropriate clinical judgment when managing RRT for AKI.

INTRODUCTION

Acute kidney injury (AKI) is one of the most common complications occurring among critically ill patients. Depending on the population studied, AKI develops in 30% to 60% of intensive care unit (ICU) patients, and approximately 5% of all ICU patients require renal replacement therapy (RRT).[1–3] AKI is independently associated with a higher risk of death, with mortalities exceeding 50% when acute dialysis is required.[1,3] This article presents current best practices for the management of RRT in critically ill patients with AKI, with an emphasis on recent developments from clinical trials. It also discusses areas in which evidence basis remains lacking.

Disclosure: The authors have nothing to disclose.
Division of Nephrology, Department of Medicine, University of Michigan, 1500 East Medical Center Drive, SPC 5364, Ann Arbor, MI 48109-5364, USA
* Corresponding author.
E-mail address: mheung@umich.edu

Crit Care Clin 33 (2017) 365–378
http://dx.doi.org/10.1016/j.ccc.2016.12.003
criticalcare.theclinics.com

PATIENT EVALUATION OVERVIEW

In the past decade, consensus definitions for AKI have been developed and adopted. At present, the most widely used definition is from the Kidney Disease Improving Global Outcomes (KDIGO) AKI guideline, which defines and classifies AKI by changes in serum creatinine or urine output.[4] Although a great deal of research has focused on identifying novel biomarkers of AKI (eg, neutrophil gelatinase-associated lipocalin, kidney injury molecule-1, interleukin-18, liver-fatty acid binding protein), serum creatinine remains the current clinical standard.

Of note, in the United States the first novel biomarker for clinical AKI risk prediction was approved in September 2014. Marketed as NephroCheck (Astute Medical, San Diego, CA), this test reports the product of the cell cycle arrest biomarkers tissue inhibitor of metalloproteinase 2 and insulin-like growth factor binding protein 7 (TIMP-2*IGFBP7) and has high sensitivity in identifying critically ill patients at risk for stage 2 or 3 AKI within the subsequent 12 hours. Clinical use of this novel biomarker has recently been reviewed.[5] Limitations to clinical implementation include poor specificity (46%) and a current lack of clinical trial data showing improved outcomes by incorporating biomarker testing into clinical decision-making protocols.

Once AKI has been identified, there should be an evaluation for underlying cause. Acute tubular necrosis (ATN) is the most common cause of severe AKI in the critical care setting, and most commonly results from renal ischemia (eg, shock, cardiopulmonary bypass), exogenous nephrotoxic insults (eg, iodinated contrast exposure, aminoglycosides, or other medications), or endogenous nephrotoxic insults (eg, rhabdomyolysis, hemolysis). ATN is suggested by a history of renal insult as well as the presence of granular casts in the urine.

Beyond ATN, several other diagnoses should be considered and explored in the ICU setting:

- Urinary obstruction can occur because of trauma (from catheterization) or medications such as narcotics that lead to bladder dysfunction.
- Intra-abdominal hypertension (defined as pressure ≥ 12 mm Hg) occurs commonly among critically ill patients and in severe cases can result in abdominal compartment syndrome, which results in AKI from impaired renal perfusion and venous congestion.[6] This condition can develop in the setting of abdominal trauma or surgery, or in patients who receive massive fluid resuscitation.
- In patients presenting with both diffuse alveolar hemorrhage and AKI, consideration should be given to autoimmune pulmonary-renal syndromes such as Goodpasture syndrome or antineutrophil cytoplasmic antibody (ANCA)–associated vasculitis (granulomatosus with polyangiitis, microscopic polyangiitis, or eosinophilic granulomatosus with polyangiitis). These conditions can be diagnosed using serologic tests (anti–glomerular basement membrane antibodies, ANCA), and require immunomodulatory therapy in addition to supportive care.[7] Plasma exchange is also indicated in severe cases.

TREATMENT OPTIONS

Regardless of underlying cause, severe AKI may necessitate the initiation of RRT. This article provides an overview of the various options to deliver RRT.

Modality

Various forms of renal replacement modalities may be used in the management of critically ill patients with AKI, including peritoneal dialysis (PD), and extracorporeal techniques such as intermittent hemodialysis (IHD), prolonged intermittent RRT (PIRRT), and continuous RRT (CRRT) (Table 1). PD is generally not used to treat AKI in adults in the developed world because of concerns with adequate clearance compared with extracorporeal techniques, although recent studies suggest that outcomes with PD may be as good as extracorporeal techniques.[8,9] The choice between various forms of RRT may be influenced by resource availability, local expertise, and clinical setting (Table 2).

- IHD offers the most rapid solute clearance and is the initial preferred option in the treatment of life-threatening hyperkalemia and many drug poisonings, such as salicylate or nonvolatile alcohol poisonings. Patients with significant potassium generation (rhabdomyolysis, tissue ischemia, and tumor lysis syndrome) even if unstable may need to be treated with hemodialysis first to sufficiently lower blood potassium levels and then maintained on CRRT to handle ongoing body potassium generation.[10]
- CRRT is in general preferred in most patients with hemodynamic instability. The KDIGO clinical practice guidelines for AKI consider CRRT and IHD as complementary therapies with consideration given to provision of CRRT in hemodynamically unstable patients and those with concomitant liver or brain injury.[4] CRRT can be performed using diffusive clearance (continuous venovenous hemodialysis [CVVHD]), convective clearance (continuous venovenous hemofiltration [CVVH]), or a combination of both (continuous venovenous hemodiafiltration [CVVHDF]). Although convective modalities offer greater clearance of middle molecules compared with diffusive clearance, this has not been shown to affect clinical outcomes in the AKI setting, and the choice between modalities should be determined by local expertise. Of note, there are no data to support survival benefit of CRRT compared with intermittent therapies. Observational studies have suggested improved renal function recovery rates with CRRT compared with IHD, but no difference is seen when only randomized clinical trials are included.[11,12]
- PIRRT, similar to CRRT, encompasses convective and/or diffusive methods of clearance delivery. PIRRT represents a hybrid therapy between IHD and CRRT, performed over 6 to 12 hours either daily or between 3 to 6 d/wk. It

Table 1
Characteristics of different modalities of extracorporeal renal replacement therapy

	IHD	PIRRT	CRRT
Mechanism of Clearance	Diffusion	Diffusion, convection, or both	Diffusion, convection, or both
Duration (h)	3–4	6–12	Continuous
Frequency (d/wk)	3	3–7	Continuous
Timing of Procedure	Usually daytime	Daytime or nighttime	Continuous
Anticoagulation	Not necessary	Not necessary	Necessary
Vascular Access	AVF, AVG, CVC	CVC	CVC
Patient Location	Ward, ICU, step-down	ICU, step-down	ICU

Abbreviations: AVF, arteriovenous fistula; AVG, arteriovenous graft; CVC, central venous catheter.

Table 2
Specific indications for each modality of renal replacement therapy

Goal	Hemodynamic Status	Preferred Modality
Urea clearance	Unstable	CRRT or PIRRT
	Stable	IHD
Severe hyperkalemia	Unstable/stable	IHD first
Metabolic acidosis	Unstable	CRRT/PIRRT or IHD first if hemodynamic instability caused by acidosis
Severe dysnatremia	Unstable/stable	CRRT
Severe hyperphosphatemia	Unstable/stable	CRRT
Brain injury	Unstable/stable	CRRT
Acute liver failure	Unstable/stable	CRRT

includes approaches such as sustained low-efficiency dialysis, extended daily dialysis with filtration, and accelerated venovenous hemofiltration. PIRRT provides the advantage of a dialysis-free period allowing daily investigations, procedures, or physical rehabilitation without compromising dialysis adequacy and hemodynamic stability.

Timing of Initiation

The decision to start RRT is unequivocal in the presence of life-threatening AKI complications such as hyperkalemia, severe acidosis, pulmonary edema, or uremic complications. However, in the absence of these factors, the optimal timing of dialysis for AKI remains uncertain.

- Several single-center non–randomized controlled studies in cardiac surgery patients[13–17] and observational cohort studies in the ICU[18–23] suggest a mortality benefit with early dialysis. These studies vary widely in their definition of early dialysis and often include arbitrary cutoffs for serum creatinine level, urea level, urine output, time from ICU admission, and duration of AKI when defining early dialysis.
- Two recently published randomized controlled trials differed in their conclusions. A single-center study, the ELAIN (Early vs Late Initiation of Renal Replacement Therapy in Critically Ill Patients With Acute Kidney Injury) trial,[24] showed greater survival over the first 90 days in patients undergoing early dialysis, whereas a larger multicenter study, the Artificial Kidney Initiation in Kidney Injury (AKIKI) study,[25] did not show survival benefit for early dialysis. Importantly, the two studies significantly differed in their definitions of early and delayed dialysis (Table 3). Also, in both studies a substantial proportion of patients randomized to late dialysis did not end up requiring dialysis (9.2% in the ELAIN trial and 49% in the AKIKI trial).

At present, there is inadequate evidence to recommend early initiation of dialysis for AKI. It is hoped that the results from ongoing randomized clinical trials addressing this issue will provide data to resolve this debate.[26,27]

Dose of Renal Replacement Therapy

By convention, dose of IHD is typically expressed by urea kinetic modeling (Kt/V, where K is dialyzer clearance, t is duration of dialysis, and V is volume of distribution). In contrast, dose of CRRT is expressed as effluent dose adjusted for body weight (in milliliters per kilogram per hour).

Table 3
Comparison between ELAIN and AKIKI randomized clinical trials examining timing of renal replacement therapy in patients with acute kidney injury

	ELAIN Trial (N = 231)[24]	AKIKI Trial (N = 620)[25]
Centers	1	31
Inclusion Criteria		
AKI Stage	Stage 2	Stage 3
Other Criteria	At least 1 of: • Severe sepsis • On vasopressors • Refractory fluid overload • SOFA score ≥2	At least 1 of: • Mechanically ventilated • On vasopressors
Biomarker	Serum NGAL >150 ng/mL	None
Dialysis Triggers		
Early Group	Within 8 h of stage 2	Within 6 h of stage 3
Delayed Group	12 h after progressing to KDIGO stage 3 AKI or any of the following dialysis triggers: • BUN >100 mg/dL • K >6 mEq/L (or ECG changes) • Mg >4 mmol/L • Urine <200 mL/24 h • Organ edema despite diuretics	Any of the following dialysis triggers: • BUN >112 mg/dL • K >6 mEq/L (or 5.5 mEq/L with treatment) • pH <7.15 (pure metabolic or mixed) • Pulmonary edema with Fio_2 >0.5 (or O_2 >5 L/min or oligo/anuria >72 h)
Outcomes		
90-d Mortality; early vs delayed (%)	39.3 vs 54.7 (P = .03)	48.5 vs 49.7 (P = .79)
Patients Needing Dialysis in Delayed Group (%)	90.8	51.0

Abbreviations: BUN, blood urea nitrogen; ECG, electrocardiogram; Fio_2, fraction of inspired oxygen; K, potassium; Mg, magnesium; SOFA, Sequential Organ Failure Assessment.

- Early small studies suggested that a higher dose of dialysis may improve outcomes in patients with AKI.[28,29]
- Subsequently, 2 large, multicenter, randomized controlled clinical trials compared standard versus more intensive dialysis dose (**Table 4**).[30,31] Both studies failed to show any difference in mortality between dosing groups. As a result, the current recommended delivered dose for RRT is a Kt/V of 1.2 to 1.4 per session 3 times per week when performing IHD, or an effluent dose of 20 to 25 mL/kg/h when performing CRRT.[4]

Importantly, delivered dose of dialysis is typically less than prescribed dose, and clinicians need to monitor dosing to ensure adequate therapy. A simplified measure of IHD clearance is the urea reduction ratio (URR), which can be performed by checking predialysis and postdialysis blood urea nitrogen (BUN) levels (URR = [(pre-BUN − post-BUN)/pre-BUN] × 100%). In general, a URR of 65% or greater correlates with Kt/V greater than 1.2 and is considered adequate clearance. Patients undergoing CRRT similarly often have less dialysis delivered than prescribed because of machine interruptions (eg, premature clotting, stoppages for procedures). As such, it is prudent

Table 4
Comparison of large clinical trials examining dialysis dose in patients with acute kidney injury

	ATN Trial (N = 1124)[30]	Renal Trial (N = 1508)[31]
Study Design		
Design and Setting	Multicenter randomized controlled trial, 27 centers in the United States	Multicenter randomized controlled trial, 35 centers in Australia and New Zealand
AKI Definition	ATN requiring RRT as determined by clinical team	AKI requiring RRT as determined by clinical team
Inclusion Criteria	Failure of ≥1 nonrenal organ system (defined as SOFA organ score ≥2), or sepsis	At least 1 of: • Oliguria unresponsive to fluid challenge • K >6.5 mEq/L • pH <7.2 • BUN >70 mg/dL • Serum Cr >3.4 mg/dL • Clinically significant organ edema
Dosing Groups		
Standard Group	IHD delivered Kt/V 1.2–1.4 for 3 weekly sessions or CVVHDF effluent dose 20 mL/kg/h	CVVHDF effluent dose 25 mL/kg/h
High-intensity Group	IHD delivered Kt/V 1.2–1.4 for 6 weekly sessions or CVVHDF effluent dose 35 mL/kg/h	CVVHDF effluent dose 40 mL/kg/h
Outcomes		
Primary Outcome (Standard vs High Intensity)	All-cause 60-d mortality 51.5% vs 53.6%, $P = .47$	All-cause 90 d mortality 44.7% vs 44.7%, $P = .99$
Renal Function Recovery (Standard vs High Intensity)	• Dialysis dependence at 28 d: 72.6% vs 75.8%, $P = .24$ • Discharged home off dialysis by 60 d: 16.4% vs 15.7%, $P = .75$	• Dialysis dependence at 28 d: 12.2% vs 14.4%, $P = .31$ • Dialysis dependence at 90 d: 4.4% vs 6.8%, $P = .14$

Abbreviation: Cr, creatinine.

to prescribe an effluent dose in the 25 to 30 mL/kg/h range in order to achieve the recommended target.[4]

Overall, dialysis dose is currently perhaps the most strongly evidence-based aspect of RRT for patients with AKI. However, it is important to remember that guidelines do not apply to all clinical situations, and there are times when higher (eg, markedly catabolic patients, tumor lysis syndrome) or lower doses (eg, morbidly obese patients) may be appropriate.

Anticoagulation

For IHD, heparin anticoagulation is the mainstay when not contraindicated (because of systemic administration); however, the high blood flow rates and shorter durations used in IHD often allow treatment without any form of anticoagulation. In contrast, clotting risk is a major consideration in CRRT, and maintaining filter patency is critical to optimizing delivered RRT dose.

Table 5 describes the advantages and disadvantages of various forms of anticoagulation used in CRRT. Regional citrate anticoagulation (RCA) uses citrate to chelate ionized calcium in the extracorporeal circuit. The unavailability of calcium as a cofactor for the coagulation cascade allows functional anticoagulation in the CRRT circuit; this is then reversed by administration of calcium with blood returning to the patient. In clinical trials, RCA has been proved to be as effective as, if not superior to, heparin for maintaining CRRT circuit patency, and is consistently associated with lower risk of serious bleeding complications.[32] As such, RCA is currently recommended as the first choice for anticoagulation in patients undergoing CRRT.[4]

Solutions

RRT solutions (ie, dialysate and replacement fluid) do not contain any waste products such as urea or creatinine, and therefore clearance of these substances is mediated by dialysis prescription parameters (eg, duration and blood flow rate in IHD; effluent dose in CRRT). For electrolytes, clearance is additionally directly proportional to the concentration gradient between the blood and RRT solution.

For IHD, dialysate is generated by the dialysis machine in real time, and composition can be changed even during treatment. Key adjustable components include sodium, bicarbonate, potassium, and calcium concentrations.

Table 5
Anticoagulation strategies for continuous renal replacement therapy

Strategy	Advantages	Disadvantages
No anticoagulation	• No bleeding risk	• Lowest filter patency rates
Regional citrate anticoagulation	• Highest filter patency rates • No systemic anticoagulation, and therefore no increased bleeding risk	• Complexity of protocols and required monitoring • Risks include citrate toxicity, metabolic alkalosis
Unfractionated heparin	• Ease of use, availability • Ability to monitor • Ability to reverse with protamine	• Systemic anticoagulation and bleeding risk
Low-molecular-weight heparin	• Can be prescribed as fixed dose or titrated to activity	• Systemic anticoagulation and bleeding risk • Expense, need for specialized monitoring (anti-Xa levels) • Less effective reversal with protamine
Thrombin antagonists	• Can be used in patients with heparin-induced thrombocytopenia	• Systemic anticoagulation and bleeding risk • Expense • No reversal agents
Prostacyclin	• Can be used alone or to augment anticoagulation with heparin	• Expense • Limited clinical experience compared with other strategies • Risk of hypotension

For CRRT, solutions can either be compounded at the institutional level or purchased commercially. The former approach can be less expensive but requires appropriate infrastructure to minimize contamination and error risk. Commercial options are typically more expensive and require significant storage space, but have long shelf lives and high reliability. There are several different options available from multiple manufacturers. Most solutions are comparable, and there have not been clinical trials to compare outcomes between different formulations. One consideration is that, when using RCA, solutions that do not contain calcium and glucose are favored because most programs use a formulation of citrate that contains dextrose (anticoagulant citrate dextrose solution, solution A [ACD-A]), and a positive glucose balance can develop without glucose removal.[33]

Drug Dosing

There remains a paucity of data regarding appropriate dosing of medications in critically ill patients undergoing RRT.[34,35] Most recommendations are empirically derived based on general pharmacokinetic principles. Some important considerations are:

- Drug levels should be used to confirm appropriate dosing whenever possible (eg, with vancomycin and aminoglycosides).
- Drug clearance can occur both via passage across the dialyzer membrane (diffusive or convective clearance) or by adherence to the dialyzer membrane (adsorptive clearance). In patients undergoing RRT who are not anuric, there can also be a component of endogenous clearance.
- Key RRT characteristics that influence drug clearance are the delivered dose, the pore size of the dialysis membrane (high flux vs low flux), and RRT modality. Convective therapies (ie, CVVH or CVVHDF) provide greater clearance of larger molecules compared with diffusive therapy; however, specific dosing recommendations based on CRRT modality are not available.
- The key drug characteristics that determine extracorporeal clearance are molecular weight (increased clearance with smaller size), degree of protein binding (less clearance with increased protein binding), and volume of distribution (less clearance with increasing volume of distribution).
- In general, it is recommended that patients undergoing IHD have medications dosed based on a creatinine clearance less than 10 mL/min, whereas for those on CRRT the medication dosing should follow guidelines based on creatinine clearance of about 30 mL/min.

Vascular Access

In contrast with patients with end-stage renal disease, in whom the preferred dialysis access is an arteriovenous fistula, patients with AKI requiring RRT need a central venous catheter placed for hemodialysis. This placement is typically performed with a temporary double-lumen dialysis catheter inserted at the bedside. Alternatively, initiating dialysis therapy via a tunneled catheter may be reasonable in select patients with AKI if the duration of the RRT is anticipated to be longer than 1 week, because such catheters are associated with lower infectious risk compared with nontunneled catheters. However, these catheters are typically inserted under fluoroscopy, and the logistics of arranging placement may lead to clinically significant delays in RRT initiation. Therefore, a more prudent approach may be to initiate RRT using temporary catheters, with later transition to a tunneled catheter.

- Basic design: several designs of double-lumen dialysis catheters have emerged over the years with no proven advantage of one design over another. The 2 lumens are arranged either in a concentric (coaxial) manner or side by side. The arterial lumen draws blood from the body and the venous lumen returns blood to the body. To decrease access recirculation, the orifice of the venous lumen is frequently about 3 cm distal to the arterial orifice.

- Catheter size: the outer diameter of the dialysis catheter varies between 11 and 14 French. The optimal length is 12 to 15 cm for the right internal jugular vein, 15 to 20 cm for the left internal jugular vein, and 19 to 24 cm for the femoral vein.[36]
- Material: the 2 blood-compatible materials used for dialysis catheters are silicone and polyurethane. Silicone catheters are soft and flexible and therefore have low risk of vessel perforation. In contrast, these mechanical properties make them harder to insert and the lumens more compressible. They are used more for tunneled catheters. Polyurethane catheters have thermoplastic properties. They are rigid at room temperature and soften when exposed to body temperature. Once these catheters bend, they are likely to remain bent and thus limit blood flow.
- Location: choice of insertion site depends on patient characteristics (eg, body habitus, coagulopathy, local infection) and the skills of the operator. KDIGO guidelines suggest the following preferential hierarchy for initial vein for dialysis access: first choice is right internal jugular (RIJ) vein, followed by femoral vein, then left internal jugular (LIJ) vein, and lastly subclavian vein (as a rescue option).[37] Catheter contact with the vessel wall is considered the primary generator for catheter-related thrombosis and vessel stenosis. RIJ vein dialysis catheter has a straight course into the right brachiocephalic vein and superior vena cava and thus the least contact with vessel walls.[38] LIJ vein or subclavian vein catheters have 1 or more angulations and considerable vessel contact, and therefore higher risk of central vein stenosis/thrombosis.[39] This risk may preclude the use of the ipsilateral arm for any future dialysis vascular access. Femoral vein and LIJ vein catheters have higher tendency for catheter malfunction than RIJ vein catheters.[40,41] Femoral catheters also limit patient mobilization, and have increased recirculation rates. In patients with the option of future kidney transplant they should be avoided to circumvent stenosis of the iliac vein, to which the transplanted kidney's vein is anatomized.[42] The tip of the catheter should be in a large vein to provide adequate blood flow and to reduce the catheter malfunction. The tip of an internal jugular catheter should ideally be at the junction of the superior vena cava and right atrium. Advancing the tip too far could perforate the right atrium or ventricle. The tip of a femoral catheter should end in the inferior vena cava.
- Catheter care: dialysis catheters should not be accessed for routine medication administration because of the associated risk of blood stream infection. Routine use of antibiotic locks in acute (temporary) dialysis catheters or topical antibiotics over the skin insertion site are not recommended by KDIGO because of their potential to promote fungal infections and antimicrobial resistance.[37]

TREATMENT COMPLICATIONS

Although serving as a potentially lifesaving therapy, RRT also carries the risk for significant treatment complications. These complications include exacerbating hemodynamic instability during therapy, bleeding risk when systemic anticoagulation is used, and medical errors related to delivery of RRT. Importantly, complications may not be recognized because of the typically high acuity and complexity of the critically ill AKI patient population. Therefore, a high degree of vigilance and use of continuous quality improvement techniques are necessary to ensure optimal care delivery.[43,44]

Complications related to dialysis catheters are another important area of consideration. These complications can include both mechanical complications related to catheter insertion, and catheter-related bloodstream infections (CRBSI):

- CRBSI are associated with increased morbidity and mortality, and should be suspected when a patient develops fever or chills without clinical evidence for another source of infection.
- Diagnosis of CRBSI requires concurrent positive blood culture from the dialysis catheter and a peripheral vein with the colony count from the catheter that is at least 5 times greater than that obtained from the peripheral vein if quantitative cultures are used. Empiric broad-spectrum systemic antibiotics should be started after blood cultures are obtained and tailored to the specific organisms when cultures are available.
- CRBSI may be caused by a broad spectrum of gram-positive bacteria, gram-negative bacteria, and yeasts.[45] Metastatic infection may lead to endocarditis, septic arthritis, osteomyelitis, and epidural abscesses and thrombophlebitis.
- With proven infection, a temporary dialysis catheter should always be removed and a tunneled catheter should be removed if any of the following are present: sepsis; metastatic infection; tunnel infection; infection with multidrug-resistant organisms, or *Staphylococcus aureus*, *Pseudomonas*, or fungi. Otherwise a tunneled catheter may be exchanged over a guidewire after 48 to 72 hours of appropriate and effective antibiotic treatment.[46] In patients with limited vascular access and/or without indications for immediate catheter removal, antibiotic lock therapy in conjunction with systemic antibiotics is an alternative to guidewire exchange or to catheter removal with delayed exchange.[47–49]

EVALUATION OF OUTCOME AND LONG-TERM RECOMMENDATIONS

AKI has consistently been shown to be an independent risk factor for mortality, both in ICU and non-ICU settings. Mortality risk increases with severity of AKI, and approaches (if not exceeds) 50% in critically ill patients requiring initiation of RRT.[1,2] However, some recent studies provide hope that AKI mortality may be decreasing.[50–52]

In addition to in-hospital mortality, AKI has several other adverse impacts on patient outcomes:

- Compared with patients with no AKI, hospital length of stay is 1.5, 1.9, and 2.2 times greater in those with increasing AKI stages 1 to 3 respectively.[53]
- Compared with patients with no AKI, readmission risk is twice as likely in patients with AKI regardless of AKI stage.[53]
- Compared with non–AKI survivors, AKI survivors have 7 times the risk of developing CKD[54,55] and 22 times the risk of developing ESRD.[54,56]
- Severity of AKI is associated with risk of both in-hospital and long-term mortality. In a large UK retrospective observational study, the in-hospital mortality was 2% for non-AKI, 8% for AKI Network stage 1 AKI (AKIN-1), 26% for AKIN-2, and 33% for AKIN-3. The 24-month survival was 90% for non-AKI, 59% for AKI stage 1, 27% for AKI stage 2, and 18% for AKI stage 3. The increased long-term mortality persists even after multiple adjustments.[53]

Therefore, follow-up care is important among survivors of an AKI episode. However, recent studies suggest that current follow-up rates with nephrology are low.[57] Considering that nephrology follow-up has been associated with lower mortality risk,[58] improving follow-up rates represents a potential significant opportunity to positively affect the long-term outcomes in this population.

SUMMARY

AKI occurs commonly among ICU patients, and is associated with increased morbidity and mortality. Regardless of underlying cause, severe cases of AKI may require initiation of RRT support. Over the last decade, clinical trial data have provided evidence-based guidance for some aspects of RRT prescription, most notably dose and anticoagulation strategy. However, there remain many unanswered areas and therefore intensivists must continue to exercise thoughtful clinical judgment in the care of these patients.

REFERENCES

1. Hoste EA, Schurgers M. Epidemiology of acute kidney injury: how big is the problem? Crit Care Med 2008;36(4 Suppl):S146–51.
2. Susantitaphong P, Cruz DN, Cerda J, et al. World incidence of AKI: a meta-analysis. Clin J Am Soc Nephrol 2013;8(9):1482–93.
3. Uchino S, Kellum JA, Bellomo R, et al. Beginning, ending supportive therapy for the kidney I. Acute renal failure in critically ill patients: a multinational, multicenter study. JAMA 2005;294(7):813–8.
4. Kidney Disease: Improving Global Outcomes (KDIGO) Acute Kidney Injury Workgroup. KDIGO clinical practice guideline for acute kidney injury. Kidney Int 2012; 2:1–138.
5. Vijayan A, Faubel S, Askenazi DJ, et al, American Society of Nephrology Acute Kidney Injury Advisory Group. Clinical use of the urine biomarker [TIMP-2] x [IGFBP7] for acute kidney injury risk assessment. Am J Kidney Dis 2016. http://dx.doi.org/10.1053/j.ajkd.2015.12.033.
6. Patel DM, Connor MJ Jr. Intra-abdominal hypertension and abdominal compartment syndrome: an underappreciated cause of acute kidney injury. Adv Chronic Kidney Dis 2016;23(3):160–6.
7. West SC, Arulkumaran N, Ind PW, et al. Pulmonary-renal syndrome: a life threatening but treatable condition. Postgrad Med J 2013;89(1051):274–83.
8. George J, Varma S, Kumar S, et al. Comparing continuous venovenous hemodiafiltration and peritoneal dialysis in critically ill patients with acute kidney injury: a pilot study. Perit Dial Int 2011;31(4):422–9.
9. Gabriel DP, Caramori JT, Martin LC, et al. Continuous peritoneal dialysis compared with daily hemodialysis in patients with acute kidney injury. Perit Dial Int 2009;29(Suppl 2):S62–71.
10. Yessayan L, Yee J, Frinak S, et al. Continuous renal replacement therapy for the management of acid-base and electrolyte imbalances in acute kidney injury. Adv Chronic Kidney Dis 2016;23(3):203–10.
11. Schneider AG, Bellomo R, Bagshaw SM, et al. Choice of renal replacement therapy modality and dialysis dependence after acute kidney injury: a systematic review and meta-analysis. Intensive Care Med 2013;39(6):987–97.
12. Bagshaw SM, Berthiaume LR, Delaney A, et al. Continuous versus intermittent renal replacement therapy for critically ill patients with acute kidney injury: a meta-analysis. Crit Care Med 2008;36(2):610–7.
13. Iyem H, Tavli M, Akcicek F, et al. Importance of early dialysis for acute renal failure after an open-heart surgery. Hemodial Int 2009;13(1):55–61.
14. Sugahara S, Suzuki H. Early start on continuous hemodialysis therapy improves survival rate in patients with acute renal failure following coronary bypass surgery. Hemodial Int 2004;8(4):320–5.

15. Manche A, Casha A, Rychter J, et al. Early dialysis in acute kidney injury after cardiac surgery. Interact Cardiovasc Thorac Surg 2008;7(5):829–32.

16. Elahi MM, Lim MY, Joseph RN, et al. Early hemofiltration improves survival in post-cardiotomy patients with acute renal failure. Eur J Cardiothorac Surg 2004;26(5):1027–31.

17. Demirkilic U, Kuralay E, Yenicesu M, et al. Timing of replacement therapy for acute renal failure after cardiac surgery. J Card Surg 2004;19(1):17–20.

18. Carl DE, Grossman C, Behnke M, et al. Effect of timing of dialysis on mortality in critically ill, septic patients with acute renal failure. Hemodial Int 2010;14(1):11–7.

19. Liu KD, Himmelfarb J, Paganini E, et al. Timing of initiation of dialysis in critically ill patients with acute kidney injury. Clin J Am Soc Nephrol 2006;1(5):915–9.

20. Bagshaw SM, Uchino S, Bellomo R, et al. Timing of renal replacement therapy and clinical outcomes in critically ill patients with severe acute kidney injury. J Crit Care 2009;24(1):129–40.

21. Wu VC, Ko WJ, Chang HW, et al. Early renal replacement therapy in patients with postoperative acute liver failure associated with acute renal failure: effect on postoperative outcomes. J Am Coll Surg 2007;205(2):266–76.

22. Shiao CC, Wu VC, Li WY, et al. Late initiation of renal replacement therapy is associated with worse outcomes in acute kidney injury after major abdominal surgery. Crit Care 2009;13(5):R171.

23. Gettings LG, Reynolds HN, Scalea T. Outcome in post-traumatic acute renal failure when continuous renal replacement therapy is applied early vs. late. Intensive Care Med 1999;25(8):805–13.

24. Zarbock A, Kellum JA, Schmidt C, et al. Effect of early vs delayed initiation of renal replacement therapy on mortality in critically ill patients with acute kidney injury: the ELAIN randomized clinical trial. JAMA 2016;315(20):2190–9.

25. Gaudry S, Hajage D, Schortgen F, et al. Initiation strategies for renal-replacement therapy in the intensive care unit. N Engl J Med 2016;375(2):122–33.

26. Smith OM, Wald R, Adhikari NK, et al. Standard Versus Accelerated Initiation of Renal Replacement Therapy in Acute Kidney Injury (STARRT-AKI): study protocol for a randomized controlled trial. Trials 2013;14(1):1–9.

27. Barbar SD, Binquet C, Monchi M, et al. Impact on mortality of the timing of renal replacement therapy in patients with severe acute kidney injury in septic shock: the IDEAL-ICU study (Initiation of Dialysis Early Versus Delayed in the Intensive Care Unit): study protocol for a randomized controlled trial. Trials 2014;15:270.

28. Schiffl H, Lang SM, Fischer R. Daily hemodialysis and the outcome of acute renal failure. N Engl J Med 2002;346(5):305–10.

29. Ronco C, Bellomo R, Homel P, et al. Effects of different doses in continuous veno-venous haemofiltration on outcomes of acute renal failure: a prospective randomised trial. Lancet 2000;356(9223):26–30.

30. VA/NIH Acute Renal Failure Trial Network, Palevsky PM, Zhang JH, et al. Intensity of renal support in critically ill patients with acute kidney injury. N Engl J Med 2008;359(1):7–20.

31. Investigators RRTS, Bellomo R, Cass A, et al. Intensity of continuous renal-replacement therapy in critically ill patients. N Engl J Med 2009;361(17):1627–38.

32. Wu MY, Hsu YH, Bai CH, et al. Regional citrate versus heparin anticoagulation for continuous renal replacement therapy: a meta-analysis of randomized controlled trials. Am J Kidney Dis 2012;59(6):810–8.

33. Stevenson JM, Heung M, Vilay AM, et al. In vitro glucose kinetics during continuous renal replacement therapy: implications for caloric balance in critically ill patients. Int J Artif Organs 2013;36(12):861–8.

34. Awdishu L, Bouchard J. How to optimize drug delivery in renal replacement therapy. Semin Dial 2011;24(2):176–82.
35. Scoville BA, Mueller BA. Medication dosing in critically ill patients with acute kidney injury treated with renal replacement therapy. Am J Kidney Dis 2013;61(3): 490–500.
36. Oliver MJ. Acute dialysis catheters. Semin Dial 2001;14(6):432–5.
37. Khwaja A. KDIGO clinical practice guidelines for acute kidney injury. Nephron Clin Pract 2012;120(4):c179–84.
38. Cimochowski GE, Worley E, Rutherford WE, et al. Superiority of the internal jugular over the subclavian access for temporary dialysis. Nephron 1990;54(2): 154–61.
39. Schillinger F, Schillinger D, Montagnac R, et al. Post catheterisation vein stenosis in haemodialysis: comparative angiographic study of 50 subclavian and 50 internal jugular accesses. Nephrol Dial Transplant 1991;6(10):722–4.
40. Hryszko T, Brzosko S, Mazerska M, et al. Risk factors of nontunneled noncuffed hemodialysis catheter malfunction. A prospective study. Nephron Clin Pract 2004;96(2):c43–7.
41. Naumovic RT, Jovanovic DB, Djukanovic LJ. Temporary vascular catheters for hemodialysis: a 3-year prospective study. Int J Artif Organs 2004;27(10):848–54.
42. Vascular Access 2006 Work Group. Clinical practice guidelines for vascular access. Am J Kidney Dis 2006;48(Suppl 1):S176–247.
43. Mottes T, Owens T, Niedner M, et al. Improving delivery of continuous renal replacement therapy: impact of a simulation-based educational intervention. Pediatr Crit Care Med 2013;14(8):747–54.
44. Sanchez-Izquierdo-Riera JA, Molano-Alvarez E, Saez-de la Fuente I, et al. Safety management of a clinical process using failure mode and effect analysis: continuous renal replacement therapies in intensive care unit patients. ASAIO J 2016; 62(1):74–9.
45. Allon M. Dialysis catheter-related bacteremia: treatment and prophylaxis. Am J Kidney Dis 2004;44(5):779–91.
46. Vanholder R, Canaud B, Fluck R, et al. Diagnosis, prevention and treatment of haemodialysis catheter-related bloodstream infections (CRBSI): a position statement of European Renal Best Practice (ERBP). NDT Plus 2010;3(3):234–46.
47. Krishnasami Z, Carlton D, Bimbo L, et al. Management of hemodialysis catheter-related bacteremia with an adjunctive antibiotic lock solution. Kidney Int 2002; 61(3):1136–42.
48. Allon M. Treatment guidelines for dialysis catheter-related bacteremia: an update. Am J Kidney Dis 2009;54(1):13–7.
49. Sychev D, Maya ID, Allon M. Clinical management of dialysis catheter-related bacteremia with concurrent exit-site infection. Semin Dial 2011;24(2):239–41.
50. Hsu RK, McCulloch CE, Dudley RA, et al. Temporal changes in incidence of dialysis-requiring AKI. J Am Soc Nephrol 2013;24(1):37–42.
51. Wald R, McArthur E, Adhikari NK, et al. Changing incidence and outcomes following dialysis-requiring acute kidney injury among critically ill adults: a population-based cohort study. Am J Kidney Dis 2015;65(6):870–7.
52. Brown JR, Rezaee ME, Hisey WM, et al. Reduced mortality associated with acute kidney injury requiring dialysis in the United States. Am J Nephrol 2016;43(4): 261–70.
53. Bedford M, Stevens PE, Wheeler TW, et al. What is the real impact of acute kidney injury? BMC Nephrol 2014;15:95.

54. Rimes-Stigare C, Frumento P, Bottai M, et al. Evolution of chronic renal impairment and long-term mortality after de novo acute kidney injury in the critically ill; a Swedish multi-centre cohort study. Crit Care 2015;19:221.

55. Thakar CV, Christianson A, Himmelfarb J, et al. Acute kidney injury episodes and chronic kidney disease risk in diabetes mellitus. Clin J Am Soc Nephrol 2011; 6(11):2567–72.

56. Ishani A, Xue JL, Himmelfarb J, et al. Acute kidney injury increases risk of ESRD among elderly. J Am Soc Nephrol 2009;20(1):223–8.

57. Siew ED, Peterson JF, Eden SK, et al. Outpatient nephrology referral rates after acute kidney injury. J Am Soc Nephrol 2012;23(2):305–12.

58. Harel Z, Wald R, Bargman JM, et al. Nephrologist follow-up improves all-cause mortality of severe acute kidney injury survivors. Kidney Int 2013;83(5):901–8.

Perioperative Acute Kidney Injury

Risk Factors and Predictive Strategies

Charles Hobson, MD, MHA[a], Rupam Ruchi, MD[b],
Azra Bihorac, MD, MS[b],*

KEYWORDS

- Acute kidney injury • AKI • Prediction scores • CEUS • BOLD MRI • DWI MRI
- Biomarkers

KEY POINTS

- Acute kidney injury is common and is associated with many adverse perioperative outcomes.
- Clinical risk factors for AKI vary in different surgical populations, and preventable risk factors are often underappreciated before surgery.
- Surgical patients should have a systematic preoperative assessment of kidney health, with an emphasis on the patient's renal reserve and susceptibility to new injury.
- The exposure to any intraoperative risk, and the extent of any renal damage, needs to be evaluated using a combination of clinical parameters, biomarkers and imaging techniques.

INTRODUCTION

Acute kidney injury (AKI) is a common and morbid complication in surgical patients and is associated with significant increases in mortality, an increased risk for chronic kidney disease (CKD) and hemodialysis after discharge, and increased cost and resource utilization.[1–11] It is characterized by inappropriate oliguria and/or an increase in serum creatinine levels beyond normal. Perioperative AKI complicates the hospital course for up to 50% of surgical patients.[1,2,12–16] Despite this impact

Conflicts of Interest and Source of Funding: No authors report conflicts of interest. A. Bihorac is supported by the P50 GM-111152 grant from the National Institute of General Medical Sciences and by the R01 GM-110240 grant from the National Institute of Health and has received research grants from the Society of Critical Care Medicine and Astute Medical, Inc. R. Ruchi and C. Hobson report no grant funding.

[a] Department of Health Services Research, Management, and Policy, 1225 Center Drive, HPNP 4151 University of Florida Gainesville, FL 32611, USA; [b] Department of Medicine, University of Florida, PO Box 100254, Gainesville, FL 32610-0254, USA
* Corresponding author.
E-mail address: ABihorac@anest.ufl.edu

Crit Care Clin 33 (2017) 379–396
http://dx.doi.org/10.1016/j.ccc.2016.12.008   **criticalcare.theclinics.com**
0749-0704/17/© 2017 The Authors. Published by Elsevier Inc. This is an open access article under the CC BY-NC-ND license (http://creativecommons.org/licenses/by-nc-nd/4.0/).

AKI remains among the most underdiagnosed and undertreated postoperative complications. Better understanding of the risk factors that contribute to perioperative AKI has led to recent advances in AKI prediction and will eventually lead to improved prevention of AKI, mitigation of injury when AKI occurs, and enhanced recovery in patients who sustain AKI. The development of advanced clinical prediction scores for AKI, new imaging techniques that enable more accurate detection of renal injury, and urinary and serum biomarkers of injury for early detection of AKI provides new tools toward these ends. Surgery provides a unique environment for the study of AKI, as the physiologic stress on the kidney at the time of surgery provides a well-defined opportunity for both risk stratification and the initiation of protective and preventive strategies.

DEFINITIONS AND EPIDEMIOLOGY

Before the development of consensus definitions of AKI, the reported incidence of AKI in the surgical population varied from 1% to 31%. The tendency was to focus on severe, and relatively rare, AKI as defined by large increases in serum creatinine and/or the need for dialysis.[17,18] In 2004 the original Risk, Injury, Failure, Loss, and End-stage Kidney (RIFLE) consensus definition for AKI was released by the Acute Dialysis Quality Initiative. The RIFLE criteria graded less severe AKI stages and provided taxonomies for both severity and recovery.[19] The current guidelines from Kidney Disease: Improving Global Outcomes (KDIGO) modified the RIFLE criteria to include changes in creatinine as small as 0.3 mg/dL[20] (Table 1). The KDIGO guidelines also provide an updated staging system from CKD (Table 2). The epidemiology of perioperative kidney disease has been almost completely redefined since the publication of these consensus definitions.

The consensus definition of AKI has not been uniformly incorporated into the clinical registries and databases used in the surgical community. The American College of Surgeons' (ACS) Committee on Trauma defines AKI as a serum creatinine increase greater or equal to 3.5 mg/dL, and the Society of Thoracic Surgeons Quality Performance Measures defines postoperative renal failure as an increase of serum creatinine to 4.0 mg/dL or greater or 3 times the most recent preoperative creatinine level. The ACS National Surgical Quality Improvement Project (NSQIP) defines AKI as an increase in serum creatinine greater than 2 mg/dL from patients' baseline or as the acute need for renal replacement therapy (RRT).[21] Studies using the ACS NSQIP database typically have high mortality associated with a low incidence of reported AKI, giving the perception that AKI in surgical patients is rare and often fatal.[22] It has been shown that the ACS NSQIP definition for AKI severely underestimates the incidence of AKI, as defined by consensus criteria, in postoperative patients.[12] The incidence of AKI in recent studies using current consensus criteria ranges from 25% in trauma patients[2] to as high as 75% for patients undergoing ruptured abdominal aortic aneurysm repair.[23]

OUTCOMES

Postoperative AKI has been demonstrated to be common and associated with increased incidence of CKD, increased incidence of other postoperative complications, increased risk for short- and long-term mortality, and much higher cost and resource utilization compared with patients with no postoperative AKI.[2,3,5,12,24–32] Two recent studies have demonstrated a continuous risk-adjusted association between postoperative increase in serum creatinine and worse clinical outcomes, and this association persisted at lower cutoffs than in the original RIFLE definition.[12,24] The adverse effects of AKI persist for years even for those patients who demonstrate partial or even full recovery in renal function by the time of hospital discharge.[3,4]

Table 1
Consensus definitions for acute kidney injury

Stage		Serum Creatinine or Glomerular Filtration Rate Criteria		Urine Output Criteria	
RIFLE	KDIGO	RIFLE	KDIGO	RIFLE	KDIGO
Risk	1	Increased sCr ≥1.5 times baseline or GFR decreased >25%	Increased sCr 1.5–1.9 times baseline or ≥0.3 mg/dL increase	Urine output <0.5 mL/kg/h for ≥6 h	Urine output <0.5 mL/kg/h for 6–12 h
Injury	2	Increased sCr ≥2 times baseline or GFR decreased >50%	Increased sCr 2.0–2.9 times baseline	Urine output <0.5 mL/kg/h for ≥12 h	Urine output <0.5 mL/kg/h for ≥12 h
Failure	3	Increased sCr ≥3 times baseline or GFR decreased >75% or sCr ≥4 mg/dL (acute increase ≥0.5 mg/dL)	Increased sCr 3.0 times baseline; or increase in sCr to ≥4.0 mg/dL; or initiation of RRT; or in patients <18 y of age, decrease in eGFR to <35 mL/min/1.73 m²	Urine output <0.3 mL/kg/h for ≥24 h or anuria for ≥12 h	Urine output <0.3 mL/kg/h for ≥24 h or anuria for ≥12 h

Abbreviations: eGFR, estimated glomerular filtration rate; GFR, glomerular filtration rate; RRT, renal replacement therapy; sCr, serum creatinine.

Table 2
Chronic kidney disease staging according to National Kidney Foundation kidney disease outcomes quality initiative guidelines

Stage	Description	Estimated GFR,[a] mL/min/1.73 m²
	At increased risk	≥90 (if CKD risk factors present)
1	Kidney damage with normal or increased GFR	≥90
2	Kidney damage with mildly decreased GFR	60–89
3	Moderately decreased GFR	30–59
4	Severely decreased GFR	15–29
5	Kidney failure	<15 (or dialysis)

Abbreviation: GFR, glomerular filtration rate.
[a] Estimated glomerular filtration rate (GFR) is an estimate of kidney function and is calculated using an equation that includes serum creatinine, age, race, and sex. Most of clinical laboratories will report a corresponding estimated GFR when reporting serum creatinine.
Data from Kidney Disease: Improving Global Outcomes (KDIGO) Acute Kidney Injury Work Group. KDIGO clinical practice guideline for acute kidney injury. Kidney Inter Suppl 2012;2:1–138.

Perioperative AKI is independently associated with a high risk for cardiovascular-specific mortality in diverse patient populations, a risk that is comparable with that observed with CKD.[33,34] In surgical patients who sustain AKI, the risk-adjusted average cost for an episode of care was $42,600 compared with $26,700 for patients with no kidney injury.[1] Recognition of the prevalence and importance of AKI in surgical patients is the first step in improving perioperative care and in developing quality measures that could translate into improved care for surgical patients.

RISK FACTORS

Many perioperative factors have been shown to be predictors of AKI after surgery. Scoring systems used to attempt to predict the risk of AKI after cardiac surgery have relied primarily on preoperative clinical and demographic variables.[35] Systems using genetic polymorphisms for selected inflammatory and vasoconstrictor genes have shown a 2- to 4-fold improvement over clinical factors alone in explaining post-cardiac surgery AKI.[36] Preoperative factors, including total lymphocyte count less than 1500 cells per microliter and elevated C-reactive protein, have been shown to be associated with postcardiac surgery AKI.[37,38] Preoperative factors related to the procedure itself increase the predictive power for patients undergoing noncardiac surgery.[39] The Norton scale score of risk for developing a pressure ulcer and preoperative use of diuretics and nonsteroidal antiinflammatory drugs (NSAIDs) have been associated with AKI following total hip arthroplasty.[40,41] The use of fenestrated grafts and high doses of intravenous contrast are associated with a higher risk for AKI among patients undergoing endovascular abdominal aortic aneurysm repair.[42] In patients sustaining severe trauma, an increase in serum creatinine, an increase in lactic acid, low body temperature, and any transfusion of blood products in the first day after admission were associated with the development of AKI[2] (see Table 1). The Model for End-Stage Liver Disease score, but not pretransplantation creatinine values, was predictive of AKI among patients undergoing liver transplantation.[43] Creating a risk score for AKI applicable to all patients has proven to be challenging.

Many important risk factors for AKI are preventable yet often ignored in surgical patients. Preoperative assessment of kidney function, combining estimated glomerular filtration rate (eGFR) using serum creatinine with albuminuria, is one of the most valuable yet often underutilized clinical resources for clinicians. It is important both to evaluate for the risk for AKI and to quantitate the risk for all postoperative morbidity and mortality. CKD, affecting 5% of the US population,[44] is an independent predictor of cardiovascular morbidity and mortality.[45] An association between CKD severity and postoperative death comparable with that seen with diabetes, stroke, and coronary disease was seen in a review of 31 studies of patients undergoing elective surgery.[46] The adjusted hazard ratio for 30-day mortality in a study using the ACS NSQIP database for patients with CKD ranged from 2.30 (stage 3 CKD) to 3.05 (stage 5 CKD) compared with patients with no CKD.[47] Preoperative proteinuria without CKD was associated with a risk for AKI and was a powerful independent predictor of all-cause mortality and end-stage renal disease after cardiac surgery.[48,49] Some perioperative risk indicator scores consider CKD an important prognostic factor in postoperative risk assessment,[50–52] whereas others do not.[53,54] One issue is that there is a complicated and poorly understood relationship between serum creatinine and the eGFR, which is calculated in many electronic health records.[55] Serum creatinine alone often does not give an accurate picture of the presence of CKD, as creatinine values within normal limits may correspond to a low eGFR, particularly in women and the elderly. Use of the eGFR, if available, can help to assure that CKD is evaluated as a risk factor for both AKI and for overall postoperative mortality.

Many potentially modifiable risk factors for AKI, in both cardiac and noncardiac surgery, include hemodilution, hemoglobin level, intraoperative transfusion, any hypotension, inadequate oxygen delivery, the use of diuretics, the use vasopressors and inotropes, and the use of cardiopulmonary bypass.[56–59] Interventions to optimize blood flow and pressure during surgery, including the use of invasive hemodynamic monitoring, showed no difference in short-term mortality; but the rates of kidney injury were significantly reduced.[60] Goal-directed intraoperative management to reduce the risk of postoperative AKI through optimizing renal perfusion is both feasible and underutilized. Preoperative medications have also been extensively evaluated as both risk and protective factors for a variety of postoperative complications. Several retrospective studies exploring any association between the preoperative use of statins and postoperative AKI have given conflicting results.[61–63] In a recent retrospective study of 98,939 patients undergoing major surgery, the preoperative use of statins was associated with a 20% to 26% reduction in the incidence of AKI as defined by consensus criteria.[64] These results, and the wide-ranging pleiotropic actions of statins, have prompted several pending prospective trials evaluating the effect of statins on perioperative complications, including AKI.

PREDICTIVE STRATEGIES

The risk for postoperative complications, including AKI, arises from the interactions between patients' preoperative health that determines the physiologic capacity to withstand surgery-related stress, modulated by the type and quality of surgery and anesthesia that patients experience. Assessment of surgical risk requires accurate and dynamic synthesis of the large amount of collected clinical information to determine both susceptibility to acute stress and the magnitude of its effect on physiologic homeostasis. During surgery, intraoperative monitors capture complex physiologic time series data reflecting ongoing response to anesthesia and surgery. Given time constraints and the increasing information load on physicians, most of the gathered data can only be screened for overt abnormalities and then discarded. With widespread adoption of electronic health records and advancements in computational power and techniques, use of real-time predictive analytics of clinical data will emerge as the most efficient initial approach for identification of patients at high risk for AKI. Once identified, the high-risk patients can be subjected to incrementally more complex and expensive evaluations with emerging biological biomarkers and imaging techniques depending on the response to initial low-cost and low-risk preventive therapies. This section outlines key clinical risk score, imaging, and biological marker techniques that can be applied in current clinical practice. The authors also provide an example of a pragmatic single-institution approach to standardized clinical assessment and management plans for AKI.

CLINICAL RISK SCORES

The utility of existing AKI scores is limited by several factors, including the use of severe AKI as an end point, restrictions in type of surgery, and lack of dynamic adjustment for preoperative and intraoperative risk factors. Huen and Parikh[35] performed a systematic review of studies among cardiac surgery patients[35] and reported 4 clinical risk scores for AKI requiring dialysis,[65–68] all of which were limited to preoperative variables, and 3 scores to predict a broader definition of AKI.[69–71] Two of the smaller studies included intraoperative data to calculate postoperative scores. The receiver operating characteristic–area under the curve (AUC) varied between 0.77 and 0.84 in both internal and validation cohorts, and most of the studies reported an array of common predictors using mainly logistic regression analysis as a computational tool. Two more recent studies in the United Kingdom and Australia used larger data registries for development and validation of predictive scores that included several intraoperative variables, although model performance remained less than 0.82.[72,73] For patients undergoing noncardiac surgery, few preoperative predictive models were developed, using either only severe AKI as an end point or limiting inclusion to a specific type of surgery.[22,32] Thottakkara and colleagues[74] recently reported a machine-learning computational approach for the development of a KDIGO AKI preoperative forecasting model, using the electronic health records of patients undergoing any type of major surgery. They used 59 variables and reported an AUC of 0.86 in the internal validation cohort.[74] Only a few studies have used intraoperative data in developing a predictive model for noncardiac surgery, and they showed only modest predictive power.[75–77]

Lack of sophistication in data access and analysis in real-time has limited the use of the large volume of complex physiologic time series data generated during surgery for the development of prediction models. To date published postoperative risk scores have used only a snapshot value for hemodynamic monitoring data, such as a mean or lowest value for blood pressure, rather than using time series data applied in their continuity and complexity. An ability to rapidly apply machine learning computational approaches to intraoperative clinical data and physiologic time series data raises the prospect of real-time risk prediction for perioperative AKI as studies using these approaches are emerging.[24,78,79]

IMAGING TECHNIQUES

Imaging techniques, including standard and Doppler ultrasound, have been used for years to help determine the cause of CKD in patients with a transplanted kidney and in patients at risk for renal artery stenosis. Three techniques have recently been developed to help assess AKI: the renal resistive index (RRI) measured using Doppler ultrasound, contrast-enhanced ultrasound (CEUS), and blood oxygenation level–dependent (BOLD) MRI.

RENAL RESISTIVE INDEX

Doppler ultrasound imaging can detect gross vascular abnormalities in the kidney as well as microvascular disorders. RRI, as determined by Doppler ultrasonography, is a measure of pulsatile blood flow that reflects the resistance to flow in the microvasculature. It quantifies changes in both renal vascular resistance and compliance, and an elevated RRI is associated with an increased risk for AKI.[80] An increased RRI has been shown to be associated with AKI associated with sepsis.[81–84] In the immediate postoperative period after cardiac surgery with cardiopulmonary bypass, the RRI predicts both the development of AKI and its severity.[85,86] The prediction of AKI by RRI as measured with intraoperative transesophageal echocardiography, for patients undergoing cardiac surgery, is comparable with that obtained by RRI through translumbar ultrasound.[87] Elevated RRI is associated with AKI in orthopedic surgery and in critically ill patients in the medical intensive care unit (ICU).[88–90] RRI has also been shown to be useful in predicting the progression of postoperative AKI.[91] Although RRI depends on renal vascular resistance and compliance, there are other factors that affect RRI, especially in unstable patients; the indications for the test are evolving.[92,93]

CONTRAST-ENHANCED ULTRASOUND

CEUS has been used for years to help assess solid and cystic lesions in the kidney.[94,95] It has more recently been used to assess renal perfusion.[96] In patients undergoing elective cardiac surgery who were considered to be at risk of AKI, renal perfusion as measured using CEUS decreased significantly within 24 hours after surgery.[97] CEUS shows early promise in assessing both the risk and prognosis of AKI in surgical patients.[98–100]

MRI

MRI is evolving as a technique to aid in diagnosis of AKI. Newer contrast agents, including ultrasmall particles of iron oxide, are less toxic and are being used to study renal blood flow and volume.[101] BOLD MRI uses deoxyhemoglobin as a nontoxic and endogenous contrast agent for the study of intrarenal oxygenation.[102] The technique of BOLD MRI has been used to demonstrate changes in renal blood flow related to the use of nephrotoxins, including NSAIDs, intravenous contrast agents, and calcineurin inhibitors.[103] It has also been used to study changes in renal blood flow associated with CKD and hypertension.[104–106] Despite the utility of BOLD MRI in studying renal oxygenation and function in animal models of AKI,[107,108] one recent study evaluating BOLD MRI in the evaluation of AKI in humans found no correlation between MRI findings and glomerular filtration rate (GFR).[109] Another recently developed MRI technique known as diffusion-weighted imaging (DWI) detects the motion of water molecules within tissue and has been used to assess renal fibrosis in both AKI and CKD.[79] As with RRI, the indications and utility of BOLD MRI and DWI MRI for predicting AKI in surgical patients are not yet characterized.

USE OF URINE AND PLASMA BIOMARKERS

A new approach for assessing kidney injury is the analysis of serum and/or urine biomarkers. Early recognition of kidney injury using serum creatinine is problematic as creatinine is a measure of renal function not injury. The ideal biomarker will reveal early evidence of cellular stress before permanent damage even occurs. Serum troponins are useful as biomarkers for cardiac injury because they rapidly reflect myocardial stress and injury. Several urine and serum biomarkers have been studied for their ability to predict kidney stress and injury.[110–115] Many biomarkers fail because of a lack of sensitivity to early cellular stress, a lack of specificity to renal injury, because they cannot differentiate AKI from CKD, and because they are also elevated by the disease process that has caused the AKI. The variety of stressors faced by surgical patients also makes the search for an effective biomarker difficult. The disease process and/or surgical procedure often results in cellular stress and injuries in several organs, complicated by hemodynamic instability requiring fluid and vasopressor support, blood transfusion, and exposure to nephrotoxic drugs.

Biomarkers to detect kidney injury have been most widely studied in cardiac surgery. Early studies identified plasma and urine neutrophil gelatinase-associated lipocalin (NGAL) as a potential biomarker.[116,117] Inflammation induces NGAL synthesis and its release from neutrophils throughout the body. A recent summary of NGAL in cardiac surgery patients demonstrated only moderate ability to discriminate AKI from other organ injury.[114] Studies of critically ill patients in both medical and surgical ICUs showed similar moderate discriminative performance.[83,118] The inability to discriminate between systemic and kidney-specific effects has limited the clinical use of NGAL.

A more kidney-specific functional biomarker that has undergone extensive evaluation, especially in pediatric patients, is cystatin C (CyC).[119,120] CyC is a protease inhibitor produced by all nucleated cells of the body, released at a constant rate, filtered by the glomeruli, and then completely reabsorbed in the renal tubules. CyC is not normally found in urine; thus, the presence of urinary CyC may reflect early kidney injury. Because of the constant rate of its production, plasma CyC concentrations may be a better marker than serum creatinine of GFR; it has recently been proposed as a replacement for serum creatinine in the routine evaluation of GFR rather than as a biomarker of AKI.[120,121] The role of CyC in risk stratification for postoperative AKI among surgical patients remains to be defined.[112]

A combination of 2 novel urinary biomarkers has recently been validated as a marker for AKI and has been approved by the US Food and Drug Administration to assess the risk of developing AKI in critically ill patients. Tissue inhibitor of metalloproteinases-2 (TIMP-2) and insulinlike growth factor binding protein 7 (IGFBP7) are cell-cycle arrest proteins, expressed by renal tubular cells and released into the urine during periods of stress due to toxin exposure, hypoxia, and inflammation, among others. Thus, these urinary biomarkers may indicate risk for injury before any actual AKI takes place.[122]

Several multicenter studies have shown that the combination of urinary TIMP-2 and IGFBP7 (TIMP-2•IGFBP7) was predictive of moderate to severe AKI in critically ill patients within 12 hours.[123–125] The power of the TIMP-2•IGFBP7 test to predict the risk of AKI in these studies was superior to serum creatinine and to other measured biomarkers. Patients with a TIMP-2•IGFBP7 higher than 0.3 (ng/mL)^2/1000 had 7 times the risk for AKI (95% confidence interval 4–22) compared with patients with lower values. A validation study confirmed the high sensitivity and high negative predictive values of 89% and 97%, respectively, for the cutoff of 0.3.[126] The development and validation of this biomarker combination is an important advance in early and accurate diagnosis of AKI.

A PRAGMATIC APPROACH

The use of standardized clinical assessment and management plans that synthesize current medical knowledge with best clinical judgment decreases practice variability and improves patient care better than clinical guidelines.[127] Considering the high prevalence of AKI, and the adverse outcomes when it occurs, efforts at the authors' institution have focused on prevention of AKI, mitigation of further injury when AKI has already occurred, treatment of negative effects on other organs, and facilitation of renal recovery in patients with established AKI.

Using KDIGO clinical guidelines as a framework, and using the authors' institutional perioperative registry outcome data,[2-4] the authors have developed a multistage approach for the determination of kidney health and risk stratification for AKI in the perioperative period and among critically ill surgical patients. This process requires assessment of patients' renal resilience and susceptibility to new injury, the extent of exposure to insult, and the resulting distress or damage sustained by that insult. The determination and management of potential causes of AKI, initiation of interventions, and reassessment of kidney distress in response to that therapy follows promptly afterward. This clinical pathway requires a medical team of experts that not only defines the standardization pathway for the institutions but also provides backup for the bedside care providers.

PREOPERATIVE PATHWAY

In the preoperative period an accurate assessment of kidney health is important because the extent of previous kidney disease significantly increases susceptibility to the acute stress of surgery. Assessment of renal resilience to acute insult requires a search for any evidence of previous functional or structural kidney damage. Review of the medical history should include diagnosis and staging of known CKD, evidence of previous AKI episodes, and presence of risk factors for CKD. The determination of functional renal reserve with a kidney stress test[128] may be indicated for more precise risk stratification among patients without apparent CKD who may be considered as high risk because of age or other comorbidities, such as hypertension, chronic obstructive pulmonary disease, vascular disease, diabetes, or liver disease.

POSTOPERATIVE PATHWAY

For those surgical patients admitted to an ICU, an assessment of kidney health is considered part of a detailed ICU admission assessment. All steps of this process, including the clinical risk stratification, the assessment of tubular distress, and the initiation of treatment, should occur within the first 12 to 24 hours of the ICU admission. Every patient admitted to the authors' ICU undergoes a simple, yet systematic assessment of kidney health. Assessment of renal resilience requires a review of the medical history for diagnosis and staging of known CKD, evidence of previous AKI episodes, and the presence of any risk factors for AKI and CKD. For each patient, the authors perform a calculation of eGFR using reference serum creatinine and, when available, a measurement of albuminuria with urine dipstick or random microalbumin/creatinine ratio tests as an inexpensive snapshot of baseline kidney function. The exposure to insult is quantified by a search of the preceding 24 hours for any evidence of hypotension, use of vasopressors or nephrotoxic medications, sepsis, severe trauma, or any other conditions associated with a high risk for AKI.

Based on this process, the authors have developed an automated algorithm built into the electronic health record note to quantify a clinical risk score for AKI (range 0–16). Patients with a low clinical risk for AKI can undergo usual ICU care. Only patients with a high score ($\geq$3) are further tested for kidney stress using the urinary biomarker TIMP-2•IGFBP7. In the authors' experience, approximately 40% of new admissions to the surgical ICU have a high clinical risk score. Only patients with both a high clinical risk score and a high urinary biomarker test result are considered to be at high risk for AKI and are subjected to the authors' *AKI bundle* of diagnostic tests and preventive measures during the subsequent 48 hours in an attempt to prevent or ameliorate kidney injury (Fig. 1).

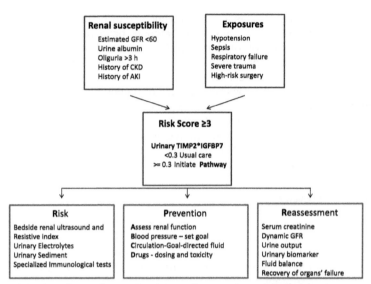

Fig. 1. A clinical pathway for evaluating and managing AKI. (*From* Bihorac A. Critical controversies: Guiding AKI prevention using biomarkers. Available at: http://www.sccm. org/Communications/Critical-Connections/Archives/Pages/Guiding-AKI-Prevention-Using-Biomarkers.aspx. Accessed August 10, 2016.)

This set of parallel clinical action pathways (risk, prevention, and reassessment) is focused on the identification of the cause of AKI, initiation of preventive therapies, and daily reassessment of the kidney response to initiated therapies. This set is more comprehensive than the KDIGO AKI management options (Fig. 2). This process

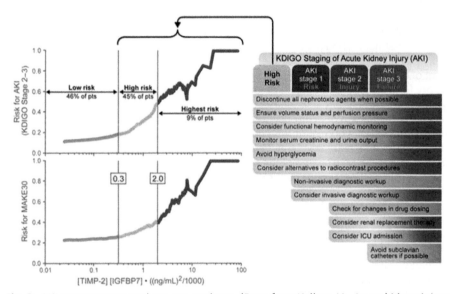

Fig. 2. AKI management options. pts, patients. (*Data from* Kellum JA. Acute kidney injury and AKI biomarkers in the ICU. Southeaster Critical Care Summit. 2016; *Adapted from* Kidney Disease: Improving Global Outcomes (KDIGO) Acute Kidney Injury Work Group. KDIGO clinical practice guideline for acute kidney injury. Kidney Inter Suppl 2012;2:1–138.)

may involve specialized clinical, laboratory, and imaging tools and represents a coordinated effort between the ICU and nephrology teams. Preventive therapies include monitoring and optimizing hemodynamic status by goal-directed fluid management and blood pressure control, strict avoidance of nephrotoxic medications, monitoring of drug levels, and avoiding side effects by adjusting drug dosing in accordance with the GFR. The goal of this phase is to prevent the progression of tubular distress toward functional decline whenever possible and to avoid the negative consequences of fluid overload and drug toxicity in patients with established tubular distress and, thus, it is hoped, to prevent any decline in renal function. The consideration for early RRT may be appropriate for patients with large levels of tubular distress and rapid functional decline, whereby impaired handling of fluids may endanger other organs.

The authors' preliminary experience with protocol implementation and compliance was excellent. One obstacle to implementation was the high cost of the TIMP-2•IGFBP7 urinary biomarker test, which the authors overcame by limiting use of the test to those indications standardized within this protocol. Whether this implementation translates into better outcomes will require further evaluation and analysis.

SUMMARY

AKI is common and is associated with many adverse perioperative outcomes. Mild to moderate AKI is much more common than severe AKI and has become much more appreciated with the introduction of consensus definitions for AKI. All stages of AKI severity are associated with increased morbidity and mortality. Clinical risk factors for AKI vary in different surgical populations, and preventable risk factors are often underappreciated before surgery. Efforts must focus on better identification of risk factors, better risk stratification and, thus, prediction of AKI in susceptible patients, and ultimately the prevention of AKI if possible or the facilitation of renal recovery in those patients who sustain AKI. Every surgical patient should have a systematic preoperative assessment of kidney health, with an emphasis on patients' renal reserve and susceptibility to new injury. In the postoperative period the exposure to any intraoperative risk, and the extent of any renal damage, needs to be evaluated using a combination of clinical parameters, novel biomarkers, and evolving imaging techniques. The prompt initiation of treatment and measures to prevent further renal injury, and to promote renal recovery, can then be instituted.

REFERENCES

1. Hobson C, Ozrazgat-Baslanti T, Kuxhausen A, et al. Cost and mortality associated with postoperative acute kidney injury. Ann Surg 2015;261(6):1207–14.
2. Bihorac A, Delano MJ, Schold JD, et al. Incidence, clinical predictors, genomics, and outcome of acute kidney injury among trauma patients. Ann Surg 2010;252(1):158–65.
3. Hobson CE, Yavas S, Segal MS, et al. Acute kidney injury is associated with increased long-term mortality after cardiothoracic surgery. Circulation 2009; 119(18):2444–53.
4. Bihorac A, Yavas S, Subbiah S, et al. Long-term risk of mortality and acute kidney injury during hospitalization after major surgery. Ann Surg 2009;249(5):851–8.
5. Wald R, Quinn RR, Luo J. Chronic dialysis and death among survivors of acute kidney injury requiring dialysis. JAMA 2009;302(11):1179–85.
6. van Kuijk JP, Flu WJ, Chonchol M, et al. Temporary perioperative decline of renal function is an independent predictor for chronic kidney disease. Clin J Am Soc Nephrol 2010;5(7):1198–204.

7. Ishani A, Nelson D, Clothier B, et al. The magnitude of acute serum creatinine increase after cardiac surgery and the risk of chronic kidney disease, progression of kidney disease, and death. Arch Intern Med 2011;171(3):226–33.

8. James MT, Ghali WA, Knudtson ML, et al. Associations between acute kidney injury and cardiovascular and renal outcomes after coronary angiography. Circulation 2011;123(4):409–16.

9. Thakar CV, Christianson A, Himmelfarb J, et al. Acute kidney injury episodes and chronic kidney disease risk in diabetes mellitus. Clin J Am Soc Nephrol 2011;6(11):2567–72.

10. Coca SG, Jammalamadaka D, Sint K, et al. Preoperative proteinuria predicts acute kidney injury in patients undergoing cardiac surgery. J Thorac Cardiovasc Surg 2012;143(2):495–502.

11. Chawla LS, Amdur RL, Shaw AD, et al. Association between AKI and long-term renal and cardiovascular outcomes in United States veterans. Clin J Am Soc Nephrol 2014;9(3):448–56.

12. Bihorac A, Brennan M, Ozrazgat Baslanti T, et al. National surgical quality improvement program underestimates the risk associated with mild and moderate postoperative acute kidney injury. Crit Care Med 2013;41(11):2570–83.

13. Borthwick E, Ferguson A. Perioperative acute kidney injury: risk factors, recognition, management, and outcomes. BMJ 2010;341:c3365.

14. Vaught A, Ozrazgat-Baslanti T, Javed A, et al. Acute kidney injury in major gynaecological surgery: an observational study. BJOG 2015;122(10):1340–8.

15. Calvert S, Shaw A. Perioperative acute kidney injury. Perioper Med (Lond) 2012;1:6.

16. Thakar CV. Perioperative acute kidney injury. Adv Chronic Kidney Dis 2013; 20(1):67–75.

17. Hoste EA, Kellum JA. Incidence, classification, and outcomes of acute kidney injury. Contrib Nephrol 2007;156:32–8.

18. Ricci Z, Cruz DN, Ronco C. Classification and staging of acute kidney injury: beyond the RIFLE and AKIN criteria. Nat Rev Nephrol 2011;7(4):201–8.

19. Bellomo R, Ronco C, Kellum JA, et al. Acute renal failure - definition, outcome measures, animal models, fluid therapy and information technology needs: the Second International Consensus Conference of the Acute Dialysis Quality Initiative (ADQI) Group. Crit Care 2004;8(4):R204–12.

20. KDOGI. Clinical practice guideline for acute kidney injury: AKI definition. Kidney Int 2012;2(Suppl 1):19–36.

21. American College of Surgeons National Surgical Quality Improvement Program. User Guide for the 2010 Participant Use Data File. 2010. Available at: http://site. acsnsqip.org/wp-content/uploads/2012/03/2010-User-Guide_FINAL.pdf. Accessed February 25, 2013.

22. Kheterpal S, Tremper KK, Heung M, et al. Development and validation of an acute kidney injury risk index for patients undergoing general surgery: results from a national data set. Anesthesiology 2009;110(3):505–15.

23. van Beek SC, Legemate DA, Vahl A, et al. Acute kidney injury defined according to the 'Risk,' 'Injury,' 'Failure,' 'Loss,' and 'End-stage'(RIFLE) criteria after repair for a ruptured abdominal aortic aneurysm. J Vasc Surg 2014;60(5):1159–67.e1.

24. Ozrazgat Baslanti T, Korenkevych D, Momcilovic P, et al. Mathematical modeling of the association between the pattern of change in postoperative serum creatinine and hospital mortality. Crit Care Med 2012;40(12):U131.

25. Dimick JB, Pronovost PJ, Cowan JA, et al. Complications and costs after high-risk surgery: where should we focus quality improvement initiatives? J Am Coll Surg 2003;196(5):671–8.

26. Dimick JB, Chen SL, Taheri PA, et al. Hospital costs associated with surgical complications: a report from the private-sector National Surgical Quality Improvement Program. J Am Coll Surgeons 2004;199(4):531–7.

27. Thakar CV, Christianson A, Freyberg R, et al. Incidence and outcomes of acute kidney injury in intensive care units: a Veterans Administration study. Crit Care Med 2009;37(9):2552–8.

28. Duran PA, Concepcion LA. Survival after acute kidney injury requiring dialysis: long-term follow up. Hemodialysis Int 2014;18(S1):S1–6.

29. Coca SG, Yusuf B, Shlipak MG, et al. Long-term risk of mortality and other adverse outcomes after acute kidney injury: a systematic review and meta-analysis. Am J Kidney Dis 2009;53(6):961–73.

30. Lafrance J-P, Miller DR. Acute kidney injury associates with increased long-term mortality. J Am Soc Nephrol 2010;21(2):345–52.

31. Amdur RL, Chawla LS, Amodeo S, et al. Outcomes following diagnosis of acute renal failure in US veterans: focus on acute tubular necrosis. Kidney Int 2009; 76(10):1089–97.

32. Bell S, Dekker FW, Vadiveloo T, et al. Risk of postoperative acute kidney injury in patients undergoing orthopaedic surgery—development and validation of a risk score and effect of acute kidney injury on survival: observational cohort study. BMJ 2015;351:h5639.

33. Ozrazgat-Baslanti T, Thottakkara P, Huber M, et al. Acute and chronic kidney disease and cardiovascular mortality after major surgery. Ann Surg 2016;264(6): 987–96.

34. Huber M, Ozrazgat-Baslanti T, Thottakkara P, et al. Cardiovascular-specific mortality and kidney disease in patients undergoing vascular surgery. JAMA Surg 2016;151(5):441–50.

35. Huen SC, Parikh CR. Predicting acute kidney injury after cardiac surgery: a systematic review. Ann Thorac Surg 2012;93(1):337–47.

36. Stafford-Smith M, Podgoreanu M, Swaminathan M, et al. Association of genetic polymorphisms with risk of renal injury after coronary bypass graft surgery. Am J Kidney Dis 2005;45(3):519–30.

37. Lomivorotov VV, Efremov SM, Boboshko VA, et al. Preoperative total lymphocyte count in peripheral blood as a predictor of poor outcome in adult cardiac surgery. J Cardiothorac Vasc Anesth 2011;25(6):975–80.

38. Kim DH, Shim JK, Hong SW, et al. Predictive value of C-reactive protein for major postoperative complications following off-pump coronary artery bypass surgery: prospective and observational trial. Circ J 2009;73(5):872–7.

39. van Kuijk JP, Flu WJ, Valentijn TM, et al. Preoperative left ventricular dysfunction predisposes to postoperative acute kidney injury and long-term mortality. J Nephrol 2011;24(6):764–70.

40. Asleh K, Sever R, Hilu S, et al. Association between low admission Norton scale scores and postoperative complications after elective THA in elderly patients. Orthopedics 2012;35(9):e1302–6.

41. Aveline C, Leroux A, Vautier P, et al. Risk factors for renal dysfunction after total hip arthroplasty. Ann Fr Anesth Reanim 2009;28(9):728–34 [in French].

42. Brooks CE, Middleton A, Dhillon R, et al. Predictors of creatinine rise post-endovascular abdominal aortic aneurysm repair. ANZ J Surg 2011;81(11): 827–30.

43. Romano TG, Schmidtbauer I, Silva FM, et al. Role of MELD score and serum creatinine as prognostic tools for the development of acute kidney injury after liver transplantation. PLoS One 2013;8(5):e64089.

44. Lamb EJ, Levey AS, Stevens PE. The Kidney Disease Improving Global Outcomes (KDIGO) guideline update for chronic kidney disease: evolution not revolution. Clin Chem 2013;59(3):462–5.

45. Matsushita K, van der Velde M, Astor BC, et al. Association of estimated glomerular filtration rate and albuminuria with all-cause and cardiovascular mortality in general population cohorts: a collaborative meta-analysis. Lancet 2010;375(9731): 2073–81.

46. Mathew A, Devereaux PJ, O'Hare A, et al. Chronic kidney disease and postoperative mortality: a systematic review and meta-analysis. Kidney Int 2008;73(9): 1069–81.

47. Gaber AO, Moore LW, Aloia TA, et al. Cross-sectional and case-control analyses of the association of kidney function staging with adverse postoperative outcomes in general and vascular surgery. Ann Surg 2013;258(1):169–77.

48. Wu VC, Huang TM, Wu PC, et al. Preoperative proteinuria is associated with long-term progression to chronic dialysis and mortality after coronary artery bypass grafting surgery. PLoS One 2012;7(1):e27687.

49. Huang TM, Wu VC, Young GH, et al. Preoperative proteinuria predicts adverse renal outcomes after coronary artery bypass grafting. J Am Soc Nephrol 2011; 22(1):156–63.

50. Fleisher LA, Eagle KA. Clinical practice. Lowering cardiac risk in noncardiac surgery. N Engl J Med 2001;345(23):1677–82.

51. Kertai MD, Boersma E, Klein J, et al. Optimizing the prediction of perioperative mortality in vascular surgery by using a customized probability model. Arch Intern Med 2005;165(8):898–904.

52. Lee TH, Marcantonio ER, Mangione CM, et al. Derivation and prospective validation of a simple index for prediction of cardiac risk of major noncardiac surgery. Circulation 1999;100(10):1043–9.

53. Detsky AS, Abrams HB, McLaughlin JR, et al. Predicting cardiac complications in patients undergoing non-cardiac surgery. J Gen Intern Med 1986; 1(4):211–9.

54. Goldman L, Caldera DL, Nussbaum SR, et al. Multifactorial index of cardiac risk in noncardiac surgical procedures. N Engl J Med 1977;297(16):845–50.

55. Levey AS, Stevens LA, Schmid CH, et al. A new equation to estimate glomerular filtration rate. Ann Intern Med 2009;150(9):604–12.

56. Karkouti K, Wijeysundera DN, Yau TM, et al. Acute kidney injury after cardiac surgery: focus on modifiable risk factors. Circulation 2009;119(4): 495–502.

57. Haase M, Bellomo R, Story D, et al. Effect of mean arterial pressure, haemoglobin and blood transfusion during cardiopulmonary bypass on post-operative acute kidney injury. Nephrol Dial Transplant 2012;27(1):153–60.

58. de Somer F, Mulholland JW, Bryan MR, et al. O-2 delivery and CO2 production during cardiopulmonary bypass as determinants of acute kidney injury: time for a goal-directed perfusion management? Crit Care 2011;15(4):R192.

59. Parolari A, Pesce LL, Pacini D, et al. Risk factors for perioperative acute kidney injury after adult cardiac surgery: role of perioperative management. Ann Thorac Surg 2012;93(2):584–91.

60. Grocott Michael PW, Dushianthan A, Hamilton Mark A, et al. Perioperative increase in global blood flow to explicit defined goals and outcomes following

surgery. Cochrane Database Syst Rev 2012;(11):CD004082. Available at: http://
onlinelibrary.wiley.com/doi/10.1002/14651858.CD004082.pub5/abstract.   http://
onlinelibrary.wiley.com/store/10.1002/14651858.CD004082.pub5/asset/CD0040
82.pdf?v=1&t=htvv4net&s=8117a1c2ac62cedf4d7e4fc5f6d9d0025614ae3d.
http://onlinelibrary.wiley.com/store/10.1002/14651858.CD004082.pub5/asset/CD
004082.pdf?v=1&t=i9cr70es&s=a62c81b3e90d1a75c74ae3d8763d6fdcf559
f8ec.

61. Liakopoulos OJ, Kuhn EW, Slottosch I, et al. Preoperative statin therapy for patients undergoing cardiac surgery. Cochrane Database Syst Rev 2012;(4):CD008493.

62. Kor DJ, Brown MJ, Iscimen R, et al. Perioperative statin therapy and renal outcomes after major vascular surgery: a propensity-based analysis. J Cardiothorac Vasc Anesth 2008;22(2):210–6.

63. Molnar AO, Coca SG, Devereaux PJ, et al. Statin use associates with a lower incidence of acute kidney injury after major elective surgery. J Am Soc Nephrol 2011;22(5):939–46.

64. Brunelli SM, Waikar SS, Bateman BT, et al. Preoperative statin use and postoperative acute kidney injury. Am J Med 2012;125(12):1195.

65. Chertow GM, Lazarus JM, Christiansen CL, et al. Preoperative renal risk stratification. Circulation 1997;95(4):878–84.

66. Thakar CV, Arrigain S, Worley S, et al. A clinical score to predict acute renal failure after cardiac surgery. J Am Soc Nephrol 2005;16(1):162–8.

67. Mehta RH, Grab JD, O'Brien SM, et al. Bedside tool for predicting the risk of postoperative dialysis in patients undergoing cardiac surgery. Circulation 2006;114(21):2208–16 [quiz: 2208].

68. Wijeysundera DN, Karkouti K, Dupuis JY, et al. Derivation and validation of a simplified predictive index for renal replacement therapy after cardiac surgery. JAMA 2007;297(16):1801–9.

69. Aronson S, Fontes ML, Miao Y, et al. Risk index for perioperative renal dysfunction/failure: critical dependence on pulse pressure hypertension. Circulation 2007;115(6):733–42.

70. Palomba H, de Castro I, Neto AL, et al. Acute kidney injury prediction following elective cardiac surgery: AKICS score. Kidney Int 2007;72(5):624–31.

71. Brown JR, Cochran RP, Leavitt BJ, et al. Multivariable prediction of renal insufficiency developing after cardiac surgery. Circulation 2007;116(Suppl 11):I139–43.

72. Birnie K, Verheyden V, Pagano D, et al. Predictive models for Kidney Disease: Improving Global Outcomes (KDIGO) defined acute kidney injury in UK cardiac surgery. Crit Care 2014;18(6):606.

73. Ng SY, Sanagou M, Wolfe R, et al. Prediction of acute kidney injury within 30 days of cardiac surgery. J Thorac Cardiovasc Surg 2014;147(6):1875–83.e1.

74. Thottakkara P, Ozrazgat-Baslanti T, Hupf BB, et al. Application of machine learning techniques to high-dimensional clinical data to forecast postoperative complications. PLoS One 2016;11(5):e0155705.

75. Rueggeberg A, Boehm S, Napieralski F, et al. Development of a risk stratification model for predicting acute renal failure in orthotopic liver transplantation recipients. Anaesthesia 2008;63(11):1174–80.

76. Kheterpal S, Tremper KK, Englesbe MJ, et al. Predictors of postoperative acute renal failure after noncardiac surgery in patients with previously normal renal function. Anesthesiology 2007;107(6):892–902.

77. Kashani K, Steuernagle JHT, Akhoundi A, et al. Vascular surgery kidney injury predictive score: a historical cohort study. J Cardiothorac Vasc Anesth 2015; 29(6):1588–95.
78. Celi LA, Galvin S, Davidzon G, et al. A database-driven decision support system: customized mortality prediction. J Pers Med 2012;2(4):138–48.
79. Bihorac A. Acute kidney injury in the surgical patient: recognition and attribution. Nephron 2015;131(2):118–22.
80. Ninet S, Schnell D, Dewitte A, et al. Doppler-based renal resistive index for prediction of renal dysfunction reversibility: a systematic review and meta-analysis. J Crit Care 2015;30(3):629–35.
81. Deruddre S, Cheisson G, Mazoit JX, et al. Renal arterial resistance in septic shock: effects of increasing mean arterial pressure with norepinephrine on the renal resistive index assessed with Doppler ultrasonography. Intensive Care Med 2007;33(9):1557–62.
82. Lerolle N, Guerot E, Faisy C, et al. Renal failure in septic shock: predictive value of Doppler-based renal arterial resistive index. Intensive Care Med 2006;32(10): 1553–9.
83. Gornik I, Godan A, Gašparović V. Renal resistive index at ICU admission and its change after 24 hours predict acute kidney injury in sepsis. Crit Care 2014; 18(Suppl 1):P366.
84. Lahmer T, Rasch S, Schnappauf C, et al. Influence of volume administration on Doppler-based renal resistive index, renal hemodynamics and renal function in medical intensive care unit patients with septic-induced acute kidney injury: a pilot study. Int Urol Nephrol 2016;48(8):1327–34.
85. Bossard G, Bourgoin P, Corbeau JJ, et al. Early detection of postoperative acute kidney injury by Doppler renal resistive index in cardiac surgery with cardiopulmonary bypass. Br J Anaesth 2011;107(6):891–8.
86. Regolisti G, Maggiore U, Cademartiri C, et al. Renal resistive index by transesophageal and transparietal echo-Doppler imaging for the prediction of acute kidney injury in patients undergoing major heart surgery. J Nephrol 2016;1–11.
87. Kararmaz A, Kemal Arslantas M, Cinel I. Renal resistive index measurement by transesophageal echocardiography: comparison with translumbar ultrasonography and relation to acute kidney injury. J Cardiothorac Vasc Anesth 2015; 29(4):875–80.
88. Darmon M, Schortgen F, Vargas F, et al. Diagnostic accuracy of Doppler renal resistive index for reversibility of acute kidney injury in critically ill patients. Intensive Care Med 2011;37(1):68–76.
89. Marty P, Szatjnic S, Ferre F, et al. Doppler renal resistive index for early detection of acute kidney injury after major orthopaedic surgery: a prospective observational study. Eur J Anaesthesiol 2015;32(1):37–43.
90. Boddi M, Bonizzoli M, Chiostri M, et al. Renal resistive index and mortality in critical patients with acute kidney injury. Eur J Clin Invest 2016;46(3):242–51.
91. Guinot PG, Bernard E, Abou Arab O, et al. Doppler-based renal resistive index can assess progression of acute kidney injury in patients undergoing cardiac surgery. J Cardiothorac Vasc Anesth 2013;27(5):890–6.
92. Viazzi F, Leoncini G, Derchi LE, et al. Ultrasound Doppler renal resistive index: a useful tool for the management of the hypertensive patient. J Hypertens 2014; 32(1):149–53.
93. Dewitte A, Coquin J, Meyssignac B, et al. Doppler resistive index to reflect regulation of renal vascular tone during sepsis and acute kidney injury. Crit Care 2012;16(5):R165.

94. Bertolotto M, Cicero C, Perrone R, et al. Renal masses with equivocal enhancement at CT: characterization with contrast-enhanced ultrasound. AJR Am J Roentgenol 2015;204(5):W557–65.

95. Chang EH, Chong WK, Kasoji SK, et al. Management of indeterminate cystic kidney lesions: review of contrast-enhanced ultrasound as a diagnostic tool. Urology 2016;87:1–10.

96. Mahoney M, Sorace A, Warram J, et al. Volumetric contrast-enhanced ultrasound imaging of renal perfusion. J Ultrasound Med 2014;33(8):1427–37.

97. Schneider AG, Goodwin MD, Schelleman A, et al. Contrast-enhanced ultrasound to evaluate changes in renal cortical perfusion around cardiac surgery: a pilot study. Crit Care 2013;17(4):1.

98. Harrois A, Duranteau J. Contrast-enhanced ultrasound: a new vision of microcirculation in the intensive care unit. Crit Care 2013;17(4):449.

99. Legrand MM, Darmon M. Renal imaging in acute kidney injury. Acute nephrology for the critical care physician. Springer; 2015. p. 125–38.

100. Göcze I, Renner P, Graf BM, et al. Simplified approach for the assessment of kidney perfusion and acute kidney injury at the bedside using contrast-enhanced ultrasound. Intensive Care Med 2015;41(2):362–3.

101. Choyke P, Kobayashi H. Functional magnetic resonance imaging of the kidney using macromolecular contrast agents. Abdom Imaging 2006;31(2):224–31.

102. Prasad PV, Edelman RR, Epstein FH. Noninvasive evaluation of intrarenal oxygenation with BOLD MRI. Circulation 1996;94(12):3271–5.

103. Hofmann L, Simon-Zoula S, Nowak A, et al. BOLD-MRI for the assessment of renal oxygenation in humans: acute effect of nephrotoxic xenobiotics. Kidney Int 2006;70(1):144–50.

104. Vink E, Boer A, Verloop W, et al. The effect of renal denervation on kidney oxygenation as determined by BOLD MRI in patients with hypertension. Eur Radiol 2015;25(7):1984–92.

105. Vink EE, de Boer A, Hoogduin HJ, et al. Renal BOLD-MRI relates to kidney function and activity of the renin-angiotensin-aldosterone system in hypertensive patients. J Hypertens 2015;33(3):597–603.

106. Pruijm M, Hofmann L, Piskunowicz M, et al. Determinants of renal tissue oxygenation as measured with BOLD-MRI in chronic kidney disease and hypertension in humans. PLoS One 2014;9(4):e95895.

107. Oostendorp M, de Vries EE, Slenter JMGM, et al. MRI of renal oxygenation and function after normothermic ischemia–reperfusion injury. NMR Biomed 2011;24(2):194–200.

108. Li L-P, Lu J, Zhou Y, et al. Evaluation of intrarenal oxygenation in iodinated contrast-induced acute kidney injury–susceptible rats by blood oxygen level–dependent magnetic resonance imaging. Invest Radiol 2014;49(6):403–10.

109. Inoue T, Kozawa E, Okada H, et al. Noninvasive evaluation of kidney hypoxia and fibrosis using magnetic resonance imaging. J Am Soc Nephrol 2011;22(8):1429–34.

110. Vanmassenhove J, Vanholder R, Nagler E, et al. Urinary and serum biomarkers for the diagnosis of acute kidney injury: an in-depth review of the literature. Nephrol Dial Transplant 2013;28(2):254–73.

111. Ostermann M, Philips BJ, Forni LG. Clinical review: biomarkers of acute kidney injury: where are we now? Crit Care 2012;16(5):233.

112. Wasung ME, Chawla LS, Madero M. Biomarkers of renal function, which and when? Clin Chim Acta 2015;438(0):350–7.

113. Charlton JR, Portilla D, Okusa MD. A basic science view of acute kidney injury biomarkers. Nephrol Dial Transplant 2014;29(7):1301–11.
114. Koyner JL, Parikh CR. Clinical utility of biomarkers of AKI in cardiac surgery and critical illness. Clin J Am Soc Nephrol 2013;8(6):1034–42.
115. Ricci Z, Villa G, Ronco C. Management of AKI: the role of biomarkers. Annual Update in Intensive Care and Emergency Medicine 2015. Springer; 2015. p. 365–77.
116. Martensson J, Bellomo R. The rise and fall of NGAL in acute kidney injury. Blood Purif 2014;37(4):304–10.
117. Hošková L, Franekova J, Málek I, et al. Comparison of cystatin C and NGAL in early diagnosis of acute kidney injury after heart transplantation. Ann Transplant 2015;21. 329–245.
118. Haase M, Bellomo R, Devarajan P, et al. Accuracy of neutrophil gelatinase-associated lipocalin (NGAL) in diagnosis and prognosis in acute kidney injury: a systematic review and meta-analysis. Am J Kidney Dis 2009; 54(6):1012–24.
119. Volpon LC, Sugo EK, Carlotti AP. Diagnostic and prognostic value of serum cystatin C in critically ill children with acute kidney injury. Pediatr Crit Care Med 2015;16(5):e125–31.
120. Lagos-Arevalo P, Palijan A, Vertullo L, et al. Cystatin C in acute kidney injury diagnosis: early biomarker or alternative to serum creatinine? Pediatr Nephrol 2015;30(4):665–76.
121. Zappitelli M, Greenberg JH, Coca SG, et al. Association of definition of acute kidney injury by cystatin C rise with biomarkers and clinical outcomes in children undergoing cardiac surgery. JAMA Pediatr 2015;169(6):583–91.
122. Gocze I, Koch M, Renner P, et al. Urinary biomarkers TIMP-2 and IGFBP7 early predict acute kidney injury after major surgery. PLoS One 2015;10(3):e0120863.
123. Bihorac A, Chawla LS, Shaw AD, et al. Validation of cell-cycle arrest biomarkers for acute kidney injury using clinical adjudication. Am J Respir Crit Care Med 2014;189(8):932–9.
124. Kashani K, Al-Khafaji A, Ardiles T, et al. Discovery and validation of cell cycle arrest biomarkers in human acute kidney injury. Crit Care 2013;17(1):R25.
125. Meersch M, Schmidt C, Van Aken H, et al. Urinary TIMP-2 and IGFBP7 as early biomarkers of acute kidney injury and renal recovery following cardiac surgery. PLoS One 2014;9(3):e93460.
126. Hoste EA, McCullough PA, Kashani K, et al. Derivation and validation of cutoffs for clinical use of cell cycle arrest biomarkers. Nephrol Dial Transplant 2014; 29(11):2054–61.
127. Farias M, Jenkins K, Lock J, et al. Standardized Clinical Assessment and Management Plans (SCAMPs) provide a better alternative to clinical practice guidelines. Health Aff (Millwood) 2013;32(5):911–20.
128. Sharma A, Zaragoza J, Villa G, et al. Optimizing a kidney stress test to evaluate renal functional reserve. Clin Nephrol 2016;86(7):18–26.

Critical Care Nutrition
Where's the Evidence?

Jayshil J. Patel, MD[a], Ryan T. Hurt, MD, PhD[b], Stephen A. McClave, MD[c], Robert G. Martindale, MD, PhD[d],*

KEYWORDS

- Critical care nutrition • Enteral nutrition • Parenteral nutrition • Nutritional risk
- Supplemental parenteral nutrition • Permissive underfeeding • Trophic feeding
- Metabolic stress response

KEY POINTS

- Critical illness takes one of three paths: the first is fulminant sepsis and end organ disease leading to death, the second; the patient returns to a preinjury or illness state and third; the patient enters a state of persistent inflammatory state.
- Enteral nutrition has numerous non-nutritional benefits including; attenuation of the metabolic response, helps maintain the gut associated lymphoid tissue and supports the gut integrity.
- The concept of defining nutritional risk and using that risk assessment to focus attention to those at greatest risk yields the optimal benefit from nutritional therapy.
- Despite the numerous benefits of enteral nutrition parenteral nutrition is still a valuable tool to support those patients in which enteral is either fully or partially unsuccessful.

INTRODUCTION

Critical illness induces a highly complex and variable metabolic response. Consequences of this metabolic response often lead to immunosuppression, reduced muscle mass, impaired wound healing, immobility, and cognitive impairment.[1] Randomized controlled trials (RCTs), observational studies, and mechanistic data suggest provision of nutrition is beneficial for critically ill patients to attenuate or

Conflicts of Interest: J.J. Patel has no conflicts. S.A. McClave is a speaker and consultant for Nestle, Abbott, Metagenics, and Covidien. R.T. Hurt has received consultant fees for Nestle. R.G. Martindale has received consultant fees from Nestle and Metagenics.
[a] Division of Pulmonary and Critical Care Medicine, Medical College of Wisconsin, 8701 West Watertown Plank Road, Milwaukee, WI 53226, USA; [b] Department of Medicine, Mayo Clinic, 200 First Street Southwest, Rochester, MN 55905, USA; [c] Division of Gastroenterology, University of Louisville, 2301 South 3rd Street, Louisville, KY 40208, USA; [d] Division of General Surgery, Department of Surgery, Oregon Health Sciences University, 3181 Southwest Sam Jackson Park Road, Portland, OR 97239, USA
* Corresponding author.
E-mail address: martindr@ohsu.edu

prevent some of the consequences of metabolic response. The purpose of this review is to (a) outline the physiologic response of critical illness, (b) describe the concept of nutrition therapy and differentiate it from nutrition support, (c) define nutritional risk and describe which critically ill patients may benefit from early aggressive nutritional optimization, (d) discuss the optimal dose of enteral nutrition (EN), (e) define the role and timing of parenteral nutrition (PN) in critical illness, and (f) define which critically ill patients may benefit from immunonutrition.

THE METABOLIC RESPONSE TO CRITICAL ILLNESS AND THE NUTRITION SUPPORT

In general, critically ill patients follow 1 of 3 clinical trajectories. The first trajectory is the patient who has an acute insult (eg, trauma, sepsis) that leads to rapid and widespread organ dysfunction. Despite aggressive resuscitation and supportive care measures, this trajectory leads to fulminant death. The second trajectory is the patient who has an acute insult, wherein resuscitation and supportive care measures follow. The underlying insult is reversed, and homeostasis is re-established; the metabolic response shifts from catabolic to anabolic. In the second trajectory, the duration of intensive care unit (ICU) stay may be a few days up to 2 weeks. The third trajectory is an extension of the second except the catabolic response persists and leads to chronic critical illness manifesting as persistent inflammation, muscle wasting, immunosuppression with propensity for nosocomial infections, and persistent organ dysfunctions (eg, dependence on mechanical ventilation and renal replacement therapy). This third phenotype is also known as persistent inflammatory immunosuppressed catabolic syndrome.[2]

What is the role of nutrition in each of these trajectories? When it is clear that patients enter the first trajectory, there is probably little or no role for early and/or aggressive nutrition support, because despite resuscitative and supportive care measures, the outcome is fulminant death. To better understand the role of nutrition in the second and third trajectories, it is important to comprehend the metabolic response to stress.

The metabolic stress response activates numerous pathways, including neuroendocrine, immune/inflammatory, and adipokine/gastrointestinal. Within seconds to minutes, sympathetic nervous system activation increases adrenergic receptor activity and adrenal medullary output of norepinephrine and epinephrine. Within seconds to hours, the neuroendocrine component turns on the sympathetic nervous systems and hypothalamic-pituitary axis. Within hours, the hypo-thalamic-pituitary axis increases anterior pituitary release of adrenocorticotropic hormone, thyroid-stimulating hormone, follicle-stimulating hormone, luteinizing hormone, and growth hormone. An immune response increases cytokines and inflammatory mediators. Tumor necrosis factor, interleukin-1 (IL-1), and IL-6 induce fevers, proteolysis, and lipolysis and trigger anorexia.[3] Adipokines, released from adipose tissue, such as leptin, resistin, and adiponectin, which are now thought to be important in the overall response, are currently being investigated for their role in modulating the metabolic stress response.[3] Gastrointestinal responses to metabolic stress are exceedingly complex and include increased cholecystokinin and peptide YY, which release digestive enzymes and reduce hunger, changes in gut integrity, and distorted motility.[3,4] The new paradigm for the human immune response to stress (eg, trauma, sepsis) includes simultaneous activation of both systemic inflammatory innate immune and compensatory anti-inflammatory responses with simultaneous adaptive immunity gene suppression.[4]

Activation of the neuroendocrine, immune/inflammatory, and adipokine/gastrointestinal pathways leads to accelerated catabolism, insulin resistance, increased energy substrate use, increased energy expenditure, a cumulative calorie deficit, and most importantly, proteolysis. In health, protein breakdown and synthesis are balanced. During metabolic stress, the ubiquitin-proteasome pathway is activated by hormones and inflammatory mediators, leading to enhanced protein degradation for supply for amino acids for acute phase proteins, immunoglobulins, and carbon skeletons gluconeogenesis.[3,5] Because metabolic stress induces accelerated catabolism, nutritional benefits of EN and PN include provision of calories and micronutrients for energy substrate to decrease muscle and tissue oxidation, increase mitochondrial function, increase protein synthesis, maintain lean body mass, and enhance muscle function and mobility. Caloric deficits of 4000 to 10,000 calories have been associated with more organ failure and increased hospital length of stay.[6,7] Negative nitrogen balance has been associated with development of ICU-acquired weakness and chronic critical illness.[8–10]

ENTERAL FEEDING AS NUTRITION THERAPY

Nonnutritional benefits of early enteral feeding include maintenance of gut integrity, reducing inflammation, and enhancing immunity. It is EN, as opposed to PN, that provides the nonnutritional benefits (ie, primary therapy). To better understand the nonnutritional benefits of EN, consider the consequences of not introducing nutrients into the lumen in a critically ill patient. At baseline, there is significant cross-talk between intestinal epithelium, the immune system, and commensal bacteria.[11–13] In the absence of luminal nutrients, there is reduced gut contractility and bacterial overgrowth. Bacteria are more likely to adhere to enterocytes, and enterocytes undergo contact-mediated apoptosis, thereby increasing enterocyte permeability. Enhanced gut permeability is a dynamic phenomenon that is time dependent (channels opening within minutes of the major insult or injury).[1] Alverdy[13] first described the interaction and relationship between intestinal bacteria and the critically ill host, proposing the "stress" of critical illness induces (normally symbiotic) bacteria to become dysbiotic bacteria.[14] Commensal bacteria sense alterations in the gut environment, particularly soluble compounds, such as catecholamines and adenosine, to activate bacterial virulence genes to promote survival.[15] The resultant dysbiotic bacteria intercept host signals via telesensing; macrophages are activated, and the inflammatory response is heightened.[14,16] Consequently, toxic mediators (eg, cytokines) migrate via lymphatics to distant organs, such as the lung, and initiate lung injury.[17,18] The "gut motor" theory of multiple organ dysfunction syndrome suggests the gut drives downstream organ dysfunction via gut-lymph activation.

Mechanistic data suggest one of the many mechanisms to explain how EN maintains enterocyte structure and function is by stimulating gut contraction to reduce bacterial stasis and overgrowth. EN enhances immunity, stimulates blood flow, and induces the release of gut trophic substances. EN promotes commensal bacteria, as opposed to conversion from a normal gut microbiome to a "pathobiome" with noted phenotypic change in bacteria normally a part of the "healthy" microbiome.[19] Virulent bacterial growth has been associated with reduced butyrin production. Butyrin production is known to reduce the inflammatory response.[16,20] The gut is responsible for 80% of immunoglobulin A (IgA) production, and EN augments immunity by increasing secretory IgA production at epithelial surfaces, increasing the anti-inflammatory Th-2 response, reducing transendothelial neutrophil and macrophage migration, and preserving intestinal blood flow.[21] EN also modulates metabolic responses to reduce insulin resistance and improve hyperglycemia.[16,21]

ENTERAL NUTRITION TIMING

To optimize nonnutritional benefits, EN must be started early in the course of critical illness. The 2016 American Society of Parenteral and Enteral Nutrition and Society of Critical Care Medicine (ASPEN/SCCM) nutrition support guidelines recommend starting early EN, defined as within 24 to 48 hours of ICU admission.[22] Multiple bodies of evidence suggest improved outcomes with early EN. In a retrospective study of prospectively collected data with propensity scoring, Artinian and colleagues[23] reported overall ICU and hospital mortalities were lower (18.1% vs 21.4%, $P = .01$; and 28.7% vs 33.5%, $P = .001$, respectively) in medical ICU patients who received EN within 48 hours, as compared with after 48 hours of mechanical ventilation. In fact, the lowest mortalities were seen in the sickest patients who received early EN. Multiple small RCTs suggest EN started within 48 hours reduces infections, hospital length of stay, and mortality, as compared with EN started after 48 hours.[1] A meta-analysis of 8 trials showed a trend toward reduced mortality (relative risk [RR] = 0.52; 95% confidence interval [CI], 0.25–1.08; $P = .08$) when EN was started within 48 hours.[1,24] A second meta-analysis of 12 trials showed significant reduction in infectious complications with early EN (RR = 0.45; 95% CI, 0.30–0.66; $P = .00006$) and hospital length of stay (mean, 2.2 days; 95% CI, 0.81–3.63 days; $P = .001$) when started on average of within 36 hours of ICU admission.[1,25] A meta-analysis of 21 trials demonstrated early EN, as compared with delayed EN, was associated with a significant reduction in mortality (RR = 0.70; 95% CI, 0.49–1.00; $P = .05$) and infectious complications (RR = 0.74; 95% CI, 0.58–0.93; $P = .01$).[1] In the patient with hemodynamic instability on vasopressor support, EN should be withheld until the patient is adequately resuscitated to ensure effective circulating volume is restored; however, vasopressor therapy is not a contraindication for EN because multiple studies have demonstrated EN tolerance, lack of complications, improvements in splanchnic hemodynamics, and improvements in clinical outcome with early EN in this subset of patients.[26–31]

ENTERAL NUTRITION DOSE

Several studies have questioned the optimal EN dose during the first week of critical illness, even suggesting a "less is more" strategy for reasons related to ease of EN delivery, improved tolerance, and preservation of autophagy.[20,32] Autophagy is a survival mechanism of the cell that serves to remove protein aggregates for cellular survival to generate energy and preserve and supply substrate for essential protein synthesis.[32] One school of thought is that aggressive feeding in critical illness disrupts autophagy, and some emerging evidence suggests meeting full energy requirements in the first week of critical illness may actually be harmful.[32,33] Permissive underfeeding is intentionally limiting non-protein calories while providing full protein requirements. Retrospective, observational, RCTs conducted between 2002 and 2014 demonstrated improvement in various outcomes with permissive underfeeding; however, heterogeneity in study design, patient populations, and methodologic flaws has limited external generalizability (Table 1).[34–40] Two observational studies placed critically ill patients into tertiles and quartiles of percentage of goal feeds received. Both studies found worse outcomes in the top tertile/quartile group (who received the most calories). These 2 studies were flawed in that the top group received more PN and more calories through propofol.[35,36] Four RCTs suggesting permissive underfeeding improved outcomes had methodologic flaws. For example, in a single-center RCT, the permissive underfeeding group achieved 59% of prescribed calories, whereas the full feeding group achieved 71% prescribed calories. The study demonstrated a 12.5% reduction

Table 1
Studies that showed improved outcomes with permissive underfeeding, as compared with full enteral feeding

Author, Year	Study Design	Study Population	No. of Patients	Comments
Ibrahim et al,[34] 2002	Single-center RCT	Medical ICU	150	Target caloric intake was not achieved and high incidence of VAP in full EN group; bolus feeding likely contributed to both
Krishnan et al,[35] 2003	Observational	Medical ICU	187	Different feeding delivery in each quartile, leading to dissimilar group comparisons
Ash et al,[36] 2005	Retrospective	Trauma ICU	120	Different feeding delivery in each quartile, leading to dissimilar group comparisons
Arabi et al,[37] 2010	Observational	Mixed ICU	523	Oral diet inclusion confounded study outcome analysis
Arabi et al,[38] 2011	Single-center RCT	Mixed ICU	240	High likelihood for type 1 error (improbable that a 12% difference in calories accounted for significant difference in mortality)
Casaer et al,[39] 2013	Multicenter RCT	Mixed ICU	4640	Post-hoc analysis showed no difference in EN between 2 groups and late PN group without suggestion of mortality by increasing percentage calories at days 3, 5, 7
Braunschweig et al,[40] 2015	Multicenter RCT	Mixed ICU	78	High likelihood for type 1 error as high death rate in full EN group limited enrollment

Abbreviation: VAP, ventilator-associated pneumonia.
Adapted from McClave SA, Codner P, Patel J, et al. Should we aim for full enteral feeding in the first week of critical illness? Nutr Clin Pract 2016;31(4):425–31; with permission.

in 90-day mortality in the permissive underfeeding group. It is difficult to surmise a 12.5% reduction in mortality based on a 12% difference in achieved calories, suggesting the study suffered from a type 1 (alpha) error.[38]

A few RCTs have also suggested permissive underfeeding is equivalent to full feeding in critically ill patients (**Table 2**).[41–44] In the largest RCT of 1000 patients, the EDEN study compared initial trophic EN (defined as 10–20 kcal/h) to full EN in patients with acute lung injury.[42] There was no difference in mortality, organ failure, ventilator-free days, or new infections between the 2 groups. Subjects were younger, had a body mass index (BMI) of 30, and had a relatively short ICU stay of 5 days. In addition, the trophic feeding group had 1.5 L less fluid balance, as compared with the full feeding group.[42] Negative fluid balance is an important tenet of acute respiratory distress syndrome (ARDS) management. In a multicenter RCT, Arabi[44] evaluated the impact of permissive underfeeding (40%–60% goal calories) versus full feeding (70%–100% goal calories) and found no difference in ICU mortality, 90-day mortality, or new infections. The study was powered to detect an 8.4% reduction in 90-day mortality;

Table 2
Studies showing equivalent outcomes with permissive underfeeding as compared with full enteral feeding

Author, Year	Study Design	Study Population	No. of Patients	Comments
Rice et al,[41] 2011	Single-center RCT	Medical ICU	200	Malnourished patients, a group that may derive greatest benefit from early aggressive EN, were excluded from the study
Rice et al,[42] 2012	Multicenter RCT	Medical ICU	1000	Younger patient population with BMI of 30 and 5 ICU days and trophic feeding group had greater negative daily fluid balance on each of the 6 study days (an important component to ARDS management)
Charles et al,[43] 2014	Single-center RCT	Trauma ICU	83	High likelihood for a type 2 error because the study only enrolled 83 of its planned 116 patients
Arabi et al,[44] 2015	Multicenter RCT	Mixed ICU	894	Study was underpowered; caloric target was not achieved in "standard" EN group, and less protein was delivered (0.7 g/kg/d)

Adapted from McClave SA, Codner P, Patel J, et al. Should we aim for full enteral feeding in the first week of critical illness? Nutr Clin Pract 2016;31(4):427; with permission.

however, the actual difference in mortality was 1.7%, suggesting the study was underpowered.

Given the variability in outcomes, heterogeneity in populations studied, and methodologic concerns, the optimal EN dose remains elusive.

NUTRITIONAL RISK

Nutritional risk is the likelihood of acquiring complications that may have been prevented by timely and adequate nutrition support.[20] As discussed earlier, the consequences of metabolic stress may predispose critically ill patients to complications and worse outcomes. Furthermore, the pre-existing nutritional state parameter may predispose the patient to complications and worse outcomes.

Classic variables, such as serum albumin or prealbumin, have not been validated tools to identify nutritional risk in critically ill patients due to the negative acute phase response to inflammation, and levels were shown to be widely variable, dependent upon timing of blood draw and metabolic and volume status of patient. Instead, scoring systems have been developed to identify nutritional risk.[45,46] In 2002, Kondrup and colleagues[46] identified pre-existing nutritional status and severity of illness variables to develop the Nutritional Risk Screening (NRS) 2002 score. To calculate a score, points from nutritional status (0–3) and severity of disease (0–3) are added together, and if the age is greater than 70 years, one additional point is added

Table 3
Nutrition risk in the critically ill score

Variable	Range	Points
Age	<50	0
	50 to <75	1
	≥75	2
APACHE II score	<15	0
	15 to <20	1
	20–28	2
	≥28	3
Sequential Organ Failure Assessment score	<6	0
	6 to <10	1
	≥10	2
Number of comorbidities	0–1	0
	≥2	1
Days from hospital to ICU admission	0 to <1	0
	≥1	1
IL-6	0 to <400	0
	≥400	1

Sum of Points	Category	Explanation
5–9	High score	• Associated with worse clinical outcomes (mortality, ventilation) • These patients are the most likely to benefit from aggressive nutrition therapy
0–4	Low score	• These patients have a low malnutrition risk

From Heyland DK, Dhaliwal R, Jiang X, et al. Identifying critically ill patients who benefit the most from nutrition therapy: the development and initial validation of a novel risk assessment tool. Critical Care 2011;15(6):R268; and Rahman A, Hasan RM, Agarwala R, et al. Identifying critically-ill patients who will benefit most from nutritional therapy: further validation of the "modified NUTRIC" nutritional risk assessment tool. Clin Nutr 2016;35(1):158–62.

to the total score. If the age-corrected score is greater than or equal to 3, then the patient is considered to be at nutritional risk and early full nutrition support is recommended.[20,46]

A second score, developed by Heyland and colleagues,[45] is the Canadian Nutrition Risk in the Critically Ill (NUTRIC) score (Table 3). The NUTRIC score takes into account 6 variables associated with nutritional risk: age, Acute Physiology and Health Evaluation II score, Sequential Organ Failure Assessment score, number of comorbidities, pre-ICU length of hospital stay, and serum IL-6 level. Emerging data suggest at-nutritional-risk patients, defined by NRS 2002 score of 3 or greater, who received early EN had fewer infectious complications.[47] Heyland and colleagues[48] analyzed 1199 patients and found a positive correlation between nutritional adequacy and 28-day survival in patients with an NUTRIC score of 6 or greater (Fig. 1). For centers that are not able to measure an IL-6 level, a modified NUTRIC score (obviating IL-6) has been validated.[49]

Therefore, barring any contraindications, the 2016 ASPEN/SCCM guidelines suggest starting a standard polymeric EN formula within 24 to 48 hours in high-nutritional-risk critically ill patients (defined as NRS 2002 ≥5 or NUTRIC ≥5 without IL-6) and titrating to more than 80% estimated energy and protein goal within 48 to 72 hours.[1] The guidelines suggest no specialized EN over the first week in those

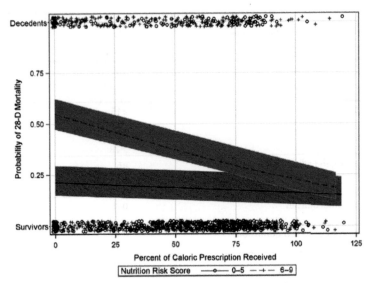

Fig. 1. Predicted probability of mortality versus nutrition received by NUTRIC score. Patients with NUTRIC score 6 to 9 (indicating at nutritional risk) that received a greater percentage of prescribed calories had a reduced 28-day mortality. (*From* Heyland DK, Dhaliwal R, Jiang X, et al. Identifying critically ill patients who benefit the most from nutrition therapy: the development and initial validation of a novel risk assessment tool. Crit Care 2011;15(6):R268; with permission.)

patients who are at low nutritional risk with normal baseline nutrition status and low disease severity (NRS $\leq$3 or NUTRIC <5)[1] (**Box 1**).

THE ROLE AND TIMING OF PARENTERAL NUTRITION

PN is delivery of nutritional components and fluid through an intravenous (IV) route. Even though EN remains the preferred route for nutrition delivery, there is still a role

---

Box 1
Nutrition bundle

- Assess patients on admission to the ICU for nutrition risk and calculate both energy and protein requirements to determine goals of nutrition therapy.

- Initiate EN within 24 to 48 hours following the onset of critical illness and admission to the ICU and increase to goals over the first week of ICU stay.

- Take steps as needed to reduce risk of aspiration or improve tolerance to gastric feeding (use prokinetic agent, continuous infusion, chlorhexidine mouthwash; elevate the head of bed; and divert level of feeding in the gastrointestinal tract).

- Implement enteral feeding protocols with institution-specific strategies to promote delivery of EN.

- Do not use gastric residual volumes as part of routine care to monitor ICU patients receiving EN.

- Start parenteral nutrition early when EN is not feasible or sufficient in high-risk or poorly nourished patients.

for PN in critically ill patients. Clearly, in a patient deemed to be high nutritional risk and unable to use the gut, early PN is recommended.[1]

When the gut is intact during critical illness, is there a difference in outcomes between early EN and PN and what is the role for supplementary PN? EN, as opposed to PN, has numerous nonnutritional benefits (as discussed earlier). Several meta-analyses have demonstrated reduced infectious complications, such as pneumonia and central line infections, in the patient with critically ill trauma, burn, head injury, major surgery, and acute pancreatitis who received EN as compared with PN.[50–56] Although the meta-analyses demonstrated improvement in infectious complications, there was a lack of consistency in demonstrating improvements in noninfectious complications, such as reduced mortality and reduced length of ICU or hospital stay. Studies included in the meta-analyses were small studies (generally <100 patients total), were older (pre-2005), and included a heterogeneous group of critically ill patients (medical and surgical). In addition, there have been improvements in preventative measures to reduce ventilator-associated pneumonia and central line–associated bloodstream infections and alterations in PN lipid emulsion delivery, suggesting the incidence of infectious complications may diminish with modern EN versus PN trials.

Indeed, in the pragmatic CALORIES trial, 2400 critically ill patients were randomized across 33 English ICUs to receive early EN or early PN. The main conclusions were no significant differences in the primary outcome of 30-day mortality or secondary outcome of infectious complications with early EN or early PN. The lack of benefit with early PN may suggest inflated estimates of benefit in previous smaller trials.[57] Regardless, the CALORIES trial suggests early PN is noninferior to early EN and can be safely administered.[58]

Importantly, lipid emulsion products available in the European Union and other parts of the world are more physiologic than those available in the United States. These products include SMOF ("soy, medium-chain triglycerides, olive oil, and fish oil") as the emulsion source. Overall, in critically ill patients who are deemed to be at nutritional risk (as defined by NUTRIC and NRS 2002) with contraindications for EN, starting early PN to achieve but not exceed 80% of the prescribed goal is reasonable.[1] In patients without nutritional risk with contraindications for EN, it is reasonable to initiate PN after 7 days. Contraindications such as "high" gastric residual volume and absence of bowel sounds should not prevent EN initiation or continuation.[22]

Supplemental PN refers to adding PN to patients receiving insufficient calories through EN, either because of intentional underfeeding (eg, trophic or permissive underfeeding) or due to EN intolerance. Recently, 3 RCTs of supplemental PN reported conflicting results (**Table 4**).[59–61] The 2 studies demonstrated that when supplemental PN was added to hypocaloric EN, there was no benefit, as compared with hypocaloric EN alone.[60,61] In the EPaNIC trial, 4640 critically ill patients were randomized to early supplemental PN (within 48 hours of ICU admission) or late PN (8 days after ICU admission). The main conclusions were the late PN group was more likely to be discharged alive from the ICU (hazard ratio for early PN, 1.06; 95% CI, 1.00–1.13; $P = .04$) and had fewer ICU-acquired infections (22.8% vs 26.2%; $P = .008$).[59] Both groups received the same amount of EN before receipt of PN, suggesting the adverse outcomes may be associated with supplementing PN. In addition, 80% of patients were not malnourished; 60% were cardiac surgery patients, and the late PN group received 20% IV dextrose, vitamins, and trace elements, limiting external generalizability.[22,59,62]

The optimal timing for supplemental PN in an at-nutritional-risk patient not achieving greater than 60% goal calories is not clear. It appears clear that if the patient is at high nutritional risk and EN is not feasible, then PN should be added soon after ICU

Table 4
Summary of recent intensive care unit studies of supplemental parenteral nutrition

Author, Year	Study Design	Study Population	No. of Patients	Comments
Casaer et al,[59] 2011	Multicenter RCT	Mixed ICU	4640	Low number of malnourished patients, >60% cardiac surgery patients, and patients in late PN group received continuous dextrose infusion
Doig et al,[60] 2013	Multicenter RCT	Mixed ICU	1372	No difference in 60-d mortality or ICU infections with early supplemental PN
Heidegger et al,[61] 2013	Multicenter RCT	Mixed ICU	305	Other nosocomial infections included respiratory tract infections, probably resulting in reported significant increased in nosocomial infection rate in EN group

admission. A reasonable strategy may be to initiate supplemental PN after the first week of critical illness in a patient not achieving at least 60% goal calories through EN; however, the 2016 ASPEN/SCCM guideline suggests the decision be made on a case-by-case basis.[1]

IMMUNONUTRITION IN CRITICAL ILLNESS

There are numerous macronutrients and micronutrients that can alter or attenuate the immune and inflammatory components to critical illness. Examples of metabolic modulating nutrients, or pharmaconutrition, include fish oils containing the omega-3 fatty acids (FA) eicosapentaenoic acid (EPA) and docosahexaenoic acid (DHA), amino acids such as glutamine, leucine, and arginine, antioxidants such as vitamin C and selenium, and probiotics, prebiotics, and synbiotics. Current literature appears to support the use of pharmaconutrition in trauma and surgical ICUs but not in the medical ICU.[1] The heterogeneity of the medical ICU population makes designing and implementing pharmaconutrition studies difficult. Although it is clear that various substrates such as fish oil, selenium, zinc, and antioxidants do not cause harm, there has been difficulty in demonstrating consistent benefit.[1]

Fish oils (EPA and DHA) have been used in critical care since the early 1990s when Gottschlich and colleagues[63] reported benefit in major burns. Multiple mechanisms have been reported and well described to illustrate how EPA and DHA affect the inflammatory and immune response, including enhancing leukocyte chemotaxis, changes in lymphocyte class, and production of series 1 and 3 eicosanoids, which are less inflammatory than omega-6 FA derived series 2 and 4 eicosanoids.[64] The use of anti-inflammatory lipids and substrates has become routine in the trauma and surgical ICUs.[1,65]

Recently, numerous human randomized clinical trials have reported that appropriate use of omega-3-FAs (EPA and DHA) in the ICU setting can partially attenuate the metabolic response to surgical and traumatic injury, abate lean body muscle loss, prevent oxidative injury in a variety of tissue beds, and improve surgical and ICU outcomes.[1] The proposed mechanisms for such benefits include modulating and limiting the synthesis of proinflammatory mediators and enhancing pathways for anti-inflammatory mediators.[65] In the acute setting, multiple mechanisms, including changes in cell membrane phospholipids ratios, alteration of membrane lipid rafts, regulating vascular integrity, modifications in inflammatory gene expression, and attenuation of endothelial expression of intercellular adhesion molecule-1, E-Selectin, and other endothelial receptors, are involved in inducing and perpetuating the inflammatory cascade. A better understanding of the observed benefits has recently been supported by discovery and elucidation of the specialized proresolving molecules. These compounds, which are endogenously produced from EPA and DHA substrates, have conclusively and consistently been shown to enhance resolution of inflammation, improve bacterial killing by macrophages, and promote tissue regeneration.[66]

Arginine use in the critical care setting has raised the most controversy in terms of specific amino acid delivery. Arginine exerts pleiotropic effects on cell metabolism, and its depletion in critical illness is associated with a wide variety of detrimental effects on critical care metabolism, including alteration in microcirculatory blood flow, impaired wound healing, and significant alterations in both macrophage and T-cell immune function.[67,68] Making generalized statements about the benefits or detriments of arginine in the critical care setting is difficult because of the heterogeneity of the "critical care population." Recently, small prospective studies have supported the use of supplemental arginine in critical care, although widespread acceptance and application remain controversial.[67] The "arginine paradox" at least partially explains these nonintuitive results.[69]

The use of glutamine and glutamine dipeptide for 3 decades was thought to be of significant benefit in the critical care setting. Eight RCTs of supplemental glutamine (most provided during emergent visceral surgery) demonstrated benefit.[70–77] However, the results of large prospective trials questioned glutamine use in critical illness. Three large multicenter randomized trials with varying doses of supplemental glutamine have failed to show benefit in regards to major outcomes.[78–81] The REDOX trial, a multinational RCT, demonstrated a trend toward increased mortality at 28 days among patients who received glutamine as compared with those who did not receive glutamine (32.4% vs 27.2%). The impact of the REDOX trial outcomes has forced a reevaluation of glutamine use in the ICU setting. A meta-analysis of supplemental glutamine on primary outcomes for elective major surgery reported glutamine did not affect overall mortality and infectious morbidity.[82] A meta-analysis of glutamine supplementation in a generic ICU population similarly reported no benefit in regards to ICU mortality, hospital mortality, or incidence of infections.[83] The 2016 ASPEN/SCCM nutrition support guidelines now recommend supplemental enteral or parenteral glutamine *not* be added to routine nutrition therapy in the ICU.[1]

SUMMARY AND FUTURE INSIGHTS

The concept of nutritional therapy for the ICU patient has changed dramatically in the last 5 decades. ICU nutrition has evolved from primarily PN in the 1970s and 1980s to primarily EN with cautious avoidance of PN, probably due to the actual and/or perceived increase in infectious complications associated with PN. Recent studies, however, have scrutinized these concepts and shown a more individualized focus using concepts, such as nutritional risk drives timing, dose, and type of nutrition therapy. What is clear is that EN should still be the primary modality for nutrition therapy and PN should be reserved for those patients in whom EN is not successful or feasible. As our technology and "omics" (genomics, proteomics, and metabolomics) expand, the impact of macronutrients, micronutrients, and immunonutrition on altering the metabolic complexity and microbiome of this population is slowly being elucidated.

Information arising from these areas will be fruitful for ongoing research and future studies.

REFERENCES

1. McClave SA, Taylor BE, Martindale RG, et al. Guidelines for the provision and assessment of nutrition support therapy in the adult critically ill patient: Society of Critical Care Medicine (SCCM) and American Society for Parenteral and Enteral Nutrition (A.S.P.E.N.). JPEN J Parenter Enteral Nutr 2016;40(2):159–211.
2. Rosenthal MD, Moore FA. Persistent inflammatory, immunosuppressed, catabolic syndrome (PICS): a new phenotype of multiple organ failure. J Adv Nutr Hum Metab 2015;1(1):e784.
3. Preiser JC, Ichai C, Orban JC, et al. Metabolic response to the stress of critical illness. Br J Anaesth 2014;113(6):945–54.
4. Rosenthal MD, Vanzant EL, Martindale RG, et al. Evolving paradigms in the nutritional support of critically ill surgical patients. Curr Probl Surg 2015;52(4):147–82.
5. Hasselgren PO. Catabolic response to stress and injury: implications for regulation. World J Surg 2000;24(12):1452–9.
6. Villet S, Chiolero RL, Bollmann MD, et al. Negative impact of hypocaloric feeding and energy balance on clinical outcome in ICU patients. Clin Nutr 2005;24(4): 502–9.
7. Dvir D, Cohen J, Singer P. Computerized energy balance and complications in critically ill patients: an observational study. Clin Nutr 2006;25(1):37–44.
8. Batt J, dos Santos CC, Cameron JI, et al. Intensive care unit-acquired weakness: clinical phenotypes and molecular mechanisms. Am J Respir Crit Care Med 2013;187(3):238–46.
9. Davidson TA, Caldwell ES, Curtis JR, et al. Reduced quality of life in survivors of acute respiratory distress syndrome compared with critically ill control patients. JAMA 1999;281(4):354–60.
10. Herridge MS, Tansey CM, Matte A, et al. Functional disability 5 years after acute respiratory distress syndrome. N Engl J Med 2011;364(14):1293–304.
11. Mizock BA. The multiple organ dysfunction syndrome. Dis Mon 2009;55(8): 476–526.
12. Alverdy J, Zaborina O, Wu L. The impact of stress and nutrition on bacterial-host interactions at the intestinal epithelial surface. Curr Opin Clin Nutr Metab Care 2005;8(2):205–9.
13. Alverdy J. The effect of nutrition on gastrointestinal barrier function. Semin Respir Infect 1994;9(4):248–55.
14. Krezalek MA, DeFazio J, Zaborina O, et al. The shift of an intestinal "microbiome" to a "pathobiome" governs the course and outcome of sepsis following surgical injury. Shock 2016;45(5):475–82.
15. Zaborin A, Smith D, Garfield K, et al. Membership and behavior of ultra-low-diversity pathogen communities present in the gut of humans during prolonged critical illness. MBio 2014;5(5). e01361-14.
16. McClave SA, Heyland DK. The physiologic response and associated clinical benefits from provision of early enteral nutrition. Nutr Clin Pract 2009;24(3):305–15.
17. Deitch EA. Bacterial translocation of the gut flora. J Trauma 1990;30(12 Suppl): S184–9.
18. Klingensmith NJ, Coopersmith CM. The gut as the motor of multiple organ dysfunction in critical illness. Crit Care Clin 2016;32(2):203–12.

19. Babrowski T, Romanowski K, Fink D, et al. The intestinal environment of surgical injury transforms pseudomonas aeruginosa into a discrete hypervirulent morphotype capable of causing lethal peritonitis. Surgery 2013;153(1):36–43.
20. Patel JJ, Codner P. Controversies in critical care nutrition support. Crit Care Clin 2016;32(2):173–89.
21. McClave SA, Martindale RG, Rice TW, et al. Feeding the critically ill patient. Crit Care Med 2014;42:2600–10.
22. McClave SA, Codner P, Patel J, et al. Should we aim for full enteral feeding in the first week of critical illness? Nutr Clin Pract 2016;31(4):425–31.
23. Artinian V, Krayem H, DiGiovine B. Effects of early enteral feeding on the outcome of critically ill mechanically ventilated medical patients. Chest 2006;129(4):960–7.
24. Dhaliwal R, Cahill N, Lemieux M, et al. The Canadian Critical Care Nutrition Guidelines in 2013: an update on current recommendations and implementation strategies. Nutr Clin Pract 2014;29(1):29–43.
25. Marik PE, Zaloga GP. Early enteral nutrition in acutely ill patients: a systematic review. Crit Care Med 2001;29(12):2264–70.
26. Berger MM, Revelly JP, Cayeux MC, et al. Enteral nutrition in critically ill patients with severe hemodynamic failure after cardiopulmonary bypass. Clin Nutr 2005; 24(1):124–32.
27. Khalid I, Doshi P, DiGiovine B. Early enteral nutrition and outcomes of critically ill patients treated with vasopressors and mechanical ventilation. Am J Crit Care 2010;19(3):261–8.
28. Berger MM, Chiolero RL. Enteral nutrition and cardiovascular failure: from myths to clinical practice. JPEN J Parenter Enteral Nutr 2009;33(6):702–9.
29. Revelly JP, Tappy L, Berger MM, et al. Early metabolic and splanchnic responses to enteral nutrition in postoperative cardiac surgery patients with circulatory compromise. Intensive Care Med 2001;27(3):540–7.
30. Patel JJ, Kozeniecki M, Biesboer A, et al. Early trophic enteral nutrition is associated with improved outcomes in mechanically ventilated patients with septic shock: a retrospective review. J Intensive Care Med 2016;31:471–7.
31. Yang S, Wu X, Yu W, et al. Early enteral nutrition in critically ill patients with hemodynamic instability: an evidence-based review and practical advice. Nutr Clin Pract 2014;29(1):90–6.
32. McClave SA, Weijs PJ. Preservation of autophagy should not direct nutritional therapy. Curr Opin Clin Nutr Metab Care 2015;18(2):155–61.
33. Jeejeebhoy KN. Permissive underfeeding of the critically ill patient. Nutr Clin Pract 2004;19(5):477–80.
34. Ibrahim EH, Mehringer L, Prentice D, et al. Early versus late enteral feeding of mechanically ventilated patients: results of a clinical trial. JPEN J Parenter Enteral Nutr 2002;26(3):174–81.
35. Krishnan JA, Parce PB, Martinez A, et al. Caloric intake in medical ICU patients: consistency of care with guidelines and relationship to clinical outcomes. Chest 2003;124(1):297–305.
36. Ash J, Gervasio JM, Zaloga GP. Does the quantity of enteral nutrition affect outcomes in critically ill trauma patients? JPEN J Parenter Enteral Nutr 2005;29:S10.
37. Arabi YM, Haddad SH, Tamim HM, et al. Near-target caloric intake in critically ill medical-surgical patients is associated with adverse outcomes. JPEN J Parenter Enteral Nutr 2010;34(3):280–8.
38. Arabi YM, Tamim HM, Dhar GS, et al. Permissive underfeeding and intensive insulin therapy in critically ill patients: a randomized controlled trial. Am J Clin Nutr 2011;93(3):569–77.

39. Casaer MP, Wilmer A, Hermans G, et al. Role of disease and macronutrient dose in the randomized controlled EPaNIC trial: a post hoc analysis. Am J Respir Crit Care Med 2013;187(3):247–55.

40. Braunschweig CA, Sheean PM, Peterson SJ, et al. Intensive nutrition in acute lung injury: a clinical trial (INTACT). JPEN J Parenter Enteral Nutr 2015;39(1):13–20.

41. Rice TW, Mogan S, Hays MA, et al. Randomized trial of initial trophic versus full-energy enteral nutrition in mechanically ventilated patients with acute respiratory failure. Crit Care Med 2011;39(5):967–74.

42. National Heart, Lung, and Blood Institute Acute Respiratory Distress Syndrome (ARDS) Clinical Trials Network, Rice TW, Wheeler AP, et al. Initial trophic vs full enteral feeding in patients with acute lung injury: the EDEN randomized trial. JAMA 2012;307(8):795–803.

43. Charles EJ, Petroze RT, Metzger R, et al. Hypocaloric compared with eucaloric nutritional support and its effect on infection rates in a surgical intensive care unit: a randomized controlled trial. Am J Clin Nutr 2014;100(5):1337–43.

44. Arabi YM, Aldawood AS, Haddad SH, et al. Permissive underfeeding or standard enteral feeding in critically ill adults. N Engl J Med 2015;373:1281.

45. Heyland DK, Dhaliwal R, Jiang X, et al. Identifying critically ill patients who benefit the most from nutrition therapy: the development and initial validation of a novel risk assessment tool. Crit Care 2011;15(6):R268.

46. Kondrup J, Johansen N, Plum LM, et al. Incidence of nutritional risk and causes of inadequate nutritional care in hospitals. Clin Nutr 2002;21(6):461–8.

47. Jie B, Jiang ZM, Nolan MT, et al. Impact of nutritional support on clinical outcome in patients at nutritional risk: a multicenter, prospective cohort study in baltimore and beijing teaching hospitals. Nutrition 2010;26(11–12):1088–93.

48. Heyland DK, Dhaliwal R, Wang M, et al. The prevalence of iatrogenic underfeeding in the nutritionally 'at-risk' critically ill patient: results of an international, multicenter, prospective study. Clin Nutr 2015;34(4):659–66.

49. Rahman A, Hasan RM, Agarwala R, et al. Identifying critically-ill patients who will benefit most from nutritional therapy: further validation of the "modified NUTRIC" nutritional risk assessment tool. Clin Nutr 2016;35(1):158–62.

50. Moore FA, Feliciano DV, Andrassy RJ, et al. Early enteral feeding, compared with parenteral, reduces postoperative septic complications. The results of a meta-analysis. Ann Surg 1992;216(2):172–83.

51. Kudsk KA, Croce MA, Fabian TC, et al. Enteral versus parenteral feeding. effects on septic morbidity after blunt and penetrating abdominal trauma. Ann Surg 1992;215(5):503–11 [discussion: 511–3].

52. Kalfarentzos F, Kehagias J, Mead N, et al. Enteral nutrition is superior to parenteral nutrition in severe acute pancreatitis: results of a randomized prospective trial. Br J Surg 1997;84(12):1665–9.

53. Everitt NJ. Enteral nutrition is superior to parenteral nutrition in severe acute pancreatitis: results of a randomized prospective trial. Br J Surg 1998;85(5):716.

54. Braunschweig CL, Levy P, Sheean PM, et al. Enteral compared with parenteral nutrition: a meta-analysis. Am J Clin Nutr 2001;74(4):534–42.

55. Gramlich L, Kichian K, Pinilla J, et al. Does enteral nutrition compared to parenteral nutrition result in better outcomes in critically ill adult patients? A systematic review of the literature. Nutrition 2004;20(10):843–8.

56. Simpson F, Doig GS. Parenteral vs. enteral nutrition in the critically ill patient: a meta-analysis of trials using the intention to treat principle. Intensive Care Med 2005;31(1):12–23.

57. Cook D, Arabi Y. The route of early nutrition in critical illness. N Engl J Med 2014; 371(18):1748–9.
58. Harvey SE, Segaran E, Leonard R. Trial of the route of early nutritional support in critically ill adults. N Engl J Med 2015;372(5):488–9.
59. Casaer MP, Mesotten D, Hermans G, et al. Early versus late parenteral nutrition in critically ill adults. N Engl J Med 2011;365(6):506–17.
60. Doig GS, Simpson F, Sweetman EA, et al. Early parenteral nutrition in critically ill patients with short-term relative contraindications to early enteral nutrition: a randomized controlled trial. JAMA 2013;309(20):2130–8.
61. Heidegger CP, Berger MM, Graf S, et al. Optimisation of energy provision with supplemental parenteral nutrition in critically ill patients: a randomised controlled clinical trial. Lancet 2013;381(9864):385–93.
62. Ziegler TR. Nutrition support in critical illness–bridging the evidence gap. N Engl J Med 2011;365(6):562–4.
63. Gottschlich MM, Jenkins M, Warden GD, et al. Differential effects of three enteral dietary regimens on selected outcome variables in burn patients. JPEN J Parenter Enteral Nutr 1990;14(3):225–36.
64. Alexander JW, Supp DM. Role of arginine and omega-3 fatty acids in wound healing and infection. Adv Wound Care (New Rochelle) 2014;3(11):682–90.
65. Martindale RG, Warren MM, McClave SA. Does the use of specialized proresolving molecules in critical care offer a more focused approach to controlling inflammation than that of fish oils? Curr Opin Clin Nutr Metab Care 2016;19(2):151–4.
66. Serhan CN. Pro-resolving lipid mediators are leads for resolution physiology. Nature 2014;510(7503):92–101.
67. Patel JJ, Miller KR, Rosenthal C, et al. When is it appropriate to use arginine in critical illness? Nutr Clin Pract 2016;31:438–44.
68. Pekarova M, Lojek A. The crucial role of l-arginine in macrophage activation: what you need to know about it. Life Sci 2015;137:44–8.
69. Tsikas D, Boger RH, Sandmann J, et al. Endogenous nitric oxide synthase inhibitors are responsible for the L-arginine paradox. FEBS Lett 2000;478(1–2):1–3.
70. Jian ZM, Cao JD, Zhu XG, et al. The impact of alanyl-glutamine on clinical safety, nitrogen balance, intestinal permeability, and clinical outcome in postoperative patients: a randomized, double-blind, controlled study of 120 patients. JPEN J Parenter Enteral Nutr 1999;23(5 Suppl):S62–6.
71. Jacobi CA, Ordemann J, Zuckermann H, et al. The influence of alanyl-glutamine on immunologic functions and morbidity in postoperative total parenteral nutrition. preliminary results of a prospective randomized trial. Zentralbl Chir 1999; 124(3):199–205.
72. Karwowska KA, Dworacki G, Trybus M, et al. Influence of glutamine-enriched parenteral nutrition on nitrogen balance and immunologic status in patients undergoing elective aortic aneurysm repair. Nutrition 2001;17(6):475–8.
73. Mertes N, Schulzki C, Goeters C, et al. Cost containment through L-alanyl-L-glutamine supplemented total parenteral nutrition after major abdominal surgery: a prospective randomized double-blind controlled study. Clin Nutr 2000;19(6): 395–401.
74. Morlion BJ, Stehle P, Wachtler P, et al. Total parenteral nutrition with glutamine dipeptide after major abdominal surgery: a randomized, double-blind, controlled study. Ann Surg 1998;227(2):302–8.
75. Neri A, Mariani F, Piccolomini A, et al. Glutamine-supplemented total parenteral nutrition in major abdominal surgery. Nutrition 2001;17(11–12):968–9.

76. Powell-Tuck J, Jamieson CP, Bettany GE, et al. A double blind, randomised, controlled trial of glutamine supplementation in parenteral nutrition. Gut 1999; 45(1):82–8.

77. Fuentes-Orozco C, Anaya-Prado R, Gonzalez-Ojeda A, et al. L-alanyl-L-glutamine-supplemented parenteral nutrition improves infectious morbidity in secondary peritonitis. Clin Nutr 2004;23(1):13–21.

78. Heyland D, Muscedere J, Wischmeyer PE, et al. A randomized trial of glutamine and antioxidants in critically ill patients. N Engl J Med 2013;368(16):1489–97.

79. Cui Y, Hu L, Liu YJ, et al. Intravenous alanyl-L-glutamine balances glucose-insulin homeostasis and facilitates recovery in patients undergoing colonic resection: a randomised controlled trial. Eur J Anaesthesiol 2014;31(4):212–8.

80. Gianotti L, Braga M, Biffi R, et al, GlutamItaly Research Group of the Italian Society of Parenteral, and Enteral Nutrition. Perioperative intravenous glutamine supplementation in major abdominal surgery for cancer: a randomized multicenter trial. Ann Surg 2009;250(5):684–90.

81. Ziegler TR, May AK, Hebbar G, et al. Efficacy and safety of glutamine-supplemented parenteral nutrition in surgical ICU patients: an American multicenter randomized controlled trial. Ann Surg 2016;263(4):646–55.

82. Sandini M, Nespoli L, Oldani M, et al. Effect of glutamine dipeptide supplementation on primary outcomes for elective major surgery: systematic review and meta-analysis. Nutrients 2015;7(1):481–99.

83. Oldani M, Sandini M, Nespoli L, et al. Glutamine supplementation in intensive care patients: a meta-analysis of randomized clinical trials. Medicine (Baltimore) 2015;94(31):e1319.

Index

Note: Page numbers of article titles are in **boldface** type.

Crit Care Clin 33 (2017) 413–421
http://dx.doi.org/10.1016/S0749-0704(17)30009-X
0749-0704/17